Blueprints Notes & Cases
Behavioral Science and Epidemiology

Blueprints **Notes & Cases**
Series Editor: Aaron B. Caughey MD, MPP, MPH

Blueprints *Notes & Cases—Microbiology and Immunology*
Monica Gandhi, Paul Baum, C. Bradley Hare, Aaron B. Caughey

Blueprints *Notes & Cases—Biochemistry, Genetics, and Embryology*
Juan E. Vargas, Aaron B. Caughey, Annie Tan, Jonathan Z. Li

Blueprints *Notes & Cases—Pharmacology*
Katherine Y. Yang, Larissa R. Graff, Aaron B. Caughey

Blueprints *Notes & Cases—Pathophysiology: Cardiovascular, Endocrine, and Reproduction*
Gordon Leung, Susan H. Tran, Tina O. Tan, Aaron B. Caughey

Blueprints *Notes & Cases—Pathophysiology: Pulmonary, Gastrointestinal, and Rheumatology*
Michael Filbin, Lisa M. Lee, Brian L. Shaffer, Aaron B. Caughey

Blueprints *Notes & Cases—Pathophysiology: Renal, Hematology, and Oncology*
Aaron B. Caughey, Christie del Castillo, Nancy Palmer, Karen Spizer, Dana N. Tuttle

Blueprints *Notes & Cases—Neuroscience*
Robert T. Wechsler, Alexander M. Morss, Courtney J. Wusthoff, Aaron B. Caughey

Blueprints *Notes & Cases—Behavioral Science and Epidemiology*
Judith Neugroschl, Jennifer Hoblyn, Christie del Castillo, Aaron B. Caughey

Blueprints **Notes & Cases**
Behavioral Science and Epidemiology

Judith Neugroschl, MD
Assistant Professor of Psychiatry
Director of Medical Student Education in Psychiatry
Mount Sinai School of Medicine
New York, New York

Jennifer Hoblyn, MB, MMSci, MRCPsych, MPH
VA Palo Alto Health Care System
Palo Alto, California
Department of Psychiatry and Behavioral Sciences
Stanford University School of Medicine
Stanford, California

Christie del Castillo, MD
Class of 2003
University of California, San Francisco, School of Medicine
San Francisco, California

Aaron B. Caughey, MD, MPP, MPH
Clinical Instructor, Division of Maternal-Fetal Medicine
Department of Obstetrics & Gynecology
University of California, San Francisco
Division of Health Services and Policy Analysis
University of California, Berkeley
Berkeley & San Francisco, California

Series Editor: Aaron B. Caughey, MD, MPP, MPH

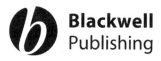
Blackwell
Publishing

Blackwell Publishing, Inc., 350 Main Street, Malden, Massachusetts 02148-5018, USA
Blackwell Publishing Ltd, 9600 Garsington Road, Oxford OX4 2DQ, UK
Blackwell Science Asia Pty Ltd, 550 Swanston Street, Carlton, Victoria 3053, Australia

03 04 05 06 5 4 3 2 1

ISBN: 1-4051-0355-8

Library of Congress Cataloging-in-Publication Data

Blueprints notes & cases. Behavioral science and epidemiology / Judith Neugroschl . . . [et al.].
        p. ; cm. — (Blueprints notes & cases)
    Includes index.
    ISBN 1-4051-0355-8 (pbk.)
    1. Psychiatry—Examinations, questions, etc. 2. Psychology, Pathological—Examinations, questions, etc. 3. Mental illness—
Diagnosis—Examinations, questions, etc. 4. Physical diagnosis—Examinations, questions, etc. 5. Psychiatric
epidemiology—Examinations, questions, etc.
    [DNLM: 1. Mental Disorders—diagnosis—Case Report. 2. Mental Disorders—diagnosis—Problems and Exercises. 3. Physical
Examination—methods—Case Report. 4. Physical Examination—methods—Problems and Exercises. 5. Physician-Patient Relations—Case Report. 6. Physician-Patient Relations—Problems and Exercises. WM 18.2 B6575 2003]   I. Title: Behavioral
science and epidemiology.   II. Title: Blueprints notes and cases. III. Neugroschl, Judith. IV. Series.
    RC457.B577 2003
    616.89′0076—dc22
                                                                                                2003018961

A catalogue record for this title is available from the British Library

Acquisitions: Beverly Copland
Development: Selene Steneck
Production: Jennifer Kowalewski
Cover design: Hannus Design Associates
Interior design: Janet Bollow Associates
Typesetter: Peirce Graphic Services in Stuart, FL
Printed and bound by Courier Companies in Westford, MA

For further information on Blackwell Publishing, visit our website: www.blackwellpublishing.com

Notice: The indications and dosages of all drugs in this book have been recommended in the
medical literature and conform to the practices of the general community. The medications
described do not necessarily have specific approval by the Food and Drug Administration for
use in the diseases and dosages for which they are recommended. The package insert for each
drug should be consulted for use and dosage as approved by the FDA. Because standards for
usage change, it is advisable to keep abreast of revised recommendations, particularly those
concerning new drugs.

Contents

Reviewers

Komal Bajaj
Class of 2004
Northwestern University Feinberg School of Medicine
Chicago, Illinois

Yen Ling Chong
Class of 2004
University of Calgary
Calgary, Alberta, Canada

Amanda Kimbrough
Class of 2004
University of Texas Health Science Center at San Antonio
San Antonio, Texas

Susan Merel
Class of 2005
University of Chicago Pritzker School of Medicine
Chicago, Illinois

Niraj Pahlajani
Class of 2004
University of Medicine & Dentistry of New Jersey—
Robert Wood Johnson Medical School
Camden, New Jersey

Jonathan Popler
Class of 2004
SUNY Stony Brook School of Medicine
Stony Brook, New York

Preface

The first two years of medical school are a demanding time for medical students. Whether the school follows a traditional curriculum or one that is case-based, every student is expected to learn and be able to apply basic science information in a clinical situation.

Medical schools are increasingly using clinical presentations as the background to teach the basic sciences. Case-based learning has become more common at many medical schools as it offers a way to catalogue the multitude of symptoms, syndromes, and diseases in medicine.

Blueprints **Notes & Cases is a new series by Blackwell Publishing designed to provide students a textbook to study the basic science topics combined with clinical data.** This method of learning is also the way to prepare for the clinical case format of USMLE questions. The eight books in this series will make the basic science topics not only more interesting, but also more meaningful and memorable. Students will be learning not only the why of a principle, but also how it might commonly be seen in practice.

The books in the *Blueprints* Notes & Cases series feature a comprehensive collection of cases which are designed to introduce one or more basic science topics. Through these cases, students gain an understanding of the coursework as they learn to:

- Think through the cases
- Look for classic presentations of most common diseases and syndromes
- Integrate the basic science content with clinical application
- Prepare for course exams and Step 1 USMLE
- Be prepared for clinical rotations

This series covers all the essential material needed in the basic science courses. Where possible, the books are organized in an organ-based system.

Clinical cases lead off and are the basis for discussion of the basic science content. A list of **"thought questions"** follows the case presentation. These questions are designed to challenge the reader to begin to think about how basic science topics apply to real-life clinical situations. The **answers to these questions** are integrated within the **basic science review and discussion** that follows. This offers a clinical framework from which to understand the basic content.

The discussion section is followed by a high-yield **Thumbnail table and Key Points box,** which highlight and summarize the essential information presented in the discussion.

The cases also include two to four **multiple-choice questions** that allow readers to check their knowledge of that topic. Many of the answer explanations provide an opportunity for further discussion by delving into more depth in related areas. An **answer key** for these questions is at the end of the section for easy reference, and **full answer explanations** can be found at the end of the book.

This new series was designed to provide comprehensive content in a concise and templated format for ease in learning. A dedicated attempt was made to include sufficient art, tables, and clinical treatment, all while keeping the books from becoming too lengthy. We know you have much to read and that what you want is high-yield, vital facts.

The authors and series editor for these eight books, as well as everyone in editorial, production, sales and marketing at Blackwell Publishing, have worked long and hard to provide new textbooks to help you learn and be able to apply what you have learned. We engaged in multiple student email surveys and many focus groups to "hear what you needed" in new basic science level textbooks to meet the current curriculums, tests, and coursework. We know that you value this "student to student" approach, and sincerely hope you like what we have put together **just for you.**

Blackwell Publishing and the authors wish you success in your studies and your future medical career. Please feel free to offer us any comments or suggestions on these new books at blue@bos.blackwellpublishing.com.

Acknowledgments

This is dedicated to Jonah, Jacob, Ari, Gerry, and Seth.
—Judith Neugroschl

Thanks to Stephanie, Patrick, and Angus.
—Jennifer Hoblyn

Thank you to my family, Mom, Dad, Roehl, Jovie, Ronin, Carlo, Michelle, Dana, Mac Mac, Arnel, Dennis, Len, and Kevin. Thank you for making my life beautiful.
—Christie del Castillo

To my parents, Bill and Carol, who have dedicated their lives to the social and mental health of others.
—Aaron B. Caughey

Abbreviations

5-HIAA	5-hydroxyindoleacetic acid	CBT	cognitive-behavioral therapy
5-HT	5-hydroxytryptamine, serotonin	CCK	cholecystokinin
AA	Alcoholics Anonymous	CD	conduct disorder
ABG	arterial blood gas	cGMP	cyclic guanosine 3′,5′-monophosphate
ACE-I	angiotensin-converting enzyme inhibitor	CHF	congestive heart failure
ACh	acetylcholine	CI	confidence interval
AChEIs	acetylcholinesterase inhibitors	CIA	Central Intelligence Agency
AD	Alzheimer's disease	CJD	Creutzfeldt-Jakob disease
ADC	AIDS dementia complex	Cl, Cl⁻	chloride
ADH	alcohol dehydrogenase	CL	contralateral
ADHD	attention deficit hyperactivity disorder	CN	cranial nerve
ADLs	activities of daily living	CNS	central nervous system
AH	auditory hallucination	CO	carbon monoxide
AIDS	acquired immunodeficiency syndrome	CO$_2$	carbon dioxide
AIMS	abnormal involuntary movement scale	COPD	chronic obstructive pulmonary disease
ALT	alanine aminotransferase (SGPT)	CPAP	continuous positive airway pressure
ApoE	apo lipoprotein E	CPK	creatinine phosphokinase
APP	Alzheimer's precursor protein	CPR	cardiopulmonary resuscitation
ASD	atrial septal defect	Cr	creatine
AST	aspartate aminotransferase (SGOT)	CRF	corticotropin releasing factor
ATPase	adenosine triphosphatase	CSF	cerebrospinal fluid
BAL	blood alcohol level	CT	computerized tomography
Beta-HCG	beta-human chorionic gonadotropin	CVA	cerebrovascular accident
BMI	body-mass index	DA	dopamine
BMR	basal metabolic rate	DDAVP	1-desamino-8-D-arginine vasopressin
BP	blood pressure	DID	dissociative identity disorder
BPD	borderline personality disorder	dL	deciliter
BUN	blood urea nitrogen	DLB	dementia with Lewy bodies
BZD	benzodiazepine	DM	diabetes mellitus
CABG	coronary artery bypass graft	DNR	do not resuscitate
Ca	calcium	DSM-IV	*Diagnostic and Statistical Manual of Mental Disorders,* 4th Edition
CAD	coronary artery disease		
cAMP	adenosine 3′,5′-cyclic monophosphate (cyclic AMP)	DTR	deep tendon reflexes
		DUI	driving under the influence
CAT	computerized axial tomography	DWI	driving while intoxicated
CBC	complete blood count	DZ	dizygotic

ECT	electroconvulsive therapy		IRS	Internal Revenue Service
EEG	electroencephalography		IV	intravenous
EKG	electrocardiogram		JVP	jugular venous pulsation
EMG	electromyogram		K	potassium
ENT	ear, nose, throat (otolaryngology)		LAAM	levo-alpha-acetyl-methadol
EPS	extrapyramidal symptoms		LC	locus ceruleus
EtOH	ethyl alcohol		LDL	low-density lipoprotein
FBI	Federal Bureau of Investigation		LFT	liver function test
FDA	Food and Drug Administration		LH	luteinizing hormone
FFS	fee-for-service		LP	lumbar puncture
FSH	follicle-stimulating hormone		LPN	licensed practical nurse
GxPy	gravida x para y		LR	likelihood ratio
GABA	gamma aminobutyric acid		LSD	lysergic acid diethylamide
GAD	generalized anxiety disorder		MAO	monoamine oxidase
GCS	Glasgow coma scale		MAOI	monoamine oxidase inhibitor
GHB	gamma-hydroxybutyrate		MBA	Master of Business Administration
GI	gastrointestinal		MCA	middle cerebral artery
HAART	highly active antiretroviral therapies		MCV	mean corpuscular volume
HCO_3	hydrogen bicarbonate		MDD	major depressive disorder
Hct	hematocrit		MDMA	3,4-methylenedioxymethamphetamine (ecstasy)
HDL	high-density lipoprotein		Mg	magnesium
Hgb	hemoglobin		MHPG	3-methoxy-4-hydroxyphenylglycol
HI	homicidal ideation		MI	myocardial infarction
HIV	human immunodeficiency virus		MMPI	Minnesota Multiphasic Personality Inventory
HMO	Health Maintenance Organization		MOA	mechanism of action
HPA	hypothalamic pituitary adrenal		MR	mental retardation
HPI	history of present illness		MRI	magnetic resonance imaging
HR	heart rate		MS	multiple sclerosis
HVA	homovanillic acid		MSE	mental status examination
IADLs	instrumental activities of daily living		MSLT	multiple sleep latency test
IM	intramuscular		MZ	monozygotic
INH	isoniazid		Na	sodium
INR	international ratio		nAchR	nicotinic acetylcholine receptor
IPA	independent practitioner association		NE	norepinephrine
IPT	interpersonal therapy		NIDDM	non-insulin dependent diabetes mellitus
IQ	intelligence quotient		NIMH	National Institute of Mental Health

NKDA	no known drug allergies	RPR	rapid plasma reagin test (for syphilis)
NMDA	*N*-methyl-*D*-aspartate	RR	relative risk
NMS	neuroleptic malignant syndrome	S1, S2	heart sounds 1 and 2
NPV	negative predictive value	Sao$_2$	arterial oxygen concentration
NSAID	nonsteroidal anti-inflammatory drug	SH	somatic hallucination
O$_2$	oxygen	SHBG	sex hormone-binding globulin
O$_2$ sat	oxygen saturation	SI	suicidal ideation
OCD	obsessive-compulsive disorder	SLE	systemic lupus erythematosus
ODD	oppositional defiant disorder	SN	substantia nigra
OR	odds ratio	SNS	sympathetic nervous system
PCP	phencyclidine	SNRI	serotonergic noradrenergic reuptake inhibitor
PD	personality disorder	SPECT	single photon emission computed tomography
PDA	patent ductus arteriosus	SSRI	selective serotonergic reuptake inhibitor
PDE	phosphodiesterase	T	temperature
PE	physical examination	T3	triiodothyronine
PERRLA	pupils equal round reactive to light and accommodation	T4	tetraiodothyronine
PET	positron emission tomography	TC	total cholesterol
PI	paranoid ideation	TCA	tricyclic antidepressant
PKU	phenylketonuria	TD	tardive dyskinesia
Plt	platelets	TENS	transcutaneous electrical nerve stimulation
PMDD	premenstrual dysphoric disorder	TFT	thyroid function test
PMH	past medical history	TG	triglycerides
PO	by mouth	THC	Δ-9-tetrahydrocannabinol
POS	point-of-service health plan	TIA	transient ischemic attack
PPO	preferred provider organization	TOF	tetralogy of Fallot
PPV	positive predictive value	TRH	thyrotropin-releasing hormone
PSHx	past surgical history	TS	Tourette syndrome
PT	prothrombin time	TSH	thyroid-stimulating hormone
PTSD	posttraumatic stress disorder	UA	urinalysis
PTT	partial thromboplastin time	UTI	urinary tract infection
RA	resident advisor	Utox	urine toxicology
RCT	randomized, controlled trial	VDRL	venereal disease research laboratory test (for syphilis)
REM	rapid eye movement	VH	visual hallucination
ROC	receiver operating characteristic	VLDL	very low-density lipoprotein
ROS	Review of Systems	VS	vital signs

Abbreviations

VSD	ventricular septal defect	**WHR**	waist-to-hip ratio
VTA	ventral tegmental area	**WISC**	Wechsler Intelligence Scale for Children
WAIS	Wechsler Adult Intelligence Scale	**XTC**	ecstasy
WBC	white blood cell		

Normal Ranges of Laboratory Values

BLOOD, PLASMA, SERUM

Alanine aminotransferase (ALT, GPT at 30 C)	8–20 U/L
Amylase, serum	25–125 U/L
Aspartate aminotransferase (AST, GOT at 30 C)	8–20 U/L
Bilirubin, serum (adult) Total // Direct	0.1–1.0 mg/dL // 0.0–0.3 mg/dL
Calcium, serum (Ca^{2+})	8.4–10.2 mg/dL
Cholesterol, serum	Rec: < 200 mg/dL
Cortisol, serum	0800 h: 5–23 μg/dL // 1600 h: 3–15 μg/dL
	2000 h: ≤ 50% of 0800 h
Creatine kinase, serum	Male: 25–90 U/L
	Female: 10–70 U/L
Creatinine, serum	0.6–1.2 mg/dL
Electrolytes, serum	
Sodium (Na$^+$)	136–145 mEq/L
Chloride (Cl$^-$)	95–105 mEq/L
Potassium (K$^+$)	3.5–5.0 mEq/L
Bicarbonate (HCO$_3^-$)	22–28 mEq/L
Magnesium (Mg^{2+})	1.5–2.0 mEq/L
Ferritin, serum	Male: 15–200 ng/mL
	Female: 12–150 ng/mL
Follicle-stimulating hormone, serum/plasma	Male: 4–25 mIU/mL
	Female: premenopause 4–30 mIU/mL
	midcycle peak 10–90 mIU/mL
	postmenopause 40–250 mIU/mL
Gases, arterial blood (room air)	
pH	7.35–7.45
Pco_2	33–45 mm Hg
Po_2	75–105 mm Hg
Glucose, serum	Fasting: 70–110 mg/dL
	2-h postprandial: < 120 mg/dL
Growth hormone—arginine stimulation	Fasting: < 5 ng/mL
	provocative stimuli: > 7 ng/mL
Iron	50–70 μg/dL
Lactate dehydrogenase, serum	45–90 U/L
Luteinizing hormone, serum/plasma	Male: 6–23 mIU/mL
	Female: follicular phase 5–30 mIU/mL
	midcycle 75–150 mIU/mL
	postmenopause 30–200 mIU/mL
Osmolality, serum	275–295 mOsmol/kg
Parathyroid hormone, serum, N-terminal	230–630 pg/mL
Phosphate (alkaline), serum (p-NPP at 30 C)	20–70 U/L
Phosphorus (inorganic), serum	3.0–4.5 mg/dL
Prolactin, serum (hPRL)	< 20 ng/mL
Proteins, serum	
Total (recumbent)	6.0–7.8 g/dL
Albumin	3.5–5.5 g/dL
Globulin	2.3–3.5 g/dL
Thyroid-stimulating hormone, serum or plasma	0.5–5.0 μU/mL
Thyroidal iodine (^{123}I) uptake	8–30% of administered dose/24 h
Thyroxine (T$_4$), serum	5–12 μg/dL
Triglycerides, serum	35–160 mg/dL
Triiodothyronine (T$_3$), serum (RIA)	115–190 ng/dL
Triiodothyronine (T$_3$), resin uptake	25–35%
Urea nitrogen, serum (BUN)	7–18 mg/dL
Uric acid, serum	3.0–8.2 mg/dL

CEREBROSPINAL FLUID

Cell count	0–5 cells/mm^3
Chloride	118–132 mEq/L
Gamma globulin	3–12% total proteins
Glucose	40–70 mg/dL
Pressure	70–180 mm H$_2$O
Proteins, total	< 40 mg/dL

HEMATOLOGIC

Bleeding time (template)	2–7 minutes
Erythrocyte count	Male: 4.3–5.9 million/mm^3
	Female: 3.5–5.5 million/mm^3
Erythrocyte sedimentation rate (Westergren)	Male: 0–15 mm/h
	Female: 0–20 mm/h
Hematocrit	Male: 41–53%
	Female: 36–46%
Hemoglobin A$_{1C}$	≤ 6%
Hemoglobin, blood	Male: 13.5–17.5 g/dL
	Female: 12.0–16.0 g/dL
Leukocyte count and differential	
Leukocyte count	4500–11,000/mm^3
Segmented neutrophils	54–62%
Bands	3–5%
Eosinophils	1–3%
Basophils	0–0.75%
Lymphocytes	25–33%
Monocytes	3–7%
Mean corpuscular hemoglobin	25.4–34.6 pg/cell
Mean corpuscular hemoglobin concentration	31–36% Hb/cell
Mean corpuscular volume	80–100 μm^3
Partial thromboplastin time (activated)	25–40 seconds
Platelet count	150,000–400,000/mm^3
Prothrombin time	11–15 seconds
Reticulocyte count	0.5–1.5% of red cells
Thrombin time	< 2 seconds deviation from control
Volume	
Plasma	Male: 25–43 mL/kg
	Female: 28–45 mL/kg
Red cell	Male: 20–36 mL/kg
	Female: 19–31 mL/kg

SWEAT

Chloride	0–35 mmol/L

URINE

Calcium	100–300 mg/24 h
Chloride	Varies with intake
Creatine clearance	Male: 97–137 mL/min
	Female: 88–128 mL/min
Osmolality	50–1400 mOsmol/kg
Oxalate	8–40 μg/mL
Potassium	Varies with diet
Proteins, total	< 150 mg/24 h
Sodium	Varies with diet
Uric acid	Varies with diet

Part I

Behavioral Science

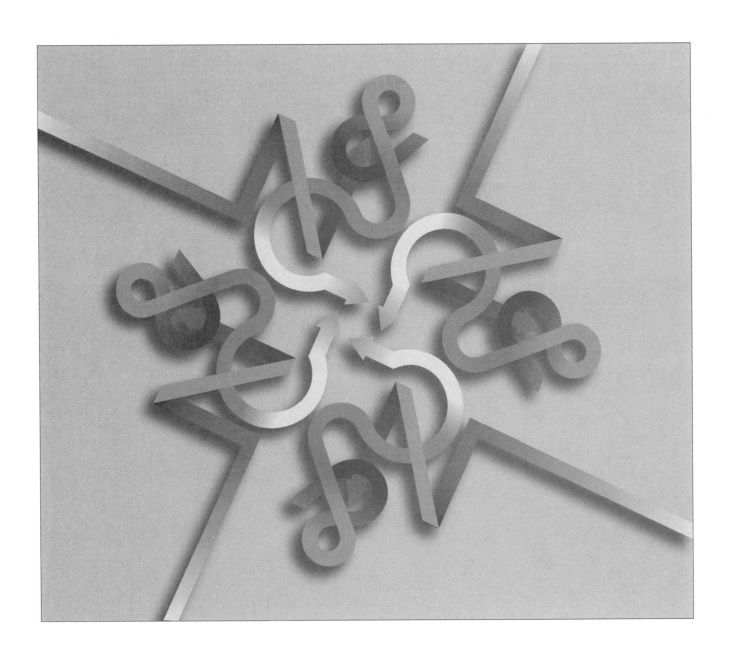

> **HPI:** Mr. and Ms. B bring in their 2-week-old to see you. Ms. B says that the baby has been eating well and sleeping on and off for much of the day, but they notice that when he's turned abruptly he has a dramatic response and begins to wail. You explain that this is a reflex and she asks you what other inborn reflexes there are, how long they will last, and whether new ones will crop up.

Thought Questions

- What is the reflex described above called?

- What other reflexes are seen in a neonate? Describe the reflex, how it is elicited, and when it is extinguished.

- What physical milestones happen in the first year?

- What about social and language milestones?

Basic Science Review and Discussion

A number of reflexes are present at birth and disappear as an infant develops normally (Table 1-1).

Early Development In the first month the child is able to lift its head and develops a social smile. By 4 months he or she may be starting to babble, can reach for objects, and can sit with assistance. By 6 months the child can sit unassisted, and soon will roll over. Between 7 and 9 months the child develops stranger anxiety, which highlights the healthy attachment to parents and the ability to differentiate others. Along with this the child develops separation anxiety. Again this is a normal response to healthy attachment to the parents.

By 1 year the child can crawl and often has taken his or her first steps. He or she can also drink from a cup, grasp things between thumb and forefinger (pincer grasp), and say his or her first word. By 18 months the child is furthering both fine and gross motor development and can climb up stairs, scribble, and use a spoon. Language also continues to develop, and the child can name common objects. Between 16 months and 2 years, the child practices moving away from the parent or caregiver and then coming back for reassurance and comfort. This practice is called rapprochement, which was described by Margaret Mahler, a developmental psychologist. In addition, between 18 months and 3 years core gender identity is established.

At age 2 the child can speak in two-word sentences, jump, and wash and dry his or her hands. By age 3 he or she can ride a tricycle, dress with supervision, speak in three- and four-word sentences, and recognize his or her whole name and some colors.

Table 1-1. Inborn Reflexes

Moro	Sudden movement stimulates extension, abduction, then adduction of arms. Disappears at about 4 to 6 months.
Babinsky	Scratching the lateral aspect of the sole (heel to toe) leads to dorsiflexion of the big toe and fanning of other toes. Disappears by 12 to 18 months
Grasp	Pressure on the palm causes infants to grasp. Disappears about 4 months.
Suck/rooting	Oral or perioral stimulation will cause orientation toward the stimulus and sucking. Disappears at 4 to 6 months.
Stepping	Hold the infant vertically, with pressure on feet; child will make stepping motions. Disappears at 2 to 3 months.

> **Case Conclusion** You do a physical exam, which is unremarkable. You review the baby's eating patterns (normal, every 2 to 3 hours). The baby is eating well, urinating and moving his bowels, and gaining weight. You discuss the parents' concerns about changing and diaper ointments. It's a light day in your practice, and as new parents, Mr. and Ms. B have many questions about what the next years will hold.

Thumbnail: Behavioral Science—Developmental Milestones in the Early Years

Physical: (Average age attained)	
1 month	Lift head
6 months	Sit unassisted
7 months	Roll over
10 months	Crawl
12 to 15 months	Walk
18 months	Walk up steps
24 months	Jump in place
36 months	Ride tricycle
48 months	Hop on one foot
Fine Motor: (Average age attained)	
4 months	Grasp object
9 months	Pincer grasp
14 months	Scribbles
18 months	Tower of 4 cubes
24 months	Imitates a vertical line
36 months	Copies an O
48 months	Copies a + (plus sign)
Social/Personal: (Average age attained)	
1 to 2 months	Social smile in response to face or voice
7 to 9 months	Stranger anxiety—Shows parental attachment and that the child can differentiate strangers
7 to 18 months (up to 3 years)	Separation anxiety (worry about being separated from parents or caregivers)
12 months	Drinks from a cup
18 months	Uses a spoon, removes a garment
24 months	Puts on clothing, washes and dries hands
36 months	Dresses with supervision, eats well with utensils
48 months	Dresses without supervision
Language: (Average age attained)	
4 to 6 months	Babbles
12 months	Speaks first real word
18 months	Names some common objects
24 months	Two-word sentences
36 months	Says first and last name, some colors

Key Points

▶ Developmental milestones are usually grouped in terms of gross motor, fine motor, social, and language skills.

▶ The age at which each milestone is reached is approximate, as each child develops differently.

▶ It is important to understand the difference between separation anxiety and stranger anxiety. Both start at about 7 months of age and indicate a secure attachment to the parents. Separation anxiety may last significantly longer. Both are normal developmental stages, and neither is pathological.

Questions

1. You are a third-year medical student doing pediatrics and you go into the waiting room to call in a patient coming in for a routine checkup. From his chart you know that he has been developing normally. You watch the child in the waiting room go away from his mother to look at a toy, quickly return for a hug, and then go off to explore further, only to return again. This behavior most typically occurs at what age and is called what?
   A. Separation anxiety—Age 4 to 6 months
   B. Rapprochement—Age 16 to 36 months
   C. Exploration—Age 4 years
   D. Insecure attachment—Age 2 to 3 years
   E. Stranger anxiety—Age 7 to 9 months

2. You go into the waiting room of your pediatric practice to call in your next patient, a little girl who has been developing normally. You see her taking a couple of wobbly steps to a table, where she picks up a crayon and scribbles. In the waiting room there are three steps going up, and she cannot walk up them, but crawls her way up. Given this information, approximately how old do you think she is?
   A. 6 months
   B. 9 months
   C. 13 months
   D. 24 months
   E. 36 months

3. FP describes his normally developing son as recently starting to speak in two-word sentences. Which of the following would you also expect him to be able to do?
   A. Copy a "+".
   B. Ride a tricycle.
   C. Wash and dry his hands.
   D. Hop on one foot.
   E. Dress without supervision.

4. You are doing a routine exam on an infant. You note that she smiles at you, grasps an object, but cannot sit independently or roll over. Given her likely age, which of the following reflexes is she most likely to have outgrown?
   A. Moro
   B. Stepping
   C. Babinsky
   D. Grasp
   E. Rooting

> **HPI:** Mr. and Mrs. B bring their 3-year-old in for his routine visit. Your physical exam is completely unremarkable. You review developmental milestones, such as climbing stairs, running, kicking a ball, identifying most common objects, and using four- and five-word sentences. You ensure that he is up to date on his immunizations and review safety concerns such as keeping medications and potentially poisonous items in locked cabinets. The family notes that he is working on his toilet training, talks about it frequently, and is focused on his ability to control his bowels. His parents are concerned that this is too great a focus and that he will become "anal" as an adult.

Thought Questions

- What are the major developmental theories of Piaget, Freud, and Erikson?

- Is the child in the case above exhibiting normal development?

Basic Science Review and Discussion

Jean Piaget Jean Piaget described four major developmental stages, which are based on the cognitive development of the child. These stages are sensorimotor, preoperational, concrete operations, and formal operations.

In the **sensorimotor stage** (0 to 2 years) the child's understanding of the world is based on sensory input and growing motor ability. Initially, it begins with basic sensory input and reflex responses. The infant lacks the idea of object permanence—that although something is out of sight or earshot, it still exists in the world. This concept is learned at about 6 to 8 months, at which time the child begins to understand that she or he is separate from the environment.

An "operation" is an action carried out through logical thinking. In the **preoperational stage** (2 to 6 years) children have not mastered logical reasoning. During these years, the child is mastering language. Piaget postulated that there are three major characteristics of the child's thought processes during this period: egocentrism (the inability to see things from another's perspective), intuitive reasoning, and failure of conservation. (For example, a liquid poured from a short, fat container into a tall, thin container is not considered to have the same amount of liquid.) They have difficulty with conceptualizing time. Thinking is also very influenced by fantasy and wishful thinking.

In the **concrete operational stage** (ages 7 to 11), thinking is logical but depends upon concrete references. Children at

this stage are unable to solve abstract or hypothetical problems but do understand conservation of matter, as in the preceding example of the liquid.

In the **formal operational stage** (ages 12 to 18), the adolescent learns to abstract, generalize, and use metaphors as well as hypothetical or deductive reasoning.

Sigmund Freud Freud's psychosexual theory posits that libido, positive or sexual energy, is primarily focused in certain anatomical areas during development. These areas are defined by the primary focus of gratification. Although babies are polymorphously perverse (they can obtain pleasure through any part of their body) their primary need is focused in the mouth. In the **oral stage** (ages 0 to 1 year) babies get their primary gratification through oral stimulation, sucking. This is followed by the **anal stage** (ages 2 to 3 years), where control and mastery of bowels and excretory functions is central. The child gets a great deal of praise and attention surrounding these activities. The **phallic phase** (which is sometimes known as the **Oedipal phase**) (3 to 6 years of age) is characterized by the child's discovery that the genitals are a site for pleasure, and this is a time of sexual curiosity. The Oedipus complex, which in its most simplistic form can be understood as a child's desire for the opposite-sex parent and therefore a conflictual wish for the same-sex parent (and any siblings) to be gone. This is resolved by identifying with the same-sex parent. The **latency phase** (6 to 12 years of age) is a time of sexual quiescence and same-sex friendships. Adolescence marks the return of sexuality and the focus on genitals for sexual gratification (12 years on).

Erik Erikson Erikson postulated that there were fundamental developmental conflicts that had to be resolved for development to proceed successfully. He divided the life cycle into eight stages and is the only one of these theorists who saw development as a process extending throughout the life span (Table 2-1).

Table 2-1. Erikson's Stages of Psychosocial Development

Age	Stage	Description
Birth to 12 months	Trust vs mistrust	Infants depend on others for food, shelter, and affection, and therefore must be able to completely trust their parents or caregivers. If needs are met, the infant will develop a secure attachment to its parents, and feel a sense of trust in the world.
12 months to 3 years	Autonomy vs shame and doubt	This is a time when the child should be gaining confidence in his or her abilities (e.g., learning to walk, and mastering bowel and bladder control). To master this stage the child needs to explore, experiment, and test limits. Parents or caregivers need to be supportive, not disapproving or inhibiting.
3 to 5 years	Initiative vs guilt	The task at this stage is to be able to initiate and carry through on tasks, to achieve a sense of competence and mastery. Children need to be encouraged and allowed to take initiative. The child sorts out the rules, expectations, and morals through pretend play. At times, however, he or she loses sight of the line between fantasy and reality. To children, if they can imagine something, they can do it. The fear of that power or impulse can turn into guilt. Another way of understanding this is that children whose initiative is considered to be a problem tend to develop a sense of guilt about pursuing their interests.
6 to 11 years	Industry vs inferiority	During this stage the child is learning the basic skills of her/his culture. The child feels a sense of competence through mastery of skills and accomplishments. If the child fails in this stage, a sense of inferiority results.
11 years to end of adolescence	Identity vs role diffusion	This is the time when the adolescent must integrate the healthy resolution of all earlier conflicts. This involves a consistent sense of oneself in any situation and the ability to ask the questions and make the decisions that are necessary to become an adult. It is also a time of separating from parents and defining personal values, beliefs, and identity. The failure to accomplish this task leads to confusion and uncertainty about one's interpersonal roles as well as one's role in society.
~ 20 to 40 years: young adulthood	Intimacy vs isolation	The developmental task is in forming lasting intimate relationships. An individual who has not developed a solid sense of identity usually will fear a committed relationship and may retreat into loneliness, isolation, or promiscuity.
40 to 65 years: middle adulthood	Generitivity vs stagnation	In this phase the adult turns his or her concerns to future generations, groups, and social institutions, passing on knowledge and skills. Failure to achieve this leads to self-absorption and stagnation.
> 65 years: older adulthood	Integrity vs despair	The task at this stage of life is to be able to review one's life and accept what it is/was as well as come to terms with death. This leads to ego integrity. Failure to achieve acceptance can lead to feelings of despair, hopelessness, guilt, resentment, and fear of death.

Case Conclusion   You ask the B's some further questions about their child's development. They state that he is very proud of his accomplishments in toilet training. He spends a great deal of time engaged in or talking about fantasy play and imagination and his parents note that they are never quite sure whether something has happened exactly as he describes. You reassure them that he is developing normally and tell them to praise him for his accomplishments and to encourage his independence.

Thumbnail: Behavioral Science—Theories of Development

Theory	Infant (0–1 yr)	Toddler (2–3 yr)	Preschool (3–6 yr)	School Age (6–12 yr)	Adolescence (12–? yr)
Freud: psychosexual	Oral	Anal	Phallic/Oedipal	Latency	Genital
Erikson: psychosocial	Basic trust	Autonomy vs shame and doubt	Initiative vs guilt	Industry vs inferiority	Identity vs role diffusion
Piaget: cognitive	Sensorimotor	Sensorimotor/preoperational	Preoperational	Concrete operations	Formal operations

Key Points

▶ **Freud** posited his theory around sexual issues in development. His stages focused on childhood.

▶ **Piaget** described cognitive development and discussed the changes in cognition in childhood development that lead to adult patterns of abstraction and thinking.

▶ **Erikson** was the only theorist of the three who conceptualized development continuing through the lifespan. He saw development as a series of eight developmental conflicts that had to be mastered successfully.

Questions

1. You observe a child being tested by a psychology graduate student. The supervisor says that the group is collecting data on normally developing children. You observe that the child is having trouble understanding that the amount of clay doesn't change if it is in a ball or rolled flat, and that the amount of water is the same if it's in a bowl or in a tall, thin beaker. The child is talking to the examiner about this question. What phase is this characteristic of, and who is the theorist?

   A. Freud—Sensorimotor
   B. Piaget—Preoperational
   C. Piaget—Concrete operational
   D. Erikson—Preoperational
   E. Erikson—Sensorimotor

2. Mrs. T brings her 4-year-old child in to see you. She is concerned because he only wants to be with her and has recently been rejecting her husband, telling him to go away. Her husband is a loving and supportive parent but has been feeling hurt by the boy's actions. Which developmental theorist might explain his behavior, and what phase is this?

   A. Freud—Latency
   B. Piaget—Preoperational
   C. Freud—Oedipal
   D. Erikson—Phallic
   E. Erikson—Sensorimotor

3. Mr. U brings his child in for a routine visit. She is able to dress without supervision, speaks in sentences, can copy an O and a + but does not write words. She has been developing normally. According to Erikson, what conflict is she most likely going through, and how old is she?

   A. Autonomy vs shame—She is between 18 months and two years.
   B. Trust vs mistrust—She is between 18 months and two years.
   C. Identity vs role diffusion—She is between 3 and 5 years.
   D. Industry vs inferiority—She is between 3 and 5 years.
   E. Initiative vs guilt—She is between 3 and 5 years.

4. Mr. and Mrs. V bring in their 11-month-old child for a routine evaluation. You are a medical student working with a developmental pediatrician who asks you to tell her in which Freudian, Eriksonian, and Piagettian stage you expect this child to be. Which one of the following selections do you tell her?

   A. Oral, Autonomy vs shame, preoperational
   B. Oral, trust vs mistrust, sensorimotor
   C. Anal, autonomy vs shame, preoperational
   D. Anal, trust vs mistrust, sensorimotor
   E. Oral, trust vs mistrust, preoperational

HPI: JB is a 13-year-old boy who has come to his pediatrician's office with his mother, who tells the doctor that she thinks something is going on with her son.

She says that she is concerned that he is depressed because he does not like to do the things he used to love, such as playing on the school soccer team. His grades have declined lately, but he is eating and sleeping as normally as any other teenager. He has become more withdrawn and has been spending more time alone in his room. He refused to go to school the day of the clinic visit. He has no significant medical history and there is no significant family medical or psychiatric history. He is the eldest of two boys. He is in the eighth grade. He denies using any alcohol or drugs. When his mother leaves the room he tells you that he has does not want to go to school because the guys in his class have been teasing him in the showers because he does not have any pubic hair yet and they call him "teeny weeny." He is frightened that he will not grow like everyone else. He also asks you to explain what happens in an orgasm.

PE: He is 5 feet tall and his vital signs are stable. He is slightly built. There is no facial hair and his voice has not broken. There is no evidence of public hair or enlargement of the penis or testes. Both testes are normal and present in the scrotum. The rest of his physical exam is within normal limits.

Thought Questions

- Is this boy normal? What are the normal stages of development for boys and girls?

- What other stages of psychological and social development are seen during adolescence?

- How do you answer his question about an orgasm?

Basic Science Review and Discussion

Adolescence is a term used to describe the phase between childhood and adulthood, whereas puberty is a **biological** event, which marks the beginning of the changes leading to a mature adult capable of reproduction. For a table describing these pubertal events please see the Thumbnail following.

Biology of Puberty Before the beginning of puberty the adrenal androgen hormones 17-ketosteroid and dehydroepiandrosterone increase. Prepubertal luteinizing hormone (LH) and follicle-stimulating hormone (FSH) are released in a nocturnal pulse fashion, but this changes at puberty to day-and-night pulses. LH stimulates the secretion of testosterone in males. Growth hormone levels directly influence height and are controlled by somatostatin (inhibits release) and growth hormone releasing factors but may be affected by glucocorticoids, thyroid hormone, and estrogen. Growth hormone directly affects the growth spurt, which occurs earlier in females.

The average age of menarche for females is 12.8 years. The average age for boys to start producing sperm is 14.3 years. Other changes seen in both sexes include an increase in muscle mass, bone density, and levels of the hormones FSH and LH. Males experience a significant increase in the width of their bones, whereas females generally do not. In girls breast development usually occurs first, but 15% may have pubic hair growth first. Usually within 2 years of breast development, the menarche occurs. In the majority of boys testicular enlargement is the first development. Pubic hair development is under the control of the adrenal androgens in both sexes. Male facial hair is affected by testosterone levels and usually begins within 2 years after the appearance of pubic hair. Enlargement of the larynx and thickening of the vocal cords leads to a deepening of the voice. During puberty females' fat stores double compared with males but their intracellular water levels decrease, whereas those of males increase. See the following Thumbnail for **Tanner's stages of puberty and development.** The actual age of onset is influenced by several factors, such as genetics, nutritional status (menarche occurs earlier with improved nutrition), general health, geographical position, and levels of exercise. Girls who live in latitudes with little light may have an earlier onset of puberty. All these physical changes are accompanied by cognitive, emotional, and social changes.

Cognitive Development The most significant cognitive development in adolescence is the ability to conceptualize ideas or theories and form more abstract thoughts. The ability to conceptualize and form abstract thoughts allows adolescents to imagine beyond their own experience. The ability to experience **empathy** also begins. The ability to understand combinations and reversibility is developed. The development of **"metacognitive" capacity** allows the adolescent to reflect upon thinking itself or another person's thinking about the adolescence's own self (also called **recursive reasoning**). They also can measure his or her own learning ability. Ideally, adolescents develop a personal value system, which balances their own needs with those of others.

Emotional Development Emotionally, adolescence has previously been described as a time of turmoil, but more recent studies report that levels of **emotional feeling do not change dramatically** from prepubertal levels. Cognitive changes described earlier enhance the adolescent's ability to think about their own emotions and those of others. Emotion influences the level of motivation for particular behaviors and relationships. Adolescents continue to resolve the struggle between their own more basic drives and what is deemed appropriate by their family and society as a whole. Conflict is considered a normal developmental milestone! There have been **increased reports of depression and anxiety in adolescents, particularly in females.** As adolescence progresses, the capacity to participate in more emotionally intimate relationships develops.

Social Development The perception of the **social** development of adolescents is defined by the surrounding social circumstances. The age for voting and enlisting for military service is 18 years, and the age in most states in the United States for legally consuming alcohol is 21 years. As with other aspects of development, ethnicity, socioeconomic circumstances, and general levels of health, education, and nutrition directly influence social development.

African American males have the highest risk of being murdered, with a homicide rate of approximately six times that of Caucasian males of the same age. Most of these homicide deaths are by gunfire. African American males also have a higher rate of suicide than Caucasian males. African American males and females are more likely to have sexual intercourse as teens than Caucasians or Hispanics. Adolescent sexual experiences are directly related to the reported increase in sexually transmitted diseases, particularly HIV, hepatitis B and C, and syphilis. Pregnant adolescent mothers are at higher risk of having infants with low birth weight and associated developmental delays. Early sexual activity has been reported to correlate with illicit substance abuse.

The rates of abuse and neglect are higher for adolescents than for younger children. Peer pressure may be more influential in younger than in older adolescents. Adolescents who have many friends are reported to have high levels of self-esteem, whereas those without friends have higher rates of academic and emotional problems. Boys may be more susceptible to group pressure to perform antisocial activities. Dropping out of school is correlated with lower incomes and higher rates of unemployment, as well as, social, behavioral, and legal problems.

Adolescence is also the time when **psychiatric disorders** may present. Such conditions may include **schizophrenia, depression, bipolar disorder, eating disorders, substance abuse, and obsessive-compulsive disorder (OCD). Personality disorders** may also become evident. Antisocial personality disorder is related to conduct disorders in earlier years.

However, delinquent behaviors may be related to low birth weight, brain damage, socioeconomic status, and poor educational achievement. Low birth weight as well as male gender, mental retardation, and intrauterine alcohol exposure are also risk factors for psychiatric disorders. Girls are more vulnerable to stressors than boys during their teens. These increased risk factors, combined with a "poor fit" with their parents, make some adolescents very vulnerable to stressors. Protective factors may include certain personality traits, a supportive family, and a healthy support system.

Sexual Response Cycle This cycle is made up of four different phases:

1. **Desire/libido:** Various hormone levels and the brain itself drive this phase. Low testosterone is associated with low libido in both genders. High levels of prolactin (can be caused by some antipsychotic agents) also decrease libido. The roles of other hormones remain unclear. The hypothalamus and the limbic system may contribute to desire. Medications (antihypertensives, digoxin, some diuretics, tricyclics, selective serotonergic reuptake inhibitors (SSRIs), and some antipsychotic agents), medical diseases, and psychiatric disorders such as depression and anxiety can all affect libido.

2. **Arousal:** In this phase the parasympathetic system causes increased blood flow to the male genitals, whereas the sympathetic system is thought to cause labial swelling and vaginal lubrication in the female. The autonomic system is responsible for increased heart rate, breathing, and hardening of the nipples. Diseases that affect blood supply to these areas, such as vascular disease, diabetes, and neurological diseases, can impair erection in the male. Levels of anxiety and various medications may also affect arousal. Medications include various antidepressants, antipsychotics, lithium, anticonvulsants, antihypertensives, beta-blockers, cimetidine, and substances such as alcohol or cocaine. If a male with erectile dysfunction cannot achieve erection with masturbation or during sleep, this suggests an organic cause.

3. **Orgasm:** In females orgasm leads to contractions in the vagina and ejaculation of fluids (in some individuals). Females are capable of multiple orgasms. In males the sympathetic system facilitates ejaculation during orgasm, which is then followed by a refractory phase. The ability to achieve orgasm may be affected by levels of anxiety, certain medications, such as antidepressants, antipsychotics, some benzodiazepines, and such substances as alcohol. Disorders of this phase in males include premature ejaculation and male orgasmic disorder (also known as inhibited male orgasm), whereas in females inhibited orgasm is referred to as female orgasmic disorder.

4. **Resolution:** This is the refractory period. During this time the individual is unable to become aroused again. The length of this phase increases with age.

Case Conclusion After a thorough examination of JB you find no evidence of any disease process that might hinder normal development. You educate him about the phases of pubertal development and sexual responses, and reassure him that he will develop normally. You encourage him to continue to participate in sports activities and to attend to his schoolwork. When he returns 6 months later for a tetanus shot after a soccer injury, he tells you "things are developing just fine."

Thumbnail: Behavioral Science—Tanner's Stages of Sexual Development

Sex Maturity Rating Stage	BOYS			GIRLS	
	Pubic Hair	Penis	Testes	Pubic Hair	Breasts
I	None	Preadolescent	Preadolescent	Preadolescent	Preadolescent
II	Scanty, long, slightly pigmented	Slight enlargement	Enlarged scrotum, pink texture altered	Sparse, lightly pigmented, straight, medial border of labia	Breast and papilla elevated as small mounds; areolar diameter is increased
III	Darker, starts to curl, small amount	Longer	Larger	Darker, starts to curl, increased amount	Breast and areola enlarged; no contour separation
IV	Like adult type, coarse and curly but less in quantity	Larger, glans and width increased in size	Larger, scrotum dark	Coarse, curly but less than adult	Areola and papilla form secondary mound
V	Adult distribution, spread to medial surface of thighs	Adult size	Adult size	Adult feminine triangle, spread to medial surface thighs	Mature, with projecting nipple and areola as part of breast contour

Key Points

► The average age of menarche for females is 12.8 years. The average age for boys to start producing sperm is 14.3 years.

► Pubic hair development is under the control of the adrenal androgens in both sexes.

► Breast development usually occurs first in females, but 15% may have pubic hair first.

► Usually, within 2 years of breast development the menarche occurs.

► Testicular enlargement is usually first in males. Male facial hair usually begins within 2 years of the appearance of pubic hair.

► Cognitive development is significant for the ability to conceptualize ideas, form more abstract thoughts, and engage in recursive thinking.

► Levels of emotional feeling do not change dramatically from prepubertal levels.

► Increased rates of depression and anxiety in adolescents have been reported, particularly in females.

► Social development is defined by the surrounding social circumstances.

► African American male adolescents have higher rates of death by suicide and homicide than Caucasian males of the same age.

► Pregnant adolescent mothers are at higher risk of having infants with low birth weight and developmental delays.

Questions

1. Which of the following syndromes is correctly matched with its genotype and phenotype?
   A. Testicular feminization syndrome—Genotype XY—Phenotype Female
   B. Congenital adrenal hyperplasia—Genotype XY—Phenotype Male
   C. Turner's syndrome—Genotype XY—Phenotype Female
   D. Testicular feminization syndrome—Genotype XX—Phenotype Female
   E. Congenital adrenal hyperplasia—Genotype XO—Phenotype Female

2. Which of the following medications is associated with a decrease in sexual functioning?
   A. Levodopa
   B. Yohimbine
   C. SSRIs
   D. Venlafaxine
   E. Sildenafil

3. A 45-year-old married male comes to your office complaining of sexual dysfunction. On further questioning he reveals that he is unable to achieve an erection either in the morning or with stimulation. Which of the following statements might you tell the patient?
   A. Between 20% and 30% of males in the United States suffer from erectile dysfunction.
   B. Treatments may include intramuscular vasodilators.
   C. It is mainly caused by psychological reasons.
   D. Organic causes include epilepsy and hypertension.
   E. Trazadone may be helpful in a third of cases.

4. TP is a 22-year-old recently married female who presents with a history of anorgasmia. She tells you that she loves her husband and was looking forward to beginning their sexual relationship. She says that she gets excited and enjoys making love with her husband but has never had an orgasm. Which of the following is accurate concerning female orgasmic disorder?
   A. It is always psychological in nature.
   B. It includes occasional orgasmic problems.
   C. It is more prevalent in older women.
   D. It is associated with certain personality disorders.
   E. Most are lifelong rather than acquired.

HPI: AB is a 29-year-old married Caucasian female who is referred to your clinic during the third month of her first pregnancy. She complains about feeling anxious and tired and has occasional insomnia as well as some nausea and vomiting. Her husband has noticed that her mood has become more erratic and that she is "quick to fly off the handle" or burst into tears. She also reports diminished sex drive and expresses concerns about her body. She is afraid that she will become less attractive as the pregnancy proceeds. She has a medical history of a tonsillectomy at age 5 and a pregnancy termination at age 17. She takes no medications other than prenatal vitamins.

Her family history includes a mother who suffered from postpartum depression and a father who has type 2 non-insulin-dependent diabetes mellitus (NIDDM). She is the youngest of three children. She graduated from college and works full-time as an accountant. She has been married for 2 years. She and her husband live in rented accommodations. She denies ever using illicit substances but before her pregnancy did drink two or three glasses of wine a couple of nights a week when socializing.

MSE: Appropriately dressed in business attire, good hygiene, eye contact, and rapport.

Speech is soft but of normal tone. She shows no abnormal movements. Her affect is tearful during the interview as she discusses her hopes and fears for the pregnancy. She describes her mood as "up and down." Thought processes are logical and goal directed. She shows no indications of psychosis and no SI or HI. Cognition, insight, and judgment are all intact.

Thought Questions

- What do you think is happening to this young woman?
- Is pregnancy associated with increased rates of psychopathology?
- How should she be treated?

Basic Science Review and Discussion

The first trimester of pregnancy can be associated with a variety of physical and psychological concerns. The physical symptoms of early pregnancy include bloating, tiredness (or even insomnia), headaches, constipation, and morning sickness. Psychological symptoms include anxiety about the pregnancy itself, whether the baby will be alright, whether her husband will find her attractive, whether she will be a good mother, and whether she can balance her own needs and career with those of a young infant. A woman's sense of mothering is often influenced strongly by her own mother as her role model. It is important to inquire about levels of support from her husband, family, and friends. Also, ask about her future aspirations for her life. Some women may experience decreased libido during pregnancy. They may have concerns about harming the fetus during intercourse or physical discomfort. Sexual intercourse is not prohibited during pregnancy and some women may find they have increased sexual interest and satisfaction during this time. This may be due to engorgement of the sexual organs, which occurs in pregnancy.

Although pregnancy is usually viewed as a healthy condition, not an illness, between 20% and 70% of pregnant women report some symptoms of depression (see Thumbnail), but only 10% to 16% meet diagnostic criteria for a major depressive episode during this time (similar to rates in nonpregnant women). It would be important to note if the women in her family had a history of postpartum depression, as this might place her at higher risk for this disorder.

Treatment of such symptoms is supportive. Both the patient and her partner may benefit from psychoeducation and supportive psychotherapy. All psychoactive medications may cross the placenta, so in general such medications are avoided unless the patient reaches diagnostic criteria for a major depressive disorder or any other *Diagnostic and Statistical Manual of Mental Disorders,* 4th edition *(DSM-IV)*, Axis 1 diagnosis.

Up to 85% of women experience some mood disturbance during the postpartum period. For the majority these symptoms are mild and do not last long, but if they are moderate or severe they can put the mother and infant at risk and have possible long-term effects on the infant's development. There is a reported increase in psychiatric admissions during this time. The majority of these conditions are mood disorders and are classified in *DSM-IV* as a subtype of depressive or bipolar disorders. Women with a history of bipolar disorder are particularly at increased risk for a relapse (between 20% and 50%) during this time. Care must be taken to rule out any medical conditions that may have psychiatric symptoms, such as hypothyroidism, Sheehan's syndrome (pituitary infarction), or delirium due to infection.

Pseudocyesis (false pregnancy) can occur in women who have an ardent desire to become pregnant and may be accompanied by many of the symptoms of real pregnancy.

Case Conclusion AB and her husband were relieved to learn that such symptoms could be normal during pregnancy. They were encouraged to attend antenatal classes offered at the hospital. During individual counseling sessions her fears and hopes for her pregnancy were explored fully and she was reassured. She was encouraged to follow the basic principles of sleep hygiene (i.e., regular exercise; avoidance of stimulating substances such as chocolate, caffeine, and alcohol; and relaxation exercises in the evening before bed). Six weeks later, she returned and was doing much better.

Thumbnail: Behavioral Science—Psychiatric Symptoms Associated with Pregnancy and the Postpartum Period

Condition	Epidemiology	Symptoms	Treatment/Prognosis
Depression during pregnancy	10% to 16%	Depressed mood, anxiety	Treatment includes psychotherapy and antidepressants if depression is severe. Increased likelihood of postpartum depression.
Baby blues	30% to 85% prevalence	Onset within 1 week postpartum. Presents with labile mood, tearfulness, anxiety, and insomnia	Treatment includes support, reassurance, and education. Symptoms tend to remit spontaneously by the tenth day.
Postpartum depression	10% to 15% prevalence	Onset within the first 3 months, may be insidious, with depression, anxiety, and insomnia	Treatment includes antidepressants and psychotherapy. Risk of recurrence is 50%.
Postpartum psychosis	0.1% to 0.2% prevalence	Onset usually within the first month, with depressed mood or manic symptoms of euphoria, irritability, agitation, disorganized behavior, depersonalization, or delusions	Treatment includes antipsychotics with mood stabilizers if bipolar in presentation and antipsychotics and antidepressants if depressed. If severe, may consider electroconvulsive therapy. Risk of recurrence is 70%.

Key Points

▶ Pregnancy can be associated with physical and psychological concerns.

▶ Between 20% and 70% of pregnant women report some symptoms of depression.

▶ Ten percent to sixteen percent of patients meet diagnostic criteria for a major depression.

▶ A family history of postpartum depression or psychosis increases the risk for developing these disorders.

▶ Treatment of psychiatric symptoms during pregnancy includes psychoeducation and supportive psychotherapy.

▶ Psychoactive medications are avoided if possible during pregnancy but may be needed if symptoms are severe.

▶ Up to 85% of women experience some mood disturbance during the postpartum period.

Questions

1. A 16-year-old female presents with her first pregnancy at 14 weeks of gestation. Aside from the usual prenatal care, you are concerned because of her age. Which of the following is associated with teenage pregnancy?
   A. It represents a small number of unmarried mothers.
   B. Low risk for obstetric complications.
   C. Depression and having divorced parents.
   D. About 50% of teenagers use contraception regularly.
   E. More than 70% of unmarried mothers are teenagers.

2. Which of the following is true concerning early adulthood (20 to 40 years)?
   A. Erikson defined this as a period of intimacy versus despair.
   B. Up to 70% of those aged 30 years are married with children.
   C. A person's role in society is envisioned.
   D. A period of reassessment does not occur.
   E. Physical development diminishes.

3. The patient from the preceding case is concerned about her risk of postpartum depression. During your discussion with her you mention all of the following but do not mention that
   A. The baby blues is a short-lived depressed mood experienced by up to 50% of women after delivery.
   B. Postpartum depression occurs in 5% to 10% of women.
   C. Postpartum psychosis develops in 1% of women.
   D. Postpartum disorders are influenced by a variety of psychosocial factors.
   E. Women with a family history of postpartum mood disorders may be at increased risk.

4. MB is a 39-year-old primigravida who had an 8-pound healthy baby boy by vaginal delivery 4 days previously. Her husband has brought her to the emergency room because he is concerned about her. Two days previously she had become restless and irritable, and had a poor appetite. She then became very agitated and confused, and appeared to be hallucinating. Which of the following would you tell him?
   A. Postpartum psychosis usually occurs in multigravida females.
   B. Family history is noncontributory.
   C. Approximately 50% recover fully.
   D. Approximately 50% have further episodes of psychosis.
   E. Approximately 10% of women commit infanticide.

HPI: TZ is a 26-year-old married woman who suffers from bipolar disorder and is well maintained on mood-stabilizing medications. At a routine follow-up appointment, she tells you that she and her husband are considering starting a family.

She was first diagnosed with bipolar affective disorder when she presented with a manic episode at age 19. She was originally stabilized on a combination of an antipsychotic haloperidol and lithium. After taking lithium for 2 years her mood stabilizer was changed to valproic acid, as she was complaining of intolerable side effects. She has been hospitalized twice for manic episodes and treated as an outpatient for depression. She has never abused substances and does not use tobacco products. She has never been suicidal. She has a family history of bipolar disorder and major depression. She graduated from college and works as a dental hygienist. She lives in a rented apartment with her husband of 2 years, who works as a mechanic. She is taking prenatal vitamins and valproic acid 750 mg by mouth twice daily.

PE: Results of a recent annual physical with Chem 7, CBC, TFT, and UA were all within normal limits. Recent valproic acid level was 80 μg/mL (reference range is 50–125 μg/mL).

MSE: She is well presented, her affect is of normal range, and her mood is euthymic. There is no evidence of psychosis and cognitive functions are intact.

Thought Questions

- What are your concerns about medications should this patient become pregnant?

- What other psychiatric medications can cause problems during pregnancy and during breast-feeding?

- What side effects of lithium may have proved intolerable?

Basic Science Review and Discussion

Care must be taken when prescribing **any medications** during pregnancy and while breast-feeding, but particular caution should be taken with psychiatric medications. The dangers to the fetus must be compared with the dangers of psychiatric illness, such as psychosis or depression. When a woman becomes pregnant her psychiatric medications and her mental state should be reviewed immediately, as the hormonal changes of pregnancy may cause changes in her psychiatric disorder.

Antipsychotic Agents   Antipsychotic agents should be avoided in the first trimester, if possible. Although there is no conclusive evidence that these agents are teratogenic, low-potency agents such as chlorpromazine may increase the risk of fetal malformations. Low-potency agents may also cause hypotension. In general, if they are needed, high-potency agents such as haloperidol should be used. Breast-feeding is not contraindicated in those taking phenothiazines. Antiparkinsonian agents should not be prescribed routinely to those who are pregnant. There have been case reports of feeding difficulties, hypertonicity, and dystonic and parkinsonian movements in infants exposed to antipsychotic agents.

Antidepressants   If possible, depressive symptoms in the first trimester should be treated with supportive measures and **psychoactive medications should be avoided,** but if severe depression develops, medications may be necessary, electroconvulsive therapy (ECT) may also be considered. Limb deformities have been reported with tricyclics, but the studies of teratogenesis remain inconclusive. Some agents such as amitriptyline, trimipramine, and trazadone have been reported to be associated with poor outcomes in animal studies. There is concern about the neurologic development of the fetus with the use of tricyclic agents in the second and third trimesters, and a withdrawal syndrome has been reported in neonates. The long-term effects of exposure to tricyclic antidepressants in breast milk are unknown and should be avoided, if possible. Monoamine oxidase inhibitors (MAOI) are contraindicated in pregnancy, as there have been reports of growth retardation in animal studies and these agents may exacerbate pregnancy-induced hypertension and affect placental perfusion. These agents are also contraindicated with the use of beta-mimetic agents in premature labor and opioids during labor itself. Selective serotonergic reuptake inhibitors (SSRI) are usually regarded as safe in pregnancy, but there is concern about possible behavioral tetratogenicity. Fluoxetine may be associated with increased minor physical anomalies, but this remains controversial. There is less information about the safety of venlafaxine, nefazadone, and bupropion.

Mood Stabilizers   Lithium should be avoided in the first trimester because of possible teratogenesis, namely Ebstein's anomaly (hypoplasia of the right ventricle and abnormalities of the tricuspid valve) which may occur in 1 in 1000 exposed. Lithium may cause neonatal goiter and impair vaginal delivery, as well as result in neurologic and cardiovascular abnormalities in the neonate. Hence, it should be avoided in the first trimester and monitored closely during the rest of pregnancy because, if it must be used, the dramatic changes in fluid volume and renal function caused by pregnancy necessitate higher doses than in the nonpregnant state. After labor, rapid fluid loss may cause toxic effects, and lithium doses should be decreased 2 weeks before delivery and carefully monitored. The physician should look for evidence of toxic effects in the neonate. Lithium is secreted in breast milk, and neonatal renal function may lead to toxicity, with cyanosis, poor muscle tone, and cardiac abnormalities. It is therefore contraindicated during breast-feeding. Other agents, such as the anticonvulsants carbamazepine and valproic acid, have been reported to be associated with a tenfold increased risk (1% to 5%) of neural tube defects such as spina bifida. There are reports of cleft palates in those exposed to these drugs in the first trimester. However, these agents may be safer than lithium in those who wish to breast-feed.

Benzodiazepines Diazepam crosses the placenta and has been reported to have a twofold increase in cleft lips and palate. The question of its teratogenesis remains unresolved; therefore it should be avoided in the first trimester. Occasional use in the second and third trimesters is not thought to have ill effects. Clonazepam may be used in the first trimester to control manic symptoms if antipsychotics cannot control symptoms. Impaired temperature regulation, apnea, low apgar scores, feeding difficulties, and hypotonicity have been reported in neonates exposed to benzodiazepines.

Miscellaneous Neonates may show withdrawal effects if the mother has been dependent on alcohol or opiates. Alcohol itself is a known teratogen and causes fetal alcohol syndrome.

Case Conclusion TZ was encouraged to plan her pregnancy carefully in close coordinated care with her obstetrician. She returns to visit you when she finds out she is pregnant. After careful discussion with both the patient and her husband, you decide to taper and discontinue the valproic acid and maintain her on low doses of haloperidol. During the second trimester, you restart the valproic acid at a lower dose and monitor her carefully throughout her pregnancy. She delivers a healthy baby boy, her medications are increased to her usual doses, and she is further carefully monitored for her high risk of postpartum relapse.

Thumbnail: Behavioral Science—Pharmacology of Lithium

Uses	Control of acute mania and prophylaxis of recurrent bipolar, unipolar disorder and schizoaffective disorder. It is used as an augmenting agent in schizophrenia.
Pharmacokinetics	Rapidly absorbed by oral route; complete within 6 to 8 hours. Peak plasma levels within 30 minutes to 2 hours. Not protein bound. Not metabolized; excreted unchanged by the kidney. **Rates of clearance depend on renal function** and follow sodium reabsorption in the proximal tubules. Increased sodium intake causes decreased reabsorption, and a sodium-restricted diet causes increased lithium reabsorption, leading to toxicity.
Therapeutic action	Exact mechanism of action remains unknown but is thought to influence sodium and calcium transfer across membranes, affecting neurotransmitter release and receptor activity; also acts via inhibiting cAMP second messenger systems. Stimulates Na and Mg-dependent ATPase. Increases uptake of tryptophan by serotoninergic neurons.
Adverse effects	Early side effects: Nausea, vomiting and diarrhea, fine tremor, dry mouth, fatigue, drowsiness, nasal congestion, and metallic taste. Long term: Nephrogenic diabetes insipidus with polyurea and polydipsia due to distal tubule becoming resistant to ADH in approximately 9% to 20% of users. Hypothyroidism in approximately 5% of users; females more commonly affected than males. Edema and weight gain. Cardiac effects include T-wave flattening and arrhythmias. Neurologic effects include choreoathetosis, ataxia, dysarthria, tardive dyskinesia, and memory impairment. Acne and alopecia. Increased risk of Ebstein's anomaly in fetuses exposed in the first trimester of pregnancy. Reported hypotonicity and cyanosis in infants.
Drug interactions	Thiazides decrease lithium clearance by 30% to 50%. Low-salt diets, pregnancy, and diarrhea/vomiting/dehydration may increase levels. NSAIDs may also increase levels. Levels and risk of neurotoxicity may be increased by neuroleptics and carbamazepine. Levels of lithium decreased by theophylline, caffeine, antacids, acetazolamide, and osmotic diuretics.
Monitoring serum levels	Sampling should be drawn 12 hours after last dose to avoid peak levels. Such peaks and troughs are avoided with slow-release preparations. In acute disorders, serum levels should range between 0.8 and 1.2 mEq/L and maintenance, 0.6 to 0.8 mEq/L. In older persons keep at 0.5 mEq/L Toxic effects occur at levels greater than 2 mmol/L and may include tremor, ataxia, slurred speech, confusion, convulsions, coma, and death.

Key Points

▶ Care must be taken when prescribing any medications during pregnancy and while breast-feeding.

▶ Antipsychotic agents should be avoided in the first trimester if possible.

▶ If possible, treat depressive symptoms in the first trimester with supportive measures and avoid medications, but, if necessary, medications or ECT may be used.

▶ Lithium should be avoided in the first trimester because of possible teratogenesis and is contraindicated during breast-feeding.

▶ Diazepam has been reported to cause cleft lips and palate, and should be avoided in the first trimester.

▶ Neonates may show withdrawal effects if the mother has been dependent on alcohol or opiates.

▶ Lithium is an effective mood stabilizer but requires monitoring to minimize adverse effects.

Questions

1. Which of the following tests would you recommend to a patient taking lithium?
   A. Urea, electrolytes, creatinine, thyroxine, TSH, and EKG monthly
   B. Follow-up lithium levels weekly
   C. EKG every 6 months
   D. Urea, electrolytes, creatinine, thyroxine, TSH, EKG, and pregnancy tests at baseline, followed by lithium levels every 8 weeks, repeat chemistry, and TFTs twice a year and EKG annually
   E. Urea, electrolytes, creatinine, thyroxine, TSH, EKG, and pregnancy tests at baseline, followed by lithium levels every 12 weeks, repeat chemistry and TFTs three times a year, and EKG twice a year

2. When discussing the possible side effects of valproic acid with the above patient and her husband which of the following do you warn her about?
   A. Nausea, vomiting, weight and hair loss
   B. Nausea, vomiting, weight gain, and hair growth
   C. Nausea, vomiting, weight gain, hair loss, agitation, neural tube defects in fetuses
   D. Nausea, vomiting, weight gain, hair loss, sedation, tremor, and neural tube defects in fetuses
   E. Nausea, vomiting, weight gain, hair loss, sedation, thyroid abnormalities, and neural tube defects in fetuses

3. In general, when prescribing medications to a patient, which of the following does not affect the distribution of a drug?
   A. Edema
   B. Pregnancy
   C. Hypoparathyroidism
   D. Obesity
   E. Age

4. Which of the following statements is correct?
   A. The therapeutic window is the ratio between the lethal dose and the clinically effective dose.
   B. The therapeutic index is the range of concentration of a drug in the serum in which the drug has a maximum clinical effect.
   C. Efficacy is a measure of a drug's maximum effect.
   D. Potency is a measure of a drug's ability to produce a desired effect.
   E. There are no drugs used in psychiatry that have a therapeutic window.

HPI: DS is an 18-year-old male who has recently moved to your area with his family due to his father's employment. He presents to your office asking "to be tested," because he has recently started in the final year at a new high school with a different curriculum and has been scoring badly on standardized tests in this new environment. He wants to have his IQ measured and to check his "personality." He denies symptoms of depression and mania but does admit to a recent onset of anxiety, which is new for him.

He denies any psychiatric history and does not use nicotine products or abuse substances. He has no significant medical history. He also denies any family psychiatric history. His father has hypertension and his mother has migraines. He is the younger of two sons, and his brother is away at college. He broke up with his girlfriend when he moved, saying that it was "pointless."

PE: Normal.

MSE: He appeared his stated age with good hygiene, eye contact, and rapport. Speech and behavior were normal. Affect was normal in range and his mood was described as "fed up." Thought processes were logical and goal directed. There was no evidence of suicidality, homicidality, or psychosis.

Thought Questions

- What kinds of IQ testing are available?

- What kinds of personality tests could he be referring to?

- Do you think such tests are indicated in this situation?

Basic Science Review and Discussion

Psychological testing may be used in various situations to assess general intelligence, personality, and neuropsychological status. Intelligence is defined as the individual's capacity to learn, recall information, integrate information constructively, and think rationally. Intelligence tests assess the current level of functioning and the capacity for adaptive behavior. Personality tests reveal enduring personality traits, and neuropsychological tests reveal the presence and degree of brain dysfunction.

IQ scores may also be used to define the subtypes of mental retardation. According to *Diagnostic and Statistical Manual of Mental Disorders,* 4th edition (*DSM-IV*), mild mental retardation is defined by an IQ score of between 50–55 and approximately 70. An IQ score ranging between 35–40 and 50–55 defines moderate mental retardation, Severe mental retardation has IQ scores ranging from 20–25 to 35–40, and those with profound mental retarda-

tion have IQ scores below 20 or 25. Approximately 2% of the population in the United States is mentally retarded. Approximately 2% have IQ scores above 130, which is considered very superior.

Psychological tests can be used to investigate the presence of organic pathology, to discriminate between functional and organic pathology, to monitor changes in functioning over time, to enhance diagnosis in psychiatric patients, to help make decisions about competency and academic placements, and to plan cognitive rehabilitation (e.g., after a stroke). All psychological tests must be standardized with regard to procedures (repeatable) and the scores related to normative data. These tests must also be reliable and valid. The advantage of such tests is that they can provide information not regularly available. This information may be obtained relatively rapidly to aid diagnosis and treatment planning and can provide objective and quantifiable information to be compared with normative data.

Psychological tests may be objective, with questions that are scored and statistically analyzed (e.g., Minnesota Multiphasic Personality Inventory [MMPI]), or subjective (e.g., the Rorschach Inkblot Test), where subjects are asked for their interpretation of a question or situation. Tests may be given to individuals or to groups of individuals (e.g., achievement tests). Achievement tests are used in schools and to provide career counseling in the industrial setting.

Case Conclusion Although DS is concerned about his current situation, it does not appear that he is suffering from any organic lesion, which could cause a change in personality or intelligence. He appears to be having difficulty adjusting to his new situation. There is no evidence of a depression, anxiety disorder, or psychosis. You counsel him with regard to your assessment and his lack of indications for such testing. You also encourage him to explore new social venues and to pursue his studies. When he returns for a follow-up visit 3 months later, his grades have significantly improved and he is doing well.

Thumbnail: Behavioral Science—Neuropsychological Tests

Type of Tests	Content and Uses
General Intelligence	
Stanford-Binet	Used to assess intellectual ability from the age of 2 to 18 years. The IQ is calculated as the ratio of mental age to chronologic age multiplied by 100. Therefore when these two ages are the same, the IQ is 100. It gives four cognitive scores, which may be compared to normative data.
Wechsler Adult Intelligence Scale (WAIS)	This has adult and other specific forms for children (Wechsler Intelligence Scale for Children [WISC] and the Wechsler Preschool and Primary Scale of Intelligence). The adult form compares normative data up to 74 years of age. It has 11 subtests, which measure verbal IQ, visual IQ, and perceptuomotor abilities. It has high validity and reliability.
Personality	
Minnesota Multiphasic Personality Inventory	A self-rating questionnaire that is used in psychiatric patients.
Rorschach Inkblot Test	A projective test used to identify thought disorders and the nature of an individual's defense systems.
Thematic Apperception Test	A projective test where subjects are asked to make up a story based on the picture shown. These responses are used to evaluate the individual's emotional state, motivations, and inner conflicts.
Sentence Completion Test	A projective test that uses sentence completion to identify an individual's problems.
Neuropsychological	
Halstead Reitan Test Battery	Can be used in children or adults. Consists of five tests that may be supplemented by ancillary individual tests. High validity. Used mainly to detect, localize, and assess the effects of localized brain lesions.
Luria-Nebraska Battery	Also has a form for adults and children. There are various clinical, localization, and summary scales, depending on the form used. Useful for assessing left-right brain dominance and for identifying specific dysfunctions, such as dyslexia.
Wechsler Memory Scale	Used to test recall, both immediate and delayed, of visual and verbal information, attention, and concentration, and associative learning. Provides information about memory.

Key Points

▶ Psychological testing may be used to assess intelligence, personality, and neuropsychological status.

▶ Intelligence is defined as the individual's capacity to learn, recall information, integrate information constructively, and think rationally.

▶ Psychological tests must be standardized with regard to procedures (repeatable) and the scores related to normative data. These tests must also be reliable and valid.

▶ Psychological tests may be objective or subjective.

▶ Achievement tests are used to evaluate how well instructed material has been learned.

Questions

1. According to the criteria of *DSM-IV*, which of the following IQ ranges is classified correctly?
   A. Borderline mental retardation: 50–55 to 70–79
   B. Mild mental retardation: 35–40 to 50–55
   C. Moderate mental retardation: 20–25 to 35–40
   D. Severe mental retardation: Below 20–25
   E. Profound mental retardation: Below 20–25

2. Which of the following sources of error that may occur when using questionnaires or interviews is correctly defined?
   A. Response set—the subject chooses answers that fit with previously chosen answers.
   B. Hawthorne effect—the subject tends to pick the middle response and avoids extreme answers.
   C. Halo effect—researchers alter the situation by virtue of their very presence.
   D. Social acceptability—the subject always tends to agree or disagree with questions.
   E. Bias towards center—the subject tends to choose the middle response and avoids extreme answers.

3. Which of the following dysfunctions is correctly paired with its associated brain location?
   A. Expressive language problems and the temporal lobe
   B. Receptive language problems and the frontal lobe
   C. Finger agnosia and the nondominant parietal lobe
   D. Constructional apraxia and the nondominant parietal lobe
   E. Dysgraphia and the nondominant parietal lobe

4. TL is a 60-year-old male who has been admitted after a hemorrhagic stroke. As part of the assessment and work-up, which of the following neuropsychological tests would you consider important?
   A. Minnesota Multiphasic Personality Inventory
   B. Sentence Completion Test
   C. Stanford-Binet
   D. Halstead Reitan Battery
   E. WAIS

HPI: The W's have brought their 6-year-old son FW to see you because he is wetting his bed several nights a week and his pediatrician thinks that you may be able to help.

FW is the eldest of three boys and is described as a "happy, normal child" by his parents. He was started on toilet training at about the age of 2 and achieved control of his bowels by the age of 3. He has never had complete control of his bladder functioning and has wet the bed at least once a week, but this has increased since the birth of his youngest brother 6 months ago. He is attending school and is doing well with no daytime wetting episodes. His pediatrician has seen him regularly since birth, and there was no evidence of structural problems, infection, or medical conditions that may be associated with bed-wetting (enuresis). He achieved all the other developmental milestones without any delay. His appetite and sleep patterns are regular and he is very social but refuses to stay over at a friend's house because of his bed-wetting.

Thought Questions

■ You decide to use the bell-and-pad technique. What is this an example of?

■ What other learning-based techniques could you consider?

■ What are other applications of behavioral techniques?

Basic Science Review and Discussion

Learning itself is the acquisition of behavior patterns and continues throughout the life cycle. Learning is divided into two major categories and includes classical conditioning and operant conditioning.

Classical Conditioning Classical conditioning is based on the work of Ivan Pavlov. Here a conditioned stimulus is associated with an unconditioned stimulus to produce a desired response. The subject is passive and the response is typically emotional or autonomic. A stimulus is a cue from an internal or external event. In Pavlov's classic experiment the unconditioned stimulus was presence of food, which caused the response of salivation. He then paired this unconditioned stimulus with a conditioned stimulus of a bell ringing. After learning occurred, the bell alone stimulated the response of salivation. There are two major phases in this type of learning. First is the **acquisition phase,** where the conditioned response is learned. Second is the **extinction phase,** where the conditioned response (salivation with the bell) fades when the conditioned stimulus is no longer followed by the unconditioned stimulus (food). Spontaneous recovery may occur when the conditioned response reappears. The link between the conditioned stimulus and conditioned response can be recovered also by repeating the pairing with the unconditioned stimulus. Stimulus generalization may also occur when a new stimulus similar to the conditioned stimulus (e.g., a buzzer instead of a bell) will provoke the conditioned response. In higher-order con-

ditioning a new conditioned stimulus can be learned by pairing it with the old conditioned stimulus, which is then acting as an unconditioned stimulus.

The bell-and-pad technique for the treatment of bed-wetting is also an example of classical conditioning. A fluid-sensitive pad is placed under the child's bedding; when urine wets the pad, a bell rings, the child wakes, and he is brought to the toilet to empty his bladder. Over time, the child learns to wake spontaneously to void his bladder.

Aversive conditioning has been used to treat unwanted behaviors (e.g., a sexual interest in children) with a noxious aversive stimulus, such as an electric shock or an agent that may cause vomiting. This type of learning also follows the preceding phases and patterns of extinction and spontaneous recovery.

Operant Conditioning B. F. Skinner did much of the initial work on operant conditioning. The frequency of a spontaneous behavior can be determined by its following consequence (or reinforcement). Reinforcement affects the probability of a response being made. This reinforcement can be a reward or a punishment. Therefore, a novel new behavior may be learned. The principles involved with reinforcement include positive reinforcements or rewards that are pleasant and increase the rate at which the desired behavior occurs (e.g., buying a present if the child achieves bladder control). These rewards can be tangible, such as a present, or intangible, such as increased attention given to the child. Negative reinforcement occurs when a negative stimulus (or unpleasant condition) is removed and it increases the rate of the desired behavior. Both types of reinforcement can be used to increase desired behavior.

There are several types of reinforcement scheduling (Table 7-1). Punishment is an aversive stimulus, which is aimed at reducing an unwanted behavior, but it may not work as well as extinction (e.g., ignoring unwanted behavior in a child). Punishment is also a negative reinforcer, as the adverse consequences of a response actually suppress a response. Escape

Table 7-1. Schedules of Reinforcement

Schedule	Features
Continuous	Reinforcement/reward given after every time desired behavior occurs. Least resistant to extinction, but although learned quickly it also disappears quickly without reinforcement.
Variable ratio	Reinforcement given after an unpredictable and random number of responses and is highly resistant to extinction.
Variable interval	Reinforcement given after an unpredictable and random amount of time. Also highly resistant to extinction.
Fixed ratio	Reinforcement given after a certain number of responses. Produces a fast response rate.
Fixed interval	Reinforcement given after a certain time. The rate of response increases as the agreed time approaches.

conditioning is a particular type of reinforcement that is very resistant to extinction, as it provides complete escape from the unpleasant situation, such as the individual with agoraphobia running out of the supermarket.

Behaviors may also be shaped or modeled. In shaping, successive approximations to the desired behavior are reinforced/rewarded until the desired behavior is reached. In modeling, behaviors of role models are observed and then adopted and are an example of observational learning. With chaining techniques more complex behaviors are broken into a sequence of steps, which are then learned. Behavior

modification is important not only in working with children or mentally retarded patients but also in social skills training and managing wards with token economy systems.

All behavioral treatments involve the principles of learning theory, with an observation of behavior, concentration on symptoms, clear goals, directive treatment methods, and an empirical approach. They can be used successfully to eliminate unwanted behaviors such as nicotine addiction. The Premack principle states that any frequently performed behavior can be used to positively reinforce a less frequent behavior.

Case Conclusion   You decide to use a combination of the bell-and-pad method and star charts. You encourage the parents to toilet FW after each awakening and to remake the bed with the pad in place. Using star charts, dry nights are rewarded with a gold star, which in turn may be used to earn a specific reward. After several weeks, FW and his parents return to report excellent results. You tell them these techniques can be reused later if the bed-wetting begins again.

Thumbnail: Behavioral Science—Other Applications of Behavioral Techniques

Phobias	Here the techniques of systematic desensitization and flooding are used to treat these irrational fears. An individual is exposed in a graded hierarchical manner either to images of a stimulus or to the actual stimulus itself in combination with relaxation exercises. This is based on the principle that when individuals are relaxed they cannot experience the fear. On the other hand, during flooding the paradoxical technique of entering the feared situation results in initially enhanced fear and arousal responses, which then decrease over time with the exposure and are extinguished.
Sexual deviancy	Here techniques of aversion (as above) and covert sensitization (e.g., ridicule, arresting, and court appearances) are used.
Chronic schizophrenia	A token economy uses positive reinforcements or rewards for good behavior, which can be exchanged for desire objects later.
Mental retardation	Techniques of behavior modification and token economy can be useful.
Obsessional conditions	Response prevention is useful in the treatment of obsessional rituals with a motor component and includes thought stopping, in which a distracting stimulus such as flicking a rubber band on the wrist is used to "break" the cycle of rumination.
Sexual inadequacy	Here behavioral techniques of Masters and Johnson can be helpful. Gradually, partners learned to relax and enjoy massage and nonsexual touching, which is gradually increased to achieve successful intercourse.
Marital difficulties	May respond to contract therapy, where spouses agree to modify certain behaviors.
Depression and anxiety	Cognitive behavior techniques are used to replace distorted, negative thoughts with more positive, enhancing ones. This is used in combination with a graded schedule of homework activities designed to enhance the patient's sense of mastery and accomplishment.
Hypertension and headaches	Biofeedback techniques
Enuresis	Bell-and-pad technique, as discussed above

Key Points

▶ Pavlov developed classical conditioning. A conditioned stimulus is associated with an unconditioned stimulus to produce a desired response. A stimulus is a cue from an internal or external event.

▶ Skinner initially described operant conditioning. The frequency of a spontaneous behavior can be determined by its consequence (or reinforcement). This reinforcement can be a reward or a punishment.

▶ There are several types of reinforcement scheduling, including continuous, variable ratio/interval, and fixed ratio/interval.

▶ Behaviors may also be shaped or modeled.

Questions

1. A child receives a course of immunizing injections from the nurse at his pediatrician's office. On a routine visit, he bursts into tears when he sees this nurse, even though he does not receive an injection. This behavior continues for several more visits before it subsides. This is an example of

   A. Operant conditioning
   B. Classical conditioning
   C. Shaping
   D. Modeling
   E. The Premack principle

2. A patient is interested in exploring nonprescription techniques that may help her migraines. When discussing biofeedback techniques you tell her which of the following?

   A. It uses classical conditioning.
   B. It uses operant conditioning.
   C. It involves learning to lower blood pressure voluntarily.
   D. It does not need high levels of motivation to learn.
   E. It does not require much practice.

3. A mother smacks her toddler when he spits food on the floor, but this does not deter his spitting behaviors; in fact, he does it more often. What is happening in this situation?

   A. Aversive conditioning
   B. Classical conditioning
   C. Punishment
   D. Negative reinforcement
   E. Positive reinforcement

4. Which of the following techniques is correctly paired with the disorder it is used to treat?

   A. Aversive therapy—Phobias
   B. Modeling—Impaired social skills
   C. Token economy—Generalized anxiety
   D. Flooding—Encopresis
   E. Systematic desensitization—Sexual inadequacy

HPI: ED is a 40-year-old married businessman who was referred to you after he contacted the chairman's office seeking a "top-notch doc."
He says he has been experiencing some depressed moods since he has difficulties with his wife recently, but he does not endorse any other symptoms of major depression. He says she wants a divorce but he does not believe that she would leave him. On further exploration, he reveals that he has always had difficulties with people but that he attributes this to others being jealous of his success. He runs his own telecommunications firm, which he tells you will be number 1 in this field in the next 5 years. He says his wife is causing all the problems in their marriage because she does not understand all the sacrifices he has to make in order to be so successful. He thinks the problems lie all with her and says that he agreed to see you to stop her complaining. He has no previous psychiatric or medical history. He denied any family psychiatric history. He has been married for 8 years and has two sons. He admits to drinking socially 2–3 nights a week and has tried cocaine twice but denies abuse of other substances.

MSE: Significant for reported depressed mood; otherwise there is no evidence of anxiety or psychosis. Cognitive functions are intact and he tells you that he is delighted to have had a "proper referral," as he was concerned that an ordinary doctor would not understand his situation.

Thought Questions

- What do you think is happening with this man?
- What is a defense mechanism?
- Which defense mechanisms does this man display?

Basic Science Review and Discussion

This man is displaying the features of a narcissistic personality disorder. Personality disorders are defined as pervasive, maladaptive patterns of behavior that are deeply ingrained and recognizable from adolescence or even earlier. These patterns of behavior continue throughout adult life, causing difficulties for either the patient or those around them. People with narcissistic personality disorder have a pervasive sense of grandiosity, need for admiration, and lack of empathy for others. They are preoccupied with fantasies of power, success, brilliance, love, or beauty. They believe that they are unique and can only be understood by those who are special or who have achieved high status. They require excessive admiration and attention. They can display a sense of entitlement, appearing arrogant or haughty. They may exploit others to achieve their own end and are often envious of others or believe that others are envious of them. Patients who have this type of personality disorder may actually threaten their physician and devalue his or her level of competence. These patients are at increased risk for developing major depression and substance abuse/dependence. They often present with marital problems and difficulties with interpersonal relationships in general.

Defense mechanisms are **unconscious** and habitual **processes** that we use to **protect the ego from conflicts between our basic desires and needs, our internalized con**trols, and the external environment. They can sometimes be pathologic (see the Thumbnail). Defense mechanisms seen in narcissistic personality disorder include denial, distortion, and projection.

As with all personality disorders, these patterns of behavior are chronic in nature. Narcissistic symptoms may diminish with age and pessimism may develop. As these individuals do not perceive that they have a problem, they may only present in a crisis of marriage, family, or career with symptoms of depression, anxiety, or substance abuse.

In general, the treatment of personality disorders involves psychotherapy and pharmacotherapy aimed at correcting behaviors (e.g., aggression, impulsivity, anxiety, psychotic symptoms and mood lability) and underlying neurobiologic mechanisms.

The different schools of psychotherapy are not mutually exclusive, complement each other, and generally fall into one of the following types:

1. **Dynamic psychotherapy:** The patient's symptoms are seen as expressions of the internal conflict between the patient's needs, emotions, and motivations (see Key Points).
2. **Behavioral therapy:** Treatment is focused on the external behaviors. The aim is to help the patient change or better control these behaviors. Types of learning include classical conditioning, operant conditioning, and cognitive behavioral and observational learning. Treatment techniques include aversive conditioning, positive reinforcement and extinction, systematic desensitization, and modeling.
3. **Cognitive therapy:** The distorted cognitive appraisals of external cues and underlying distorted beliefs are corrected or restructured and maladaptive behaviors are treated.

Psychoanalysis Psychoanalysis is both a psychological theory of the mind and a therapeutic treatment. It is based on the work of Sigmund Freud. He described the topographic theory of the mind and the structural theory of the mind (Table 8-1).

The main strategy of psychoanalysis is to uncover these unconscious feelings and memories and to integrate them into the conscious mind. Several techniques are used and they include free association of words and thoughts, interpretation of the therapeutic relationship, dreams, and parapraxes (apparent errors in everyday life that symbolize underlying attitudes). For psychoanalysis to be suitable for a patient the problem must be understandable in psychological terms and the patient must be willing to understand these problems in psychological terms, must not be psychotic, must have enough ego strength to deal with the tensions caused by these inner conflicts, must have a stable life situation, and must be able to sustain a psychotherapeutic relationship. Psychoanalysis usually consists of three to five sessions a week for several years.

Table 8-1. Freud's Theories of the Mind

Topographical theory	1. The **unconscious** mind contains the repressed thoughts and feelings, and contains primary process thinking, which is associated with the primary drives; pleasure and wish fulfillment, and dreams, which represent the gratification of basic impulses and wish fulfillment. 2. The **preconscious** mind contains memories that can be accessed by the conscious mind. 3. The **conscious** mind does not have access to the unconscious mind and contains the thoughts and feelings that the individual is aware of.
Structural theory	The component parts of the mind operate mostly on an unconscious level. 1. The **id** represents the instinctual aggressive and sexual drives, is controlled by primary process thinking, and is not affected by external reality. 2. The **ego** is in direct contact with reality; it controls the drives of the id and adapts to the environment using reality testing to develop sustaining relationships. It also has cognitive and defensive functions. 3. The **superego** also controls the drives of the id, regulating moral values and functioning as the conscience.

Case Conclusion ED is not currently experiencing significant symptoms of depression or anxiety. You counsel him about the potential dangers of alcohol and substance abuse, and recommend a course of psychotherapy. He refuses to accept that he needs psychiatric treatment, because the problem is his wife, not him. He does not return for follow-up.

Thumbnail: Behavioral Science—Defense Mechanisms

Acting out	A direct expression of an unconscious impulse in order to avoid awareness of the accompanying affect (e.g., the patient throwing furniture because the dinner cart is late).
Altruism	Using a constructive service to others to provide vicarious satisfaction (e.g., the unhappy divorcee volunteering in a soup kitchen).
Denial	A conscious refusal to accept external reality (e.g., the patient who has been diagnosed with cancer and leaves the hospital against medical advice).
Distortion	Grossly reshaping external reality to accommodate internal needs (e.g., the substance abuser who believes that amphetamine helps clear his/her thinking).
Displacement	The shifting of feelings onto a less cared for object (e.g., the disgruntled employee who returns home and kicks the cat)
Dissociation	Temporary change of character or identity to avoid distress (e.g., the man who becomes bankrupt and develops amnesia).
Identification	Behavior patterns changed to emulate another (e.g., medical students wearing white coats on the wards).
Intellectualization	Excessively using reason to avoid affective experiences (e.g., the physician who has a terminal illness and constantly discusses the details with colleagues).
Isolation	An idea is separated from its associated affect (e.g., an abused woman calmly plans to kill her husband).
Projection	Unacceptable feelings are attributed to others, may become delusional (e.g., the person who wants to have an affair accuses his or her spouse of infidelity).
Projective identification	Unacceptable aspects of the personality are dissociated and projected onto another, who is then identified with (e.g., the person who wishes to have an affair projects this onto an admired close friend).
Rationalization	Reason is used to justify unacceptable emotions and feelings (e.g., the individual who had an indiscretion blames it on a single martini).
Reaction formation	An unacceptable impulse is transformed into its opposite (e.g., the televangelist who rails against illicit sex was caught on film with a prostitute).
Regression	Attempts to return to earlier behaviors to avoid anxiety (e.g., the child who returns to wetting the bed when his parents separate).
Repression	Refusal to accept into consciousness a feeling or instinct. It is the most basic defense mechanism (e.g., the wife of the traveling salesman who says that she does not need intimacy).
Splitting	Positive and negative aspects of relationships are separately and alternatively conscious (e.g., the patient who thinks that his/her physician is wonderful until one day the physician is late for an appointment and is then perceived as dreadful).
Sublimation	An unacceptable impulse is directed in a socially acceptable manner (e.g., the male with aggressive impulses becomes a surgeon).
Suppression	Ideas or feelings are consciously suppressed to minimize discomfort (e.g., the patient who has a life-threatening illness and decides to worry about it for a limited time each day).
Turning against the self	Unacceptable aggression toward others is expressed indirectly toward the self (e.g., the teenager who dislikes her step-father cuts herself superficially).

Key Points

▶ Defense mechanisms are unconscious and habitual processes that we use to protect the ego from conflicts between our basic desires and needs, our internalized controls, and the external environment. They can sometimes be pathologic.

▶ The main strategy of psychoanalysis is to uncover these unconscious feelings and memories and to integrate them into the conscious mind.

▶ Personality disorders are defined as pervasive, maladaptive patterns of behavior that are deeply ingrained and recognizable from adolescence or even earlier.

▶ Schools of psychotherapy include dynamic, behavioral, and cognitive.

▶ Sigmund Freud described his topographic and structural theories of the mind. Topographic theory describes the unconscious, preconscious, and conscious mind. Structural theory describes the id, ego, and superego.

Questions

1. Which of the following is a mature defense mechanism?
   A. Repression
   B. Isolation
   C. Denial
   D. Acting out
   E. Suppression

2. Which of the following conditions is correctly paired with its associated defense mechanisms?
   A. Hysteria—Displacement of affect
   B. Obsessional conditions—Denial, projection, and identification
   C. Paranoia—Turning on the self
   D. Phobias—Displacement of affect
   E. Depression—Isolation, reaction formation, and magical undoing

3. Which of the following examples is correctly paired with its associated defense mechanism?
   A. A woman who was sexually abused as a child develops multiple personalities as an adult: Splitting
   B. A man who is attracted to his sister-in-law begins to believe that his wife is having an affair: Reaction formation
   C. A woman who was physically abused as a child begins to physically abuse her own children: Identification
   D. A teenager whose parent has been diagnosed with cancer begins to neglect his schoolwork and becomes argumentative at home: Regression
   E. A man with bowel cancer tells you that he only worries about it for 20 minutes a day: Denial

4. Which of the following is correctly paired with its definition?
   A. Transference describes the therapist's attitude and response to the patient.
   B. Countertransference describes the shifting of a past person or object in the patient's life onto the therapist.
   C. Primary process thinking is unconscious and is based on the basic pleasure principle of the id; both logic and the sense of time are absent in this type of thinking.
   D. Secondary process thinking is also unconscious and unassociated with reality.
   E. Dream work is the process that examines only the manifest content of dreams.

HPI: FB is a 25-year-old single graduate student who presents with excessive sleepiness. This began about 2 months previously with increased daytime somnolence. He has been trying to get about 8 hours sleep during the night, but this has not made any difference. He is concerned because last week while in traffic he fell asleep suddenly and crashed into the car in front of him. He also reports strange experiences, "almost like hallucinations," as he wakes up, which he perceives as very vivid dreams. He has no significant psychiatric or medical history.

In his family history, his father had a myocardial infarction (MI), and his mother has hypothyroidism. He is the eldest of three sons. He is in his final year of an MBA program, does not smoke, and drinks moderate amounts of alcohol at social occasions about once a week. Although he admits to having smoked marijuana while an undergraduate, he denies use of other illicit substances. No legal history. Lab tests Utox, CBC, and Chem 7 were all normal.

MSE: Appropriately dressed young male, good eye contact and rapport. Speech and behavior within normal limits. Affect reactive, normal range. Mood "a little worried." Thought process logical and goal directed. Denies AH/VH/SH, SI/HI, or PI. Cognitive functions intact; insight and judgment intact.

Thought Questions

- Are there any additional investigations that you would like to perform and why?

- What are the characteristic features of this condition? How does this disorder differ from insomnia or sleep apnea? What are the other sleep disorders?

- What is the normal architecture of sleep? How does this change as we age? How does this change in depression?

Basic Science Review and Discussion

FB appears to be suffering from narcolepsy. A sleep study with EEG known as the multiple sleep latency test (MSLT) may reveal short rapid eye movement (REM) latency during multiple naps. Other characteristic features of this condition include **hypnagogic hallucinations** (on going to sleep), **hypnapompic hallucinations** (on waking up), **sleep paralysis** (episodes of being unable to move for a few seconds after waking), and **cataplexy** (episodes of complete loss of muscle tone provoked by strong emotions such as laughter or anger). The hallucinations are actually vivid dreams that occur while the patient is conscious. Other symptoms that may occur include disturbed nighttime sleep with multiple awakenings; nightmares; and leg jerks, tossing, and turning in bed. It usually presents in young adults.

Insomnia, on the other hand, is defined as difficulty falling asleep (initial insomnia) or staying asleep at least three times a week for at least 1 month, causing difficulties performing usual social or occupational functions. It can be associated with stress, anxiety, excessive caffeine intake, substance abuse, and depression (early morning wakening may be reported). It affects up to one-third of Americans. It is usually treated by avoiding alcohol, caffeine, or illicit substances by appropriate treatment of any associated psychiatric condition, and by other sleep hygiene techniques. These include regular exercise, avoidance of overstimulation before bedtime, relaxation, and going to bed and getting up at a consistent, regular time.

Breathing-related sleep disorders include those caused by obstructive or central sleep apnea or central alveolar hypoventilation. These disorders cause disruption of sleep with insomnia or more commonly excessive sleepiness, which can be uncontrollable.

Obstructive sleep apnea is the most common type and is caused by upper-airway obstruction in overweight individuals and causes excess sleepiness. Characteristically, there are very loud snores and silent periods of apnea lasting 20 to 30 seconds. Breathing can be suppressed for up to 90 seconds and cause cyanosis.

In central sleep apnea there is no airway obstruction or breathing movement. It is caused by neurologic or cardiac conditions that affect ventilation regulation. Patients with this condition present with insomnia due to multiple awakenings but do not have significant snoring.

Central alveolar hypoventilation tends to occur in those who are very overweight, leading to abnormally low blood oxygen levels that drop further during sleep, but their lungs are normal.

Sleep disorders are divided into four different types in the *Diagnostic and Statistical Manual of Mental Disorders,* 4th edition *(DSM-IV):*

1. Primary sleep disorders, which include

   a. Dyssomnias: These disorders are characterized by disturbances in the quality, quantity, or timing of sleep, such as primary insomnia, primary hypersomnia, narcolepsy, breathing-related sleep disorder (see above), and circadian rhythm sleep disorder (includes jet lag and shift work types).

b. Parasomnias: In these disorders there are abnormal behavioral or physiological events, which occur during sleep-wake transitions or during specific stages of sleep itself. These patients usually present with complaints about unusual behaviors during sleep, such as nightmares, night terrors, or sleepwalking.

Nightmares tend to occur only during REM sleep, particularly during the second half of the night, when REM periods are longer. **Sleep terrors,** on the other hand, tend to occur during the first third of the sleep and the individual wakes abruptly with a scream, intense autonomic arousal (elevated blood pressure (BP), heart rate, breathing, and increased sweating), relative unresponsiveness to the comfort of others, and amnesia for the episode.

Sleepwalking also tends to occur during the first third of sleep. Those who sleepwalk are also relatively unresponsive to others and have amnesia for the episode.

2. Sleep disorders related to another mental disorder include subtypes of insomnia or hypersomnia.

3. Sleep disorders due to a general medical condition, which includes insomnia, hypersomnia, parasomnia, or mixed subtypes.

4. Substance-induced sleep disorder: These disorders can occur during withdrawal or intoxication and may include insomnia, hypersomnia, and parasomnia or may be mixed in subtype.

Architecture of Sleep   Sleep studies using EEG tracings reveal the normal architecture of sleep. Sleep is cyclical in nature, moving from stage I, the lightest phase, to stage IV, the deepest phase. During a normal night's sleep there are four or five periods of emergence from stages III and IV into REM sleep (which is also known as paradoxical or desynchronized sleep). Each period of REM sleep lasts approximately 20 minutes. The amount of time usually spent in the different phases differ by age and according to whether psychiatric disorder (e.g., major depression) is present. Babies spend approximately 50% of their total time asleep in non-REM sleep, and young adults spend 75% of their time asleep in non-REM sleep.

As we age, the amount of time spent in stages 3, 4, and REM decreases. There may also be multiple awakenings. In major depression sleep studies reveal short REM latency (< 90 minutes), a longer first REM phase; stages 3 and 4 are decreased with multiple awakenings followed by early morning wakening (1 to 2 hours earlier than usual).

Case Conclusion   A sleep study was performed and the results confirmed the diagnosis of narcolepsy. FB was started on a course of methylphenidate, which was titrated; when he returned a month later he reported that he was doing much better. He had not fallen asleep during the day for the previous 2 weeks, was no longer experiencing hallucinations, and could concentrate on his coursework much better.

Thumbnail: Behavioral Science—Stages of Sleep

Sleep Stages	EEG Pattern	Percent of Sleep	Characteristics
Awake	Alpha and beta waves		Alpha seen when relaxed with eyes closed. Beta seen when actively concentrating
Stage 1	Theta waves appear	5	Pulse and breathing slow, BP decreases, and there may be episodic body movements. This is the lightest stage of sleep.
Stage 2	Sleep spindles (13 to 15 Hz) and high-voltage κ-complexes	45	Majority of sleep spent in this stage
Stages 3 and 4	Delta (also known as slow-wave sleep)	25	It is during this deepest stage of sleep that enuresis, sleepwalking, or night terrors may occur.
REM sleep	Alpha, beta, and theta in a sawtooth pattern	25	These phases of rapid conjugate eye movement occur approximately every 90 minutes. In this stage, there is increased blood flow to the penis and clitoris, increased cerebral blood flow and gastric motility, increased cardiovascular activity, irregular respiration and an absence of skeletal muscle movement with absent tendon reflexes. Vivid and bizarre dreams.

Key Points

▶ Insomnia is a symptom, which may be experienced by 35% of the population and may be clinically significant in 17% of the population.

▶ Insomnia is worse in women, older persons, those with depression and anxiety, and those with health problems.

▶ Forty percent of insomniacs self-medicate with over-the-counter medications or alcohol. Twenty percent take hypnotics or sedatives.

▶ Narcolepsy consists of a tetrad of symptoms: hypersomnia, sleep paralysis, hypnagogic or hyp-

napompic hallucinations and cataplexy, but only 25% of patients have all the symptoms.

▶ Dyssomnias are characterized by disturbances in the quality, quantity, or timing of sleep, such as primary insomnia, primary hypersomnia, narcolepsy, breathing-related sleep disorder, and circadian rhythm sleep disorder.

▶ Parasomnias involve abnormal behavioral or physiologic events, which occur during sleep-wake transitions or during specific stages of sleep itself such as nightmares, night terrors, or sleepwalking.

Questions

1. When educating FB about narcolepsy, which of the following are you *least* likely to tell him?
   A. It affects approximately 250,000 Americans.
   B. The first symptoms usually appear between 15 to 30 years of age.
   C. It affects men and women at different rates.
   D. The etiology of this disorder may have been identified.
   E. Narcolepsy may place the sufferer in danger.

2. The treatment of narcolepsy includes which of the following?
   A. Avoiding daytime naps
   B. Monoamine oxidase A inhibitors
   C. Anxiolytics
   D. Hypnotics
   E. Dextroamphetamine

3. Which of the following is true concerning sleep disorders?
   A. Parasomnias include insomnia, narcolepsy, and sleep apnea.
   B. Dyssomnias include somnambulism, nightmares, and sleep terrors.
   C. Sleep terrors are usually treated with hypnotics.
   D. Treatment of sleep apnea includes continuous positive airway pressure.
   E. Increased risk of sleep apnea in females.

4. Which of the following neurotransmitters is correctly matched with its effect on sleep?
   A. Acetylcholine decreases REM sleep.
   B. Dopamine blockade causes poor sleep.
   C. Noradrenaline decreases REM sleep.
   D. Serotonin decreases slow-wave sleep.
   E. Histamine decreases wakefulness.

HPI: RC is a 29-year-old single Caucasian female who was brought in to the medical emergency room 5 days ago by her housemate, after she found her unconscious with an empty bottle of acetaminophen and vodka at her side. She was treated with gastric lavage, *N*-acetylcysteine, was monitored in the medical intensive care unit, and then transferred to the medical floor with one-to-one observation. She is now stable. You are asked to evaluate her for transfer to psychiatry.

RC, a biology graduate student, has been depressed for the last month after the breakup of a relationship. She says that she's been feeling "horrible," is barely able to keep up with her duties as a teaching assistant in an undergraduate biology class, and has great difficulty focusing enough to grade the problem sets. She had not been able to make herself go to the lab for the last 2 weeks and had her bench mate feed and split her cells. She was waking up at 5 A.M. and would worry about the things that she wasn't doing, unable to sleep. She has been feeling worthless and increasingly hopeless. She was seen in the psych emergency room last week and was referred for outpatient therapy and medication, saying that if she felt suicidal she would return to the emergency room. Over the past week things did not go well. She slept through her appointment with the psychiatry outpatient service. The evening of the attempt she finally went to her lab, only to find that her cells were overgrown and infected and that she would have to begin the complex experiment again. As she was walking home, she saw her ex-boyfriend across the quadrangle, walking hand in hand with someone else. She felt humiliated, worthless, and hopeless; went home; and took the acetaminophen and drank the vodka. She said that her housemate had been away for a few days and she thought no one would find her.

Thought Questions

- How serious was this suicide attempt?
- Should she be transferred to psychiatry?
- What if she refuses hospitalization?

Basic Science Review and Discussion

This was a very serious **suicide attempt.** Acetaminophen overdoses are potentially lethal, may cause fulminant hepatic failure, and can be associated with significant hepatic damage. In addition, she thought her housemate was away and wouldn't find her, adding to her lethal intent. At this point there is no question that she requires hospitalization.

In general, in assessing safety and potential suicidality, one needs to ask directly about **plans** (hanging, overdose, crashing a car), **means** (pills, firearms, a vehicle), and **intent** to carry suicide out. It is also crucial to explore previous ideation and attempts, substance abuse history, and family history of completed suicide or attempts.

In this case, if she were to refuse hospitalization, even if she stated that she had "learned her lesson," she would still require hospital-level care and would meet criteria for involuntary hospitalization. She has an untreated major depression (depressed mood, impaired sleep with early-morning awakening, decreased energy/motivation and concentration; see Case 20: Depression) and has just had an extremely serious suicide attempt. She is therefore a continuing danger to herself. In addition, although she had said in her initial evaluation that she would seek help if her suici-

dality worsened, she had not done so. The criteria for involuntary hospitalization in most states include being a significant danger to oneself or others or being so gravely impaired that one cannot provide the basics of self-care.

Suicide Although suicide can be the unfortunate outcome in a number of psychiatric disorders, it is most commonly seen in the context of **mood disorders.** The diagnosis of a current mood disorder is a risk factor for suicide; however, there are other risk factors as well. Substance abuse alone or especially when it is comorbid with another psychiatric disorder is a significant risk factor for suicide.

Another psychiatric disorder with high prevalence rates of suicide attempts or completions is **schizophrenia.** Approximately 25% to 50% of schizophrenics attempt suicide, and about 10% die from it. Risk factors for suicide in schizophrenia include having made previous attempts, being male, being young, being hopeless (especially in the context of lost expectations, such as a college education and significant ambitions), having multiple relapses, being in a depressed mood, living alone, and using drugs.

In general, suicide attempts are more common in women than in men (by a factor of approximately 3:1), but completed suicide is more common in men than in women (by a factor of 4:1). There are an estimated eight to 25 attempted suicides to one completion. Of all firearm suicides, 79% are committed by Caucasian men. During the year following an attempt, patients are at high risk for another attempt.

Other risk factors include age greater than 60, current medical illness, comorbid substance abuse, and divorce. In 1999, suicide was the eleventh leading cause of death in the

United States. Suicide outnumbered homicides by 5 to 3. Suicide by firearms was the most common method for both men and women, accounting for 57% of all completed suicides. The highest rates of completed suicide, when categorized by gender and race, are for white men over the age of 85, who had a rate of 59/100,000. (For more information, see the NIMH suicide research consortium and fact sheet: http://www.nimh.nih.gov/research/suifact.htm.)

Case Conclusion RC was admitted to psychiatry voluntarily after her discharge from the medical intensive care unit. She was started on a course of antidepressants and began to have some individual psychotherapy to understand her suicide attempt. During the course of her 2-week hospitalization, she tolerated the medication well, was titrated up to a therapeutic dose, and met a therapist who she would continue to work with after discharge. At the time of discharge she was less dysphoric and more hopeful, and was able to describe alternate ways of coping should she become suicidal again.

Thumbnail: Behavioral Science—Medications in Overdose

Medications are potentially lethal. Of course patients can overdose on any medication with varying potential lethality, depending on the amount ingested and the combination of medications and/or other drugs involved.

Medication in Overdose	Effects/Comments
Acetaminophen	Hepatic failure
Aspirin	Metabolic acidosis, and bleeding complications
Tricyclic antidepressants	Prolonged Q-T interval and A-V block, may lead to ventricular tachycardia or torsade de pointes.
Selective serotonin reuptake inhibitors	Rarely lethal if taken alone, may be associated with drowsiness, tremor, nausea, vomiting, seizures, electrocardiogram changes, and decreased consciousness.
Nonsteroidal anti-inflammatory drugs (NSAIDs)	Disorientation, dizziness, lethargy, confusion, nausea, vomiting, abdominal pain, seizures, increased blood urea nitrogen (BUN) and serum creatinine, tachycardia, and coma.

Key Points

▶ Suicide is between the eighth and the eleventh leading cause of death in the United States.

▶ In 2000 it accounted for 1.2% of all deaths. The three leading causes of death were heart disease (29.6%), cancer (23%), and stroke (7%).

▶ In young people (aged 15 to 24) suicide was the third leading cause of death, following unintentional injuries and homicide.

▶ The 2000 age-adjusted rate was 10.6/100,000, or 0.01%. (Age-adjusted rates are adjusted by population norms and allow for comparisons across time and among risk groups.)

▶ The rate among elderly white men over the age of 85 was close to 60/100,000.

▶ Women attempt suicide much more frequently than men (3:1), but men succeed more frequently (4:1).

▶ Approximately 50% of people who attempt suicide will have a second attempt, and 10% will succeed. The risk is greatest in the 3 months following the initial attempt.

▶ Patients can be admitted involuntarily if they are deemed a danger to themselves or others or are so gravely disabled that they cannot provide adequate self-care. The exact requirements vary from state to state. Usually either one or two licensed physicians must sign commitment papers that are valid for a finite time.

▶ Patients should always be asked about suicidal thoughts, intent, and possible plans. An assessment also needs to be made of the accessibility of the means.

Questions

1. KH is a 30-year-old married female who presented to the emergency room after trying to poison herself with carbon monoxide in her car. She was found by her husband, who called for emergency services. Which of the following is true about people who attempt suicide?

   A. She says she is remorseful. She is unlikely to make another attempt.

   B. Approximately 75% of people who attempt suicide have another attempt.

   C. She is at serious risk for trying again, particularly in the next 3 months, and 80% of such attempts are subsequently successful.

   D. She is at serious risk for trying again, particularly in the next 3 months, and 10% of such attempts are subsequently successful.

   E. Approximately 5% of people who attempt suicide make another attempt.

2. LC is an 80-year-old, recently widowed African American male with chronic congestive heart failure, renal insufficiency, and osteoarthritis. He was in the military and has a gun collection.

   Which of the following characteristics does not increase his risk for suicide?

   A. Ethnicity—African American

   B. Age—80

   C. Chronic medical illnesses

   D. Access to a gun

   E. Male gender

3. JG is a 16-year-old boy who has taken an overdose of a medication from his parents' medicine cabinet. Which of the following is safest in overdose?

   A. Fluoxetine

   B. Ibuprofen

   C. Acetaminophen

   D. Aspirin

   E. Imipramine

4. BP is a 29-year-old schizophrenic who has recently been hospitalized after a suicide attempt. His parents want to know more about suicide. Which of the following is true?

   A. Seventy percent of schizophrenics attempt suicide.

   B. Ten percent of schizophrenics will die from suicide.

   C. The fact that he had completed 2 years at an Ivy League college decreases his risk of suicide.

   D. Men are at less risk of completed suicide than women.

   E. His current use of alcohol and marijuana does not affect his risk.

HPI: ST is a 78-year-old man whose wife died 6 months ago at home with hospice care from a prolonged case of breast cancer. He admits that he is finding it very difficult to cope, as they were married for 55 years. He says he is surviving on take-out food and can barely manage minimal housework. His sleep is poor and he admits that he has experienced a "vision" of his wife in their bedroom and that she spoke to him. He also says that he is feeling helpless and hopeless and that he cries nearly every day. He has no significant psychiatric history, but he suffered a myocardial infarction (MI) at the age of 70 and has had hypertension since his 40s, for which he takes metoprolol. ST lives alone in the family home. He retired as a lawyer at 65 years of age. He has three sons, who all live far away. His only remaining sibling is his sister, who is in a nursing home in the next state. He says he has an occasional glass of whiskey "to cheer myself up" but has never smoked. There is no significant family history.

MSE: He is disheveled, his clothing is stained with food, and his hygiene is poor. His eye contact is poor and his speech is low in tone and volume. He becomes tearful when talking about his wife. His affect is dysphoric and he describes his mood as "very down." His thought processes are logical and goal directed. Apart from the previously described "vision" of his wife, he denied other hallucinations or psychotic symptoms. He admitted that some days he has thought that he would be "better off dead" but denied any plans for suicide. Cognitive functions were intact, with a mini-mental state examination of 30/30.

Labs: CBC, Chemistry, TFT, vitamin B_{12}, and folate levels all within normal limits.

Thought Questions

- Is ST's reaction normal?

- Does he need treatment?

- Are you concerned about any of his behaviors?

- What are the differences between normal and abnormal grief?

Basic Science Review and Discussion

Bereavement refers to a loss through death, and grief refers to the feelings and behaviors associated with the awareness of this loss. Grieving is completed when the bereaved is able to invest emotionally in new directions. The various manifestations of grief reflect the individual's own personality, coping mechanisms, previous experiences, level of psychosocial supports, health, and relationship with the deceased. Although we expect the bereaved to be able to return to previous function within a few weeks or months, it may last a lot longer for particular individuals (Table 11-1). Normal grief usually resolves within 1 to 2 years, but some symptoms may continue. Treatment of bereavement includes supportive therapy and groups, with short-term treatment of insomnia if needed. Antidepressants are generally not needed. In the year following the death of a spouse there is increased incidence of psychiatric referral, suicide, and death, however the majority of older persons adjust to the loss.

Grief may be provoked by the loss of a body part (e.g., mastectomy, amputation), divorce, death of a pet, or retirement. Loss of youth, health, and roles can provoke grief reactions. Some studies have suggested that divorce may be a greater risk factor for depression than the actual death of a spouse.

Atypical grief may include chronic grief with features of a depressive episode, inhibited or delayed grief, or even a mixed nonspecific reaction with symptoms of neurosis or psychosis. Atypical grief may also be referred to as complicated, distorted, abnormal, or morbid grief. Prolonged grief

Table 11-1. Phases of Grief

1. Shock and denial	This can last days or weeks and involves disbelief, a feeling of being stunned, and numbing of emotions. The bereaved may protest and exhibit searching behaviors.
2. Anguish	This phase may last weeks or months and may involve feelings of distress (may have somatic symptoms), anger, guilt, preoccupation, identification with the bereaved (adoption of behaviors and traits of the deceased), and changes in behavior that may vary from irritability, agitation to a loss of motivation. Transitory hallucinations may occur.
3. Resolution (acceptance and readjustment)	This phase may also take months or years. Here the bereaved is able to recognize the extent of the loss and can move on to resuming work or previous responsibilities, experience pleasure again, and acquire needed roles or develop new relationships with others.

These are in contrast to Kübler-Ross's Stages of Death and Dying: Denial, Anger, Bargaining, Depression, and, finally, Acceptance.

is seen more commonly in those who are socially isolated, poor, and had limited experience of death in earlier years.

Most bereaved persons do not require treatment and obtain support from friends and family. Support groups may help others deal with the grief process. Those with a history of mental illness or who have lost someone in a traumatic way (e.g., homicide or suicide) may need brief psychotherapy. Grief may be complicated by a major depressive episode (see Thumbnail).

Depression is the most common psychiatric disorder in the elderly and occurs in approximately 15% of those over 65 years of age (roughly 3% may meet criteria for major depression). Risk factors include loss of spouse, friends, and poor health. Suicide is twice as common in older persons as in the general population. Risk factors include being older, male, white, widowed; having poor psychosocial support; being unemployed; and having poor physical health, particularly chronic pain and alcohol dependence. Depression requires treatment with psychotherapy and/or antidepressants, and may require antipsychotic agents or electroconvulsive

therapy (ECT). Depression associated with grief should be treated with medication if psychotherapy fails, if the depression is more severe, or if there is a history of major depression, suicidal ideation, morbid guilt or feelings of worthlessness, impaired functioning, or psychomotor retardation. If posttraumatic stress disorder occurs with grief, the posttraumatic stress disorder (PTSD) should be treated first.

A mnemonic for remembering the risk factors for suicide is "SADPERSONS":

S-Sex male

A-Age less than 19 and more than 45 years

D-Depression, clinical

P-Previous attempts

E-Ethanol and illicit substances

R-Rational thinking absent (i.e., psychotic)

O-Organized plan

N-No spouse: single, divorced, or widowed

S-Sick: medical illness (e.g. chronic pain)

Case Conclusion   You are concerned about ST. His symptoms indicate depression and abnormal grief. You also explore his drinking history further, as between 10% and 15% of the elderly have problems with alcohol that often go undetected. ST was treated with an antidepressant, citalopram, and attended a bereavement support group; 6 months later he was doing much better.

Thumbnail: Behavioral Science—Characteristics of Normal and Abnormal Grief

Bereavement (Normal Grief)	Depression (Abnormal Grief)
Minor sleep disturbances	Significant sleep disturbances
Insignificant weight loss	Significant weight loss
Normal sadness	Suicidal ideations or attempts
May have some guilt about deceased	May feel worthless or hopeless
Illusions	Hallucinations and delusions
Severest symptoms last less than 2 months	Severest symptoms may last more than 2 months
Symptoms last less than 1 year	Symptoms last for more than 1 year
Normal attention to hygiene	Poor attention to hygiene

Key Points

▸ Normal grief usually resolves within 1 or 2 years, but some symptoms may continue.

▸ After the death of a spouse there is increased incidence of psychiatric referral, suicide, and death.

▸ Grief may be chronic, inhibited, or delayed.

▸ Depression is the most common psychiatric disorder in the elderly. Risk factors include loss of spouse, friends, and poor health.

▸ Suicide is twice as common in older persons as in the general population. Risk factors include being older, male, Caucasian, widowed; having poor psychosocial support; being unemployed; alcohol dependence; and having poor physical health, particularly chronic pain.

▸ Phases of grief include shock/denial, anguish, and resolution.

Questions

1. Which of the following is true concerning grief?
   A. Grief does not begin before the actual death.
   B. Anniversary reactions may occur.
   C. Grief usually becomes chronic in nature.
   D. Feelings of loneliness are usually short-lived.
   E. Guilt always indicates abnormal grief.

2. Which of the following is a risk factor for developing complicated grief?
   A. A long, happy, secure relationship with the deceased
   B. Expected deaths
   C. Female gender
   D. Age
   E. Impaired personality in the bereaved

3. Which of the following statements is correct concerning complicated grief?
   A. It may be hypotrophic.
   B. Chronic forms are rarely seen.
   C. It may be delayed.
   D. It is not associated with increased medical complications.
   E. It is not associated with increased psychiatric illness.

4. MO is a 67-year-old recently widowed female who has come for her annual physical exam. Which of the following would be considered typical of normal bereavement?
   A. Feeling worthless
   B. Loss of appetite
   C. Suicidal ideation
   D. Poor attention to self-hygiene
   E. Significant insomnia

HPI: OP is a 76-year-old patient of yours who comes to your clinic concerned that she is going to die soon. She has not experienced any change in her physical condition lately, is still living alone, and attends a local senior center regularly. She has her groceries delivered and has help with her heavier housekeeping chores. She still cooks for herself and knits extensively for her many grandchildren. She has noticed that she has become a little more forgetful lately and is very concerned that she will end up being incapacitated, residing in a nursing home, and being a "burden" to her family. She has no psychiatric history but her medical history is significant for hypertension, osteoarthritis, and non-insulin-dependent diabetes mellitus (NIDDM). She takes lisinopril, celecoxib, and metformin.

Her father died of a myocardial infarction (MI) in his 60s and her mother died of "old age" at 85 years. OP is the eldest of two daughters; her sister is 2 years younger and lives in the next state. OP was a homemaker and the mother of four children, two sons, and two daughters, all of whom are alive and well. She has 15 grandchildren and two great-grandchildren. Her husband was an accountant who died 10 years previously at the age of 72 from lung cancer. She nursed him at home until his death with hospice support.

PE: Her PE is unchanged since you last saw her 6 months previously. There is no evidence of abnormality on her general mental state examination. On cognitive testing using the Mini Mental State Examination she scored 28 out of a possible 30, as her short-term recall at 3 minutes was one of three objects.

Thought Questions

- Are these concerns normal for a person of her age?

- What are the changes that can be expected with aging?

- How can you advise OP to help organize her concerns for her future care?

Basic Science Review and Discussion

It is quite normal for older persons to be concerned about their health (see Table 12-1 for changes associated with aging) and their ability to maintain their independence. If these concerns were causing impairment in her functioning, you would be concerned about her developing depression or an anxiety disorder. Although she does not have a significant psychiatric history, older persons remain at risk for developing these conditions, particularly those who suffer from bereavement, physical illnesses, and chronic pain and who have poor psychosocial support systems.

Depression may cause cognitive impairments and cause a "pseudodementia." Both of these conditions can be treated successfully with psychotherapy and pharmacotherapy. Severe depression may require electroconvulsive treatment. (Table 12-2)

It has been estimated that more than 60% of all deaths occur in hospitals (see Table 12-3 for life expectancies in the United States) and that another 20% occur in nursing homes. Hospice care may help those wishing to die at home. Often these patients are dying from chronic illnesses, and advances in technology such as assisted respiration can prolong an individual's life beyond the hope of regaining any meaningful autonomous existence. Advanced directives are documents that allow competent individuals to state in advance what type of medical care they wish to receive if they become unable to participate in such decisions in the

Table 12-1. Changes Associated with Aging

Physical	a. Impairments in vision, hearing
	b. Impaired immune functioning
	c. Loss of muscle mass and increased body fat
	d. Osteoporosis
	e. Decreased functioning of the lungs cardiovascular system, gastrointestinal tract, and kidneys
	f. The brain decreases in weight with increased ventricle size and widened sulci.
	g. Sleep may decrease in amount with multiple awakenings.
	h. Physiologic changes may cause changes in drug effects.
	i. Frequency and intensity of sexual activity may decrease but some individuals remain interested and active sexually into their 90s.
Psychological	a. IQ remains approximately the same but recall and new learning may be impaired.
	b. Coming to terms with loss of spouses and friends and facing one's own mortality
	c. Mild memory problems may be present but do not impair functioning.
	d. Anxiety can arise due to concerns about health and being alone.
	e. Depression

Table 12-2. Comparing Features of Dementia and Pseudodementia

Dementia	"Pseudodementia" due to depression
Family vaguely aware of onset	Family usually aware of onset of symptoms
Progression of symptoms usually slow	Rapid progression of symptoms
Tend not to complain of deficits	Tend to complain in detail of deficits
Memory deficits usually affect short-term memory and learning of new material	Memory deficits appear to affect both short-term and long-term memory
Minimize their failures	Highlight their failures, emphasize difficulties, and communicate distress
Will dismiss failures on testing as unimportant	Made little effort to perform on testing Often answer "I don't know"
Consistent levels of difficulty seen on similar tasks	Marked variability in performance of similarly difficult tasks
Past Medical History may be contributory	Past Psychological History may be contributory
Nocturnal exacerbation with confusion may occur	Nocturnal exacerbation is not uncommon
May have areas of cortical atrophy on scanning or EEG changes consistent with dementia such as increased slow waves	No cortical atrophy or EEG changes consistent with dementia
May have focal findings on physical exam particularly in vascular dementias	Generally do not have focal findings on physical exam

future. Another form of instruction is the living will, in which the patient may decide to accept or refuse treatments that may prolong life, such as resuscitation, artificial respiration, parenteral nutrition, fluids, or even pain medications. These are legally valid in most states in the United States. A durable power of attorney can appoint someone to make medical decisions for the patient in case he or she cannot do so. These options should be explored with patients and their families.

Kübler-Ross studied dying patients and reported that they know when they are dying even if not told and need to be able to talk about it and maintain some hope. The physician's role is to help and support the patient through this transition. Not every patient may reach all these stages, and he or she may fluctuate between them rapidly. Different patients may use different coping mechanisms, such as humor and compassion. The physician must be sensitive to the cultural and religious needs of the dying patient and his or her family. Physicians must also come to terms with their own feelings about their dying patients. They may feel that they have failed in their care of the patient or, alternatively, the patient may remind the physician of a loved one or of his or her own mortality.

Table 12-3. Life Expectancy at Birth in the U.S. by Gender and Race (in Years)

	Overall	African American	Caucasian
Males	72.0	64.6	72.9
Females	78.9	73.8	79.6

Thumbnail: Behavioral Science—Kübler-Ross's Stages of Death and Dying

1. Denial	In this initial stage the patient cannot believe that he or she is terminally ill; it can be a defense against overwhelming anxiety.
2. Anger	This may be aimed at themselves, caregivers, friends, family, and/or God. Patients may become demanding, irritable, bitter, confused, and difficult to care for.
3. Bargaining	During this stage the patient may rediscover religious beliefs and attempt to "bargain" by promising various things, such as donating organs, in order to buy extra time.
4. Depression	Here the patient fully realizes that he or she is dying and depression and despair may set in. Patients may detach themselves from friends and family and become reflective about the meaning of life itself.
5. Acceptance	In this final stage the patient accepts his or her death and may become more calm or detached.

Case Conclusion   After reviewing her current physical status and mental state, you reassure OP that she is doing well. You encourage her to pursue any legal arrangements that she wishes to make concerning end-of-life care, and she decides to formalize her will and to give her eldest daughter power of attorney for health care decisions. Her level of anxiety decreases and when she returns for a follow-up visit she is doing well.

Key Points

- Older people are at risk for developing psychiatric disorders, particularly those who suffer from bereavement, chronic physical illnesses, and chronic pain and who have poor psychosocial support systems.
- Depression may cause cognitive impairments and cause "pseudodementia."
- More than 60% of all deaths occur in hospitals and another 20% take place in nursing homes.

- Advanced directives, living wills, and powers of attorney can all be used to plan for health care if a person should lose capacity to make such decisions.
- Aging is associated with physical and psychological changes.
- Kübler-Ross described five stages of dying: denial, anger, bargaining, depression, and acceptance.

Questions

1. Which of the following is associated with increased longevity?
   - A. Divorce
   - B. Early retirement
   - C. Less education
   - D. Late retirement
   - E. Sleeping 4 to 6 hours a night

2. Which of the following statements is correct?
   - A. The age specific death rate in the United States is 90 deaths per 100,000.
   - B. Deaths from heart disease are currently increasing.
   - C. Since the 1980s deaths from diabetes have increased.
   - D. Life expectancy at birth has increased since 1980.
   - E. By the year 2020 more than 35% of the population will be more than 65 years of age.

3. Which of the following is correct concerning age and health?
   - A. Twenty percent of people > 65 require nursing home care.
   - B. Fifty percent of all heath care costs are from the elderly.
   - C. The most common medical conditions in the elderly are arthritis, hypertension, and heart disease.
   - D. The likelihood of physical illness increases in the elderly but that of mental illness does not.
   - E. Cognitive decline is inevitable.

4. A 70-year-old female presents with symptoms of major depression. You decide to prescribe her antidepressants. Which of the following is a concern when prescribing medications to older persons?
   - A. Drug distributions remain unchanged
   - B. Increased protein binding
   - C. Decreased renal tubular functioning
   - D. Poor compliance
   - E. Unimpaired absorption

HPI: RT is a 67-year-old male who has been feeling very fatigued lately. He went to his internist, who did routine laboratory tests that revealed a low hematocrit with a low mean corpuscular volume (MCV). He is sent to you for a colonoscopy and further work-up. The colonoscopy reveals a malignant lesion in the ascending colon. The abdominal CT does not show any evidence of metastases. The day after the scan, he calls you to ask about the results.

Thought Question

- How do you break bad news? Is the phone appropriate?
- How should this be handled?

Basic Science Review and Discussion

The theme behind all doctor-patient communication is eliciting or giving information in a way that fosters the relationship with the patient. In terms of giving information the key is in listening to what your patients already know, want to know, and are able to hear. The physician must then communicate important information in a way that the patient can absorb. Lecturing the patient on what you want him to know is often counterproductive and makes it harder for him to hear your message. For example, telling your patient that he is 40 pounds overweight and needs to lose weight without talking to him about his concerns about weight and lifestyle, and finding out what he has tried and what he wants to do about his weight will probably alienate him. This may make him less likely to return, and if he does, make him embarrassed or defensive about his failure to lose. In this section we will review some of the techniques used in interviewing, and then the paradigm for breaking bad news, one of the hardest things to do in medicine. The themes are really the same as in any doctor-patient interaction.

A number of techniques are used in interviewing. Some of these techniques help to foster the physician-patient relationship, and some are more in the service of obtaining information. Both are important. Maybe even more important is being able to listen well. Having the patient participate by asking questions may also improve patient compliance. Use clear, precise language that is not "medicalese." Patients may be confused, frightened, or intimidated by medical terms and may not feel comfortable asking for clarification. Use open-ended questions that allow the patient to elaborate on the issues that have prompted him to seek treatment. They yield much more information than a closed-ended question, which can be answered in one or two words, and do not further rapport. Clarification, in which the examiner repeats what the patient has said, helps the patient feel heard and understood, and allows the examiner to clarify any uncertainties. Other useful techniques are

also useful. These include facilitation (asking questions or making gestures that encourage the patient to continue talking) and reflection (putting the patient's emotional experience into words). In some settings sign posting (i.e., letting the patient know what is expected in the subsequent part of the interview) helps the patient to feel comfortable with the process of the interview. In general, all these techniques serve to elicit important information while helping the patient feel comfortable and cared for.

Discussing Bad News It is important to discuss test results, particularly bad news, with patients in a respectful and appropriate manner. In general, having a discussion about the diagnosis of cancer over the phone is not appropriate, although occasionally it may be unavoidable. It is always better to set up a face-to-face interview. It is also important to ask who the patient wants to participate in the discussion and to try to ensure some privacy (if it is taking place in the context of a hospital room). Patients may or may not want their grown children, friends, or relatives in the room.

The next questions are, "What does the patient know?" and "What does he want to know?" First, one needs to find out what the patient already knows or is thinking about. What are the fears, expectations, and desire for disclosure? What is the patient's emotional state? The level of understanding and information that the patient has will inform you where to begin your discussion. If the patient says that he's concerned that this is a stage IV adenocarcinoma, he is clearly in a different place than if he were to say "I hope it's not cancer" or even "What does my colon have to do with my being tired?"

Family members may well tell you that the patient *cannot* know this diagnosis because it would be too overwhelming, "would kill him." Despite their desire to protect their relative, it is important to address this directly with the patient. Of course if the patient tells you that he or she does not want to know anything, you must respect that. However, the lines of communication must also be left open and the question revisited at a later time. This does not imply that the treatment and planning cannot be discussed.

In framing a discussion, one first starts from where the patient is and then offers small bits of information about diagnosis, treatment, and prognosis. Studies show that patients remember less than 50% of what their doctors tell them. Use language that is appropriate to the individual and give him or her time to ask questions. This is useful to assess what information has been absorbed and what words or concepts may have been too complicated. This also gives the patient a way to participate in the conversation instead of hearing a mini-lecture. Offer to write things down so that the patient can look them up or discuss them with friends or family. In addition, the patient may have concerns that are not on your immediate agenda. For instance, the patient may be concerned with whether the chemotherapy is associated with impotence, or hair loss, or whether he or she should tell friends about the diagnosis, or whether there will be adequate pain medication. Taking time to find out about and address these concerns is crucial in creating an ongoing, effective relationship with the patient.

There are a few other important things to consider in talking to the patient. One is that he needs to feel that you will not abandon him and will see him through the treatment, that there are ways to prepare and plan that take into account the worst-case scenario (making a will, advanced directives, eldercare attorneys) yet allow continued hope for the best-case scenario (the condition will remit, or stabilize, or the progression will be very slow). It is also important to help the patient think about how to cope with this situation, support systems, need for social interventions (e.g., direct services because of his or her condition), supportive therapy, and so on. Of course all these issues cannot be addressed and resolved in the initial discussion, but they should be considered as part of treatment planning.

Case Conclusion   You arrange with RT to come in the following day to discuss the results of his evaluation, and ask if he would like his wife to be present. They come in and before you start he says, "I have cancer, don't I." Starting from that point, you discuss his diagnosis, prognosis, and treatment options. His wife tells you that his cousin was recently diagnosed with colon cancer, had undergone a resection, and was now starting chemotherapy. He remains quiet during most of the discussion, and each time you stop and ask about questions, his wife follows up with a number of appropriate and well-focused questions and she jots down the answers in a notebook. At the end of the session, you give them an appointment with a surgeon and arrange to see them in the hospital postoperatively. You comment to RT that he has been quite quiet. He says, "This is going to take some adjusting to . . . I was hoping that I was wrong. I'm sure in the next few days I'll start to have lots of questions." You suggest that you speak to him again later in the week, or the following week, whenever he feels ready.

Thumbnail: Behavioral Science—Communication Techniques

Technique	Example	Use, Comments
Closed-ended questions	"Where does it hurt?" "Do you feel sad?" "Is the pain worse when you take a deep breath?"	To get brief, focused information in a timely manner. Does not yield detail; if used too much makes the patient feel interrogated.
Open-ended questions	"What brings you in today?" "Tell me about the pain.	Allows the patient to express his or her concerns and elaborate on issues. Promotes rapport.
Clarification, or checking	"So as I understand it, your compulsion to wash had decreased with therapy, but last Tuesday when you learned of the financial disaster, the symptoms came back in full force. Is that correct? Have you noticed that your symptoms usually increase in times of stress?" "The pain started on Monday, but this morning it changed in quality and became sharp and worse when you coughed."	Reflects what the patient has said. It clarifies for you what has been said, may elicit new information, and lets the patient know that you have heard his or her concerns. It may also be used as a way to expand or probe.
Facilitation	"What happened next?" "Uh huh" Nodding	Encourages the patient to elaborate. A general question is asked or another gesture, sound, or even silence may encourage a patient to bring up concerns or participate in the interview.
Empathic responses	"I understand that you are feeling sad in talking about this." "Discussing this diagnosis is very frightening."	Help the patient feel understood as a person.
Reflection	"You looked very sad just now. What were you thinking about?" "You looked really angry when you talked about. . . ."	Put into words the patient's emotional experience. This serves a number of functions, including validating how the patient feels, helping him or her realize that you are interested and responsive, and giving the patient permission to talk about the emotion or experience.

Key Points

There are many techniques to use in communicating with patients:

▶ For the physician, acknowledging his or her reaction to the patient (anger, wanting to avoid the patient, attraction, etc.) allows him or her to *not* act out those feelings with the patient.

▶ In general, techniques like open-ended questions, facilitation, clarification (checking), empathic responses, and reflection of the patient's emotional state help the patient to feel heard and understood.

▶ In discussing diagnosis and treatment or other clinical issues with patients, it is important to find out what the patient already knows, is afraid of, and wants to know.

▶ Setting up clinical interactions considering privacy, and with the persons present with whom the patient feels comfortable, will facilitate the process.

▶ Working with the patient to identify and create goals increases compliance.

▶ Setting manageable goals and writing information and instructions down improves compliance.

▶ Explaining the treatment plan and helping to identify sources of support (including interpersonal and community) also improve the patient's ability to cope with acute or chronic illness.

Questions

1. KL is a 40-year-old-businessman who comes in for evaluation of a large mole on his arm, which has grown and changed color and shape. He says he has been noticing this over the last year but he only came in this week when his girlfriend insisted.
   The most likely reason that he did not seek treatment is
   A. Time constraints
   B. Major depression
   C. Suicidal ideation
   D. Denial
   E. Apathy

2. A 35-year-old patient comes in to your office for a routine physical. As always, this patient is suggestive and seductive, and suggests that you continue your conversation over coffee. Of the following choices, which is the most effective way of responding to this?
   A. Do not do a physical exam, as it might be misinterpreted.
   B. You both are single, you find the patient attractive, so you arrange dinner.
   C. You both are single, you find the patient attractive, but you lie and tell the patient that you are married.
   D. Since this is consistent behavior, as always you ask your assistant to join you in the room during the exam, and ignore the behavior.
   E. You confront the patient, saying, "Why are you trying to seduce me? Are you looking for some stability in your life?"

3. BR comes into your office with an erythematous rash on his ankles. He appears extremely anxious about showing you the rash. Upon examination it looks like a contact dermatitis due to poison ivy. You take a history, which confirms that he was clearing out the shrubs in his back yard. A good way to approach this patient would be to
   A. Laugh and say, "This is nothing, just some poison ivy."
   B. Ask the patient what he thinks it is, and then explain the probable cause of the rash.
   C. Tell him that it is dermatitis from urushiol and will require topical steroids.
   D. Say, "Don't worry, this cream will help."
   E. Tell him that he needs to burn all of his clothes that might have come in contact with the plant and that he's lucky that he came in today before it got worse.

4. CL is a 56-year-old woman who has new-onset, non-insulin-dependent diabetes mellitus. She is obese, has high cholesterol, is sedentary, and smokes. You have done a glucose tolerance test and are meeting with her to discuss her diagnosis. After you have explained the diagnosis and prognosis, which of the following is most likely to increase her chances of compliance with your treatment regimen:
   A. Tell her that she needs to take medications, stop smoking, change her diet, lose weight, and exercise in order to get her medical conditions under control.
   B. Tell her that if she doesn't make major life changes she is going to die of a heart attack, lose her kidney function, or go blind.
   C. Tell her what your goals of treatment are and then discuss with her which aspect of the plan she wishes to address first and how she might achieve it.
   D. Tell her what your goals of treatment are and then give her a plan to address them one at a time, including a preprinted diet.
   E. Tell her what your goals of treatment are and then say you know that she feels OK now, but when her medical conditions worsen she'll regret not listening to you.

HPI: PS is a 70-year-old retired postman with a history of schizophrenia who lives with his sister and her family. He has not been attending the outpatient clinic for his depot antipsychotic medication for a couple of months.
After the clinic staff called the sister several times, the patient came to the clinic. You decide to check his blood pressure; when you roll back his sleeve you notice burn marks. You ask the patient to remove his shirt and you notice significant yellow and green bruises across his chest wall. You ask the patient what happened and he says that he must have fallen. He has a long history of schizophrenia, has been hospitalized several times, and was first diagnosed when he was 20 years old. However, he had managed to maintain his job as a postman for approximately 40 years. He finished high school. He lives in his deceased parents' house with his sister, who is widowed, and her two children, who attend college locally. He never married and has no children. He has a small pension and says that his sister takes care of his finances. He does not drink alcohol or abuse substances. He has no forensic history.

MSE: He appeared older than his stated age. His clothing was worn but generally clean. He was badly shaven. Eye contact and rapport were fair. He was a little anxious at times during the interview, though his affect was generally blunted. He described his mood as "alright." Thought processes were linear and there was no evidence of psychosis. He denied suicidal or homicidal ideation. Cognitively, he scored 28/30 on the Mini Mental, missing two of three items on delayed recall. Insight and judgment were fair.

PE: Vital signs were stable. He was a thin, frail male; with superficial healing burn marks on both forearms and multiple fading bruises across the chest. No bony tenderness. Otherwise the rest of the examination was within normal limits.

Labs/Studies: CBC and Chem 20 within normal limits. X-rays of his chest reveal a dozen circular fractures of several ribs.

Thought Questions

- What do you think has been happening to this man?

- What should you do? Should you file a report?

Review and Discussion of Abuse and Neglect

Abuse of elders and children is increasing across the United States. It has been reported that 4% of those more than 65 years of age may be abused. Sexual abuse of children is reported more nowadays than in the past. It has been reported that up to 25% of females and 12% of males report sexual abuse. Between 5% and 20% of families have an abused member. Abuse of an elder may include physical abuse, sexual abuse, emotional abuse, financial abuse, and active and passive neglect.

First of all, this gentleman should be given a comprehensive physical evaluation, looking for signs of missed or other old injuries. Questions should be placed in a non-judgmental manner. Investigate the possibility of sexual abuse, which could involve bruising of the genitals or in females vaginal bleeding. Look also for evidence of malnutrition. Neglect is also a form of abuse, which can be both physical and psychological. In this particular case there may be concern that the patient's sister may misappropriate his funds.

The most common type of abuse in the elderly is financial abuse, followed by physical abuse and active neglect. Signs of physical abuse in an elderly person include signs of neglect and signs of physical abuse. Look out for signs of poor hygiene, self-care, and malnutrition. Other forms of neglect may include the withholding of needed equipment (such as a cane, hearing aids, dentures, eyeglasses, or even medication). Evidence of physical abuse includes evidence of old fractures, burns, and bruising, particularly on the arms, where the elder may have been grasped.

Signs of abuse or neglect in a child also include poor personal care, such as diaper rash, malnutrition, bruises in areas not normally injured, old or healing fractures (including spiral fractures from rotating/twisting limbs), burns (including burns on the bottom or limb extremities from dipping the child in scalding water), and marks from whipping or beating the child with an instrument (e.g., a cane or belt). Mental and emotional abuse can be as harmful as physical abuse in children and may be more difficult to detect. See the Thumbnail for signs of sexual abuse in children.

There is no increase in the rate of psychiatric disorders among parents who abuse their children. They may be isolated in a community without close friends and may seem unwilling to provide for the child's basic needs. They may make excessive demands of their children and fail to teach them how to correct their behavior. When asked about the child's injury, they do not provide an explanation or else they provide a conflicting one.

Mandatory reporting to Child Protective Services or Adult Protective Services of the local Department of Social Services is required by law throughout the United States. All doctors, nurses, hospital personnel, dentists, medical examiners, coroners, mental health professionals, researchers, social workers, teachers, school personnel, child care workers, and law enforcement officials must report suspected abuse of an individual. Some states require that all individuals report suspected cases of neglect and of physical and sexual abuse. Failure to report suspected abuse and malicious false reporting can lead to prosecution.

Forty-five states have physician-mandated reporting requirements for injuries sustained by knives, guns or other weapons, crimes, or domestic violence. Physicians working in each state should check the state's regulations and requirements.

Case Conclusion PS was admitted to the hospital for his own safety. When told about the results of the chest x-rays, he confessed that his sister had hit and poked him with the end of a broomstick. She had also placed his forearms on the hot radiator because of his "bad table manners." His stay in the hospital was uneventful but significant for a 20-pound increase in weight. He did not wish his sister to be prosecuted, even though half of his pension money had been removed. A guardian was appointed and PS was placed in an independent living facility. A year later he was doing well.

Thumbnail: Behavioral Science—Sexual Abuse in Children

Physical signs	Signs of sexual abuse in a child include recurrent urinary tract infections, bruising or injury to the genitals or anus, or presence of a sexually transmitted disease.
Psychological signs	From a psychological perspective the children may show signs of having inappropriate knowledge of sexual acts or may start sexual activities with their friends. There may be a change in behavior ranging from showing increased disruptive behavior to becoming more withdrawn and passive. Children's sleep may be disrupted, with nightmares, bed–wetting, the need for a nightlight, or fear of sleeping alone.
Characteristics of the abuser	Most abusers are male and are known to the child. The abuser may abuse alcohol or illicit substances and may lack a suitable sexual partner or actually be a pedophile.
Characteristics of the victim	The majority of abused children are between 9 and 12 years of age, but some are younger. The children often report that they were afraid that the abuser would punish them or not care for them any longer if they reported the abuse. They may feel ashamed and guilty about the abuse.

Key Points

▶ Four percent of those more than 65 years of age may be abused.

▶ Twenty-five percent of females and 12% of males report sexual abuse. Five percent to twenty percent of families have an abused member.

▶ Twenty-five percent of murders occur among family members.

▶ The most common type of abuse in the elderly is financial abuse.

▶ There is no increase in the rate of psychiatric disorders among abusive parents.

▶ The law requires mandatory reporting to Child Protective Services or Adult Protective Services of the local Department of Social Services.

Questions

1. Which of the following characteristics are found in abusers of the elderly?
   A. They tend to be physically dependent on the victim.
   B. They usually have dementia.
   C. They are usually financially dependent on the victim.
   D. They often do not have a personal history of abuse.
   E. They are often the closest family member.

2. Which of the following are characteristics of physically abused children?
   A. Mostly these children reached full term.
   B. They have been in good health previously.
   C. The majority are over 5 years of age.
   D. They may be described as "slow."
   E. They usually report their injuries.

3. Which of the following statements is correct concerning the structures of family units in the United States today?
   A. Approximately 50% of families involve a single parent.
   B. Approximately 80% of children under 18 years of age have parents that both work outside the home.
   C. The number of children being born to married couples is declining.
   D. Approximately 55% of couples are childless.
   E. The majority of new marriages will divorce within 2 years.

4. TP is a 32-year-old married female who presented to the emergency room with a black eye. She told the emergency room physician that she had fallen in her home against the door of a kitchen cabinet. On examination you find evidence of red marks and recent bruises on her arms and legs. She tells you that she is 2 months pregnant. Which of the following is appropriate to tell her?
   A. She should leave home immediately.
   B. Dangers to the unborn child include low birth weight and premature birth.
   C. She does not need to report this to the police.
   D. Counseling should involve both partners together.
   E. Most female murder victims are killed by their partners.

HPI: MT is a 29-year-old Caucasian male who is brought to the emergency room in handcuffs by the police after he assaulted another patron in a bar. The policeman reports that MT was extremely agitated when approached and had been restrained by several patrons at the bar. Witnesses told the policeman that MT had been watching a football game on the television when he began to argue with his neighbor at the bar. He suddenly stood up and started to beat up the other fellow. The other fellow wished to press charges. When you ask MT about this incident he drunkenly tells you that the other fellow "deserved it . . . bad mouthing my team." He is not very cooperative with the assessment and tells you to "buzz off . . . busy bee." He does tell you that he has no serious medical or psychiatric history. He cannot tell you if he hit his head in the fight or if he lost consciousness at all. The policeman tells you that MT has a history of arrest for driving while intoxicated (DWI) and assault, for which he has spent time in jail.

PE: His breath smells of alcohol and his finger stick reveals a blood glucose of 100. His BP is 130/82, pulse is 100, and RR are 16 per minute. He has multiple tattoos across his torso and arms. No needle marks. He has some fresh red marks in his abdomen, where he was recently punched, but otherwise the examination is normal.

MSE: He is disheveled, has a torn shirt, but is generally clean. His eye contact and rapport are limited. No evidence of abnormal movements. His speech is loud at times. His affect is labile and irritable, and his mood is described as "P_ off." Thought process is generally goal directed. He denies SI but does endorse HI+ "I'll kill that guy when I get my hands on him." He denies AH/VH/SH. He shows no evidence of remorse for his recent behaviors. He is oriented to person but refuses to answer questions about time or place. He has no insight into his condition and his judgment is obviously impaired.

Labs/Studies: CBC and Chem. 20 wnl. Utox negative but blood alcohol level was 0.8. CT scan of his head without contrast was normal.

Thought Questions

■ What is the most likely cause of this man's aggressive behavior?

■ What other conditions may cause aggressive behavior?

■ Do you need to warn the other fellow about this patient's threat?

Basic Science Review and Discussion

Aggression involves the expression of anger when provoked by a perceived threat. Different temperamental, developmental, and cultural influences may affect the individual's expression of aggression. Genetics and environmental factors both play a role in the development of aggressive temperaments. Aggression can be directed toward others or toward the self.

It is most likely that this patient's impulsive aggressive outburst is due to alcohol intoxication, but several possible causes and conditions should be considered.

Antisocial Personality Disorder The *Diagnostic and Statistical Manual of Mental Disorders,* 4th edition (*DSM-IV*), defines antisocial personality disorder as a pervasive pattern of disregard and violation of the rights of others, which has been present since the age of 15. They also have three of the following features: **failure to conform to social norms** with respect to lawful behaviors, deceitfulness, **impulsivity** and failure to plan ahead, **irritability** and aggressiveness (with physical assaults), **reckless disregard** for the safety of others, consistent **irresponsible** behaviors, and a **lack of remorse.** The individual must be at least 18 years old with **a history of conduct disorder** (onset before 15 years) in order to receive this diagnosis. The antisocial behavior does not occur exclusively during the course of a manic or schizophrenic illness.

Epidemiology Approximately 3% of males and 1% of females in the general population have antisocial personality disorder, but between 3% and 30% in clinical settings are affected, and the number may be higher in forensic or substance abuse treatment environments.

Associated Features Antisocial personality disorder may be associated with low socioeconomic status and urban settings. Individuals tend to be callous and show lack of empathy for others; may appear arrogant, with inflated self-esteem; or may be superficially charming. They can also be irresponsible in their relationships.

Differential Diagnosis Substance abuse, narcissistic, histrionic, or borderline personality disorders. Antisocial and borderline personality disorders are both associated with a lifelong pattern of impulsive aggression and violence. Persons with antisocial personality disorder do not feel remorse for their aggressive actions. Individuals with narcissistic personality disorder may lack empathy for others and have an exploitative interpersonal style. Borderline individuals may have unstable intense relationships with impulsive, possibly self-damaging behaviors and inappropriate anger, but they have unstable self-images. Borderlines have a history of intense, unstable relationships, affect, and self-image, with impulsive behaviors. Individuals with histrionic personality disorder have pervasive patterns of excess emotionality and may be excessively attention seeking, seductive, and shallow, with dramatic theatrical behaviors.

Course and Prognosis Antisocial personality disorder follows a chronic course; some may show evidence of improvement in their 40s. They are more likely than the general population to die prematurely from violent means. Treatment involves self-help techniques, careful use of anticonvulsants if indicated, and substance abuse treatment.

Conduct disorder is usually diagnosed in children who have a persistent pattern of behavior, which violates the rights of others or the age-appropriate norms or rules of society. The disturbance in behavior causes significant impairment in functioning. The diagnostic criteria also include at least three of the following behaviors:

1. Aggression to people or animals
2. Destruction of property
3. Deceitfulness or theft
4. Serious violation of rules.

Conduct disorders are reported in between 1% and 16% of children and adolescents. It is more common in boys at all ages.

Intermittent explosive disorder is a rare disorder defined in the *DSM-IV* as a condition in which there are **several discrete episodes of failure to resist aggressive impulses that result in serious assault acts or destruction of property.** The degree of expressed aggressiveness is out of proportion to the precipitating stressors. These episodes are not better accounted for by another psychiatric disorder or substance use. It has been described as a diagnosis of exclusion. This condition is assumed to occur more often in Caucasian men, who generally are treated in forensic facilities. On the other hand, women may commit less severe aggressive acts and be treated in a psychiatric setting. These patients may be genuinely distressed by these violent episodes. Those close to them may provoke violent episodes.

The exact prevalence of this disorder is unknown; it is described as starting between late adolescence and the third decade. People with intermittent explosive disorder may have **nonspecific findings on EEG** (slowing) **and neurologic exam** (impaired coordination or reflex asymmetry) or a history of childhood head injuries without a loss of consciousness. Many of those who have this disorder report personal or family histories of **significant substance abuse,** particularly alcohol. This condition may be related to impaired ability to anticipate frustration and delay gratification, which is a normal developmental achievement. Impulsive aggression may also be related to **low** levels of the neurotransmitter **serotonin.**

Other psychiatric causes of impulsive aggressive/violent behavior include a **psychotic illness, substance intoxication** (alcohol, PCP), **mania, attention deficit/hyperactivity disorder, conduct disorder, mental retardation, and borderline personality disorders.** Medical causes include substance intoxication, dementias, complex partial seizures, and certain inborn errors of metabolism and head trauma. Other medical conditions associated with a personality change with aggression include stroke, normal-pressure hydrocephalus, encephalitis, brain abscess, and subarachnoid hemorrhage.

A particular culture-bound syndrome of episodic aggression is called **amok.** It was originally described in Malaysia and refers to a situation in which an individual suddenly attempts to attack or kill others and even themselves. Those who survive report no memory of the attacks.

Several different types of medications have been used to treat intermittent explosive disorder and other forms of impulsive aggressive behavior. These agents include carbamazepine, lithium, valproate, tricyclics, selective serotonergic reuptake inhibitors (SSRIs), beta-blockers, buspirone, and benzodiazepines.

Tarasoff Principle If a therapist discovers that his or her patient intends to harm or kill another individual, then the therapist has an obligation to warn the intended victim or to tell others who will warn the intended victim, such as the police. This is called the **Tarasoff principle,** which was named after the California university student who was murdered by a fellow student in 1976. This principle applies in the state of California. The **Tarasoff I** ruling refers to the original case of *Tarasoff vs Regents of University of California.* The court ruled that a physician or psychotherapist who has reason to believe that a patient may injure or kill someone must notify the potential victim, their relatives, or the authorities. The **Tarasoff II** ruling broadened the duty to warn to include the duty to protect in the case of imminent potentially serious harm to another person. Thus the patient may be held involuntarily.

Case Conclusion   MT was monitored closely in the emergency room until he sobered up and his assessment was completed. He had a significant history of behavioral disturbance in his youth, which met criteria for conduct disorder. He blames this behavior on the divorce of his parents. He said he "liked to set fire to cats." He denied any intention to harm his fellow patron in the bar. He had also been arrested twice previously for DWIs and was assaultive toward police officers while intoxicated. He was divorced with two young children with whom he has no contact, and he admitted that he does not pay child support. He was advised to abstain from alcohol and illicit substances and was escorted to the county jail for processing.

Thumbnail: Behavioral Science—Antisocial Personality Disorder

Diagnostic criteria	Pervasive pattern of disregard and violation of the rights of others, which may include a failure to conform to social norms with respect to lawful behaviors, deceitfulness, impulsivity and failure to plan ahead, irritability and aggressiveness (with physical assaults), reckless disregard for the safety of others, consistent irresponsible behaviors, and lack of remorse.
Epidemiology	Approximately 3% of males and 1% of females in the general population.
Etiology	Genetic and environmental causes.
Associated features	May be associated with low socioeconomic status and urban settings.
Differential diagnosis	Substance abuse, narcissistic, histrionic or borderline personality disorders.
Course and prognosis	Follows a chronic course, some may show evidence of improvement in their 40s.

Key Points

- Approximately 3% of males and 1% of females in the general population have antisocial disorder.
- Individuals with antisocial personality disorder have a pervasive pattern of disregard and violation of the rights of others and a significant lack of remorse.
- Intermittent explosive disorder is a condition in which there are several episodes of failure to resist aggressive impulses that result in serious assault acts or destruction of property.
- The aggressiveness is out of proportion to the precipitating stressors.

- Other causes of impulsive aggressive/violent behavior include psychosis, substance intoxication, mania, attention deficit/hyperactivity disorder, conduct disorder, mental retardation, antisocial/borderline personality disorders.
- Carbamazepine, lithium, valproate, tricyclics, SSRIs, beta-blockers, buspirone, and benzodiazepines have been used to treat impulsive aggression.
- The Tarasoff principle includes the duty to warn potential victims of serious threat and to protect the patient.

Questions

1. Which of the following is associated with increased risk of impulsive aggression?
   A. High CSF levels of 5-HIAA
   B. Low CSF levels of 5-HIAA
   C. High serotonergic response on challenge testing
   D. Bilateral temporal lobe lesions
   E. A dominant frontal lobe lesion

2. Which of the following are risk factors for divorce?
   A. A long courtship
   B. A previous history of divorce
   C. Premarital pregnancy
   D. Older age at marriage
   E. Overly similar backgrounds

3. A 10-year-old boy is brought by his parents for assessment, as they are concerned about him. He was caught painting graffiti slogans on the school wall with two classmates 6 months ago and torturing a cat previously. His grades are going down and he slipped out of the house during the night to meet "someone." Moreover, he will not do anything his parents ask him to. The final straw was when his teacher called to tell his parents that he had been caught bullying younger boys for their lunch money. Which of the following is the most likely diagnosis?
   A. Oppositional defiant disorder
   B. Attention-deficit hyperactivity disorder
   C. Adjustment disorder
   D. Conduct disorder
   E. Mania

4. Which of the following is characteristic of antisocial personality disorder?
   A. Fast waves on the EEG
   B. Focal neurologic deficits
   C. Increased rates of somatization disorder in relatives
   D. Increased risk of developing OCD
   E. A need for excessive admiration

HPI: You are called on to assess capacity of a 63-year-old single Caucasian female with schizophrenia who is refusing chemotherapy. JK has a 40-year history of paranoid schizophrenia and was diagnosed with colon cancer 3 weeks ago. She underwent a resection, and at that time was found to have stage IV adenocarcinoma with multiple metastases to the liver and carcinomatosis. On chest x-ray it appears that she has lung metastases as well. She is refusing chemotherapy. Her oncologist says that she is delusional and he questions her capacity to decide on a treatment. On exam you find her to be cooperative with the interview, sometimes digressing about her delusional material, but basically understanding that she has metastatic cancer and that her prognosis is poor with a less than 5% chance of 5-year survival. On further exam of her psychiatric symptoms, she believes that when she was on a high school field trip to the museum, someone implanted an accessory uterus for use in experimentation and for control of her thoughts. Somehow this is connected to both the Hare Krishnas and the Kennedy assassinations. She believes that the Krishnas can implant thoughts in her mind, especially about politicians and TV newscasters. In discussing her treatment options, she explains that given her prognosis and the fact that she has had relatives die of this and other cancers, she feels that the morbidity from the chemotherapy outweighs the potential benefits. She has had numerous psychiatric hospitalizations and at present her medication is "optimized." She is not depressed or suicidal.

Thought Question

■ Do you think she has the capacity to decide whether to accept chemotherapy?

Basic Science Review and Discussion

Competence vs Capacity   It is important to understand that competence is a legal concept and can only be decided in the courts. Capacity is a clinical judgment about the patient's ability to make a decision. Capacity can be assessed by any physician, although psychiatrists are often called to make that assessment.

Decision-making capacity is based on four things. First, patients must be able to evidence a choice. They must understand that there is a choice to be made. Next, they must understand the relevant information. Often this involves being able to "explain back" what the doctor has said about the treatment or the procedure. Third, they should be able to understand the risks and benefits. Again this can be evidenced by seeing if they can repeat or explain in their own words what was told to them. Finally, the highest level of capacity is to be able to manipulate the information and to explain the rationale behind the decision.

It is important to note that, depending on the risk of the treatment or procedure, physicians will expect different levels of capacity. For example, a low-risk procedure like drawing blood has no informed consent, and the patient basically just has to evidence a choice (i.e., letting the blood be drawn or refusing). When prescribing an antihypertensive with few side effects, physicians may document that they explained the risks of untreated hypertension and the potential side effects of the medication. Patients are rarely asked to sign consent about accepting a specific medication. Most often if patients are compliant and take the medication, they are evidencing a choice, and if they understand the purpose of taking the medication ("to treat my high blood pressure"), they are demonstrating that they understand the relevant information. When the stakes are greater (e.g., accepting an invasive procedure or potentially toxic treatment, or refusing a treatment that could be lifesaving), the expectations for the capacity of the patient are higher.

In terms of psychiatric symptoms the greatest concern is that the symptoms are somehow influencing the person's decision. A severely depressed patient who believes there is no hope may refuse treatment because of his fatalistic outlook and severe depression. For example, a patient with a major depression may refuse to have a malignant melanoma removed because, "There is no hope; I will die anyway, and I deserve to die." With treatment and remission of the depression the patient would feel quite different, and probably would regret having let a potentially curable lesion evolve into a fatal one. Psychotic patients may have delusions that, for example, surgery is actually a plot to hurt them or a way for a governmental agency to implant a device. In this example the delusion is clearly influencing the patient's ability to think through the treatment decision.

Patients without capacity either can have health care proxies (if they have designated one) or have court-appointed guardians make health care decisions. In some states a family member may make decisions on a patient's behalf if he or she lacks capacity, whereas in others only a court-appointed guardian or health care proxy can make decisions, unless the patient has clear documentation of his or her wishes. Although these concepts are used in all states, the details of the laws differ.

Case Conclusion You review the prognosis with the oncologist, who confirms the survival rates. Her prognosis is worse because of the distant metastases and the multiple intrahepatic and peritoneal lesions. The oncologist still believes that chemotherapy may improve the patient's quality of life. In your examination of this patient, although she is quite psychotic, her delusions do not appear to be related to or involve her illness. She understands that there is a choice to be made, can explain the risks and benefits of accepting the treatment, and can explain why she has decided not to accept treatment. Patients do not have to agree with their doctor's recommendations about treatment, quality of life, and so on, as long as they have the capacity to make their own decisions.

Thumbnail: Behavioral Science—Decisions Involving Minors

Decision or Situation	Parental Consent Needed?
Children under 18	Parents have the right to sign consent for their minor children
Abortions	Parental consent required in approximately 50% of states
Prenatal care, treatment of sexually transmitted diseases, or treatment of substance abuse	Generally does not require parental consent
Emergency treatment	Generally does not require parental consent. Parents cannot refuse life saving medical treatment. (Christian Scientists have been brought to court to ensure medical intervention for their children.)
Emancipated minors (i.e., those who are self-supporting or are married)	Are treated as adults and do not require parental consent

Key Points

▶ Competence is a legal standard.

▶ Capacity is a clinical judgment about the patient's ability to make a decision that can be assessed by any physician.

▶ Capacity is based on the ability to

  ▶ Evidence a choice.

  ▶ Understand the relevant information.

  ▶ Understand the risks and benefits of the treatment or procedure.

  ▶ Manipulate the information and explain the rationale behind the decision.

Questions

Questions 1 and 2 refer to the following case.

MS is an 88-year-old woman with dementia who presents to the emergency department with productive cough and shortness of breath. At baseline she has severely impaired short- and long-term memory and cannot manage her activities of daily living, such as bathing, grooming, and toileting without assistance. She has a receptive and expressive (fluent) aphasia and will talk "endlessly" without making much sense. She is diagnosed with pneumonia by the emergency department physician.

1. Which of the following statements is true about her ability to make medical decisions:
   A. A physician cannot declare her incompetent to make decisions.
   B. If she refuses a procedure, her health care proxy cannot accept on her behalf.
   C. As long as she goes along with the treatment recommendations of her doctor, she does not have to demonstrate capacity.
   D. Although she had made a living will and discussed her preferences with her doctor prior to her dementia, her cousin's husband can decide that she needs to be resuscitated if she has a cardiac arrest, despite her wishes to the contrary.
   E. Only a psychiatrist can determine her decisional capacity.

2. MS wants to leave the emergency room before being admitted. She is very briefly evaluated and the inexperienced physician says, "She is an adult; she can decide to leave the hospital without treatment." She is allowed to leave and somehow manages to get home by showing her ID and giving $20 to a cab driver. The following day she becomes hypoxic, goes into respiratory arrest, and dies. In suing for malpractice, which of the following concepts is important:
   A. Demonstrating malicious intent
   B. Demonstrating that a crime was committed
   C. Demonstrating that there was a duty by the physician
   D. Demonstrating that the physician was paid by the insurance company
   E. Demonstrating that the hospital verified the physicians credentials

3. Which of the following clinical scenarios is absolutely true?
   A. A patient with a stroke and hemiplegia does not have capacity.
   B. A Jehovah's Witness who is cognitively intact cannot refuse a transfusion in an emergency.
   C. A Christian Scientist who is cognitively intact may refuse surgery for appendicitis.
   D. A patient with early-stage Alzheimer's disease does not have capacity to accept a skin biopsy.
   E. A Christian Scientist who is cognitively intact may refuse an emergency appendectomy for his or her child.

4. Which of the following patients probably has capacity?
   A. A patient with a severe major depression who refuses treatment for a skin cancer because "it's all hopeless."
   B. A 35-year-old patient with widely metastatic ovarian cancer who has had no response to four trials of chemotherapy and says "no more."
   C. A patient with anorexia nervosa who is less than 60% of her ideal body weight, is bradycardic, and says she can gain on her own and doesn't need admission.
   D. An 85-year-old man with moderate Alzheimer's disease who requires 8 hours of home care daily, states that he wants to have a rhinoplasty, and can manage the postoperative care himself.
   E. A schizophrenic who believed that chemotherapy was used as "mind control" by the CIA.

HPI: AG is a 27-year-old single white female who presents to the outpatient clinic complaining of fatigue and "an inability to do anything." She has early-morning awakening, poor appetite, low energy, and poor concentration; does not enjoy anything; and is feeling passively suicidal. She states that she doesn't have any plans to kill herself, but if she didn't wake up tomorrow, that would be "just fine."

MSE: She is mildly disheveled and her hair is unbrushed. She is sitting in her chair, shoulders hunched, making poor eye contact. She is psychomotorically retarded. Her speech is somewhat slow, quiet, and lacks normal prosody. Her mood is "bad" and her affect is constricted to the dysphoric. Her thought process is linear and goal-directed, and her thought content is ruminative about how worthless she is and how her life is "going nowhere." However, she has no active suicidal ideation, intent, or plan. She has no perceptual changes. Her cognitive functioning is grossly intact, and she is oriented to time and place. Her insight is fair (she knows that she is depressed and needs help, but she thinks that everything is hopeless and that nothing *will* actually help) and her social judgment is intact.

Thought Questions

- What are the basic components of a mental status exam?
- What is the diagnostic framework currently used in psychiatry?
- How would you apply it to this case?

Basic Science Review and Discussion

Diagnostic Frameworks in Psychiatry Psychiatric diagnoses are formulated in accordance with the multiaxial scheme of the *Diagnostic and Statistical Manual of Mental Disorders,* 4th edition (*DSM-IV*). The American Psychiatric Association developed this for use in clinical work, education, and research. The term mental disorder is defined as a "clinically significant psychological or behavioral condition that causes distress or disability in an individual or increased risk of disability, loss of important freedom, pain, or death." It is not merely an understandable response to an event such as death.

The *DSM-IV* is categorical in nature and divides mental disorders into groups according to defining features and criteria. Because the etiology of most psychiatric illnesses is not well defined, the *DSM-IV* defines illnesses by symptom clusters, not etiology. The categories therefore may not be discrete entities, and even those who have the same disorder may be heterogeneous. That said, it is a comprehensive and widely used system of classification.

The *DSM-IV* provides for a "multiaxial" diagnosis, in appreciation of the fact that psychiatric illnesses are complex and have multiple influences (see Thumbnail).

The Mental Status Exam In psychiatry, physicians are expected to do physical and neurologic exams in the assessment of their patients, but the specialized exam in psychiatry is called the mental status exam. In doing a mental status exam, there are number of terms that are important to learn. In addition, many disorders have classic presentations on mental status. The woman described above has a classic major depression. Not only do her symptoms reflect a major depression—depressed mood, decreased sleep, energy, appetite, concentration, etc.—but her exam is also reflective of that. Her grooming is only fair, she is slowed down and her eye contact is poor.

Another classic case example would be that of mania. In that disorder the classic exam might be as follows:

SH is a 24-year-old woman, dressed in bright shirt with an unmatching scarf, wearing a great deal of hastily applied makeup. She is psychomotorically agitated, getting up, walking, and sitting down. Her speech is pressured and rapid. Her mood is "great, fantastic, fabulous" and her affect is expansive. Her thought process is circumstantial with flight of ideas. She has grandiose delusions, thinks that she has been chosen to star in a feature-length film about her own life and that she has discovered a new scientific theory that "will unify the world." She has no hallucinations or other altered perceptions; she is cognitively intact, although extremely distractible. Her insight is poor, as she thinks that nothing is wrong. Her judgment is impaired—she has impulsively spent $5000 on new clothing for "the film and the opening," has had sex with three strangers in the last 2 days, and was brought in by the police because she was wearing only a bikini and a flowing wrap in 40-degree weather. (She explained that she felt "free.")

Box 17-1 contains a glossary of terms used in describing a mental status exam. This should be helpful in describing psychiatric patients and in understanding the cases.

Box 17-1. Terms Used in Describing a Mental Status Exam

Appearance
Dress, grooming, hygiene, general behavior, facial expression

Attitudes/Relatedness
Indifference–lack of concern, interest or feeling
Passive–taking no part; offering no opposition; submissive
Dependent–relies excessively on examiner for support or aid
Hostile–unfriendly; adverse; antagonistic
Suspicious–mistrusting; questions motives
Manipulative–artful management or control by shrewd use of influence or handling
Dramatic–vivid, highly emotional, action oriented

Psycho/Motor Behavior
Agitation–excessive bodily movements, hand-wringing, pacing
Retardation–poverty of bodily movements
Abnormal movements: tremors, movements associated with tardive dyskinesia, etc.

Speech
Volume, rate: slow, fast, pressured
Prosody: normal fluctuation in tone of speech

Mood
Usually refers to the patient's self-described mood

Affect
External appreciation of the patient's affective state
Inappropriate–patient's affect appears inconsistent with the situation, content of material or his subjective mood
Lability–inordinate variability in moment-to-moment feeling tone
Blunted–lack of emotional sensitivity
Flat–limitation of expression of emotion
Constricted–decreased range of emotion
Expansive–broad range of emotion

Thought Process
Linear, goal directed
Perseverations: involuntary pathologic persistence of a single response or idea
Incoherence: thinking processes so disrupted that they do not result in a complete idea
Circumstantiality: proceeding indirectly to goal with many tedious details and irrelevant additions
Tangentiality: divergent and does not come to grip with central issue

Loose associations: lack of logical relationships between contiguous thoughts or ideas
Blocking: sudden cessation in a train of thought that is unexplainable to a patient
Flight of ideas: rapid skipping from one idea to another. Associations are still evident.
Poverty: decreased content
Racing or slowing of the thought process

Thought Content
Obsessions: a persistent unwanted thought that cannot be eliminated
Ruminations: repetitive, often circular speculations, which are voluntary—excessive worries
Doubting and indecision: excessively time-consuming uncertainties
Ideas of reference: incorrect interpretation of incidents and events as having direct reference to oneself
Delusions: fixed false belief, out of keeping with educational and cultural background. (Specify type—e.g., paranoid, religious, grandiose, guilty, etc.)
Helplessness/Hopelessness
Hyperreligiosity: detrimental, excessive concern with spiritual and religious matters. Not of delusional nature.
Suicidality or **Homicidality**

Disorders of Perception
Illusions: misinterpretation of a real sensory experience
Hallucination: a false sensory perception in the absence of an actual external stimulus (specify type and content: auditory, visual, olfactory, gustatory, tactile)
Hypnagogic: disorders of perception occurring in semiconscious state going to sleep
Hypnopompic: disorders of perception occurring in semiconscious state upon awakening

Intellectual/Cognitive Functioning
Folstein's Mini Mental Status Exam covers orientation to time, place, immediate and delayed recall, naming, repeating, copying, attention, and concentration. Orientation to person (self and examiner) and long-term memory should be assessed in the interview.

Insight/Judgment/Plans
Insight: awareness of illness, psychological nature of illness, and need for treatment
Judgment: may encompass judgment about social, financial, planning, and other issues

---

Case Conclusion As mentioned earlier, AG met criteria for major depression. She was started on an antidepressant and a course of psychotherapy, and did well. One month later her exam is as follows:
Well groomed, good eye contact, no psychomotor agitation or retardation. Her speech is normal in rate, rhythm, and tone. Her mood is "better, not perfect," and her affect is much more reactive. Her thought process is linear and goal directed, and her thought content is no longer ruminative. She is hopeful. She has no suicidal or homicidal ideation, and no perceptual changes. Her cognitive functioning is intact, and she is oriented to time and place. Her insight is good and her judgment is intact.

Thumbnail: Behavioral Science—Diagnostic Frameworks in Psychiatry

Axis	Definition	Examples
Axis I	Clinical disorders or conditions requiring clinical attention [course specifiers (i.e., degree of remission or severity) may be used]	Major depression, bipolar disorder, schizophrenia
Axis II	Personality disorders and mental retardation	Antisocial personality disorder, dependent personality disorder, mental retardation
Axis III	General medical conditions	Hypertension, cerebrovascular accident, gout
Axis IV	Psychosocial and environmental problems and stressors	Divorce, death of spouse, occupational problems, legal problems
Axis V	Global assessment of the patient's functioning (100-point scale)	91 to 100: superior functioning, no symptoms 61 to 71: some mild symptoms, or difficulties, but generally functioning pretty well 21 to 30: behavior considerably influenced by delusions; serious impairment in communication or judgment

Key Points

▶ The mental status exam encompasses the description of the psychiatric patient and uses a vocabulary that reflects the patient's presentation.

▶ In general, the key components are appearance; attitude/relatedness; psycho/motor behavior; speech; mood (usually refers to the patient's self-described mood); affect (external appreciation of the patient's affective state); thought process; thought content; disorders of perception; intellectual/cognitive functioning; insight/judgment.

▶ The *DSM-IV* uses a multiaxial formulation with five axes. Those axes represent acute clinical disorders (Axis I), personality disorders and mental retardation (Axis II), general medical conditions (Axis III), psychosocial stressors (Axis IV), and global assessment of functioning (Axis V).

Questions

Questions 1 and 2 refer to the following case:

HP is a 35-year-old man living in a group home; he has hypertension and an IQ of 60. His mother died last year, and over the past few months he has been depressed, has been anhedonic, and has had poor sleep, low energy, and reduced appetite. Recently, he has been talking about wanting to die, to be with his mother. He is brought to the emergency room for evaluation.

1. According to the *DSM-IV,* which is the correct way to categorize his diagnoses?
   A. Axis I: major depression, mental retardation. Axis II: none. Axis III: hypertension
   B. Axis I: major depression. Axis II: mental retardation. Axis III: hypertension
   C. Axis I: major depression, mental retardation. Axis II: hypertension. Axis III: none
   D. Axis I: hypertension. Axis II: major depression. Axis III: mental retardation
   E. Axis I: major depression. Axis II: hypertension. Axis III: mental retardation

2. Which of the following findings on mental status is most likely to be associated with major depression?
   A. Pressured speech
   B. Flight of ideas
   C. Psychomotor retardation
   D. Circumstantiality
   E. Suspiciousness

3: AQ is a 23-year-old woman who is brought to the emergency room for evaluation. Her old chart says that she has bipolar disorder, and the nurse comes in to tell you that she's "back, off her meds, and manic." Which of the following is a correct pairing likely to be seen in her mental status exam?
   A. Thought content: circumstantiality
   B. Thought process: grandiose delusions
   C. Speech: loosening of associations
   D. Thought process: flight of ideas
   E. Affect: flat

4. BT is a 31-year-old woman with schizophrenia that is only fairly controlled with medications. You are discussing symptoms of thought content and perceptions with the resident. Which of the following is most associated with schizophrenia?
   A. Hypnagogic hallucinations
   B. Illusions
   C. Intrusive ego dystonic thoughts
   D. Hypnopompic hallucinations
   E. Fixed false beliefs

HPI: CF is a 15-year-old female who has been brought to the family doctor by her mother, who is concerned that she has been losing too much weight.

Her mother had noticed a more dramatic change in her daughter over the previous 3 months. Mrs. F said that her daughter had always been a little "chubby" until approximately 1 year earlier but had gradually begun to lose weight. Lately she had been making excuses to eat alone and wanted to prepare her own "healthy" food. She began exercising more with daily workouts of about 2 hours on top of her regular ballet training. When you ask CF about her weight loss she tells you that she needed to lose weight because the ballet teacher has been posting their weights on the wall and making comments about her size. She is actually 5 feet, 5 inches and weighs 100 pounds. She admitted that she had been restricting her food intake but denied that she had been inducing vomiting or abusing laxatives. She has no psychiatric history and there is no significant family history. She is the middle of three girls. She is in her first year of high school and maintains an A average in her grades. Her mother had discovered that she had been accessing a website called "Ana," which apparently is for anorexics, and she was concerned that her daughter had anorexia.

PE: Vitals signs were significant for a BP of 110/70 and a pulse of 50 beats per minute. Revealed a thin young female with dry, yellow-colored skin and fine lanugo hair on both her face and back. There was some swelling of the parotid glands. She had a sinus bradycardia but no murmurs. Neurologic exam was intact.

Thought Questions

■ What types of eating disorders are there? What signs would you look for in anorexia?

■ What kind of treatments would you recommend?

■ What are the principles of family and group therapy?

Basic Science Review and Discussion

There are two major types of eating disorders: anorexia nervosa and bulimia nervosa. Both are divided into two specific types. Anorexia subtypes include restricting and binge eating/purging types, whereas bulimia is divided into purging and nonpurging subtypes. For a description of the associated features of both disorders see Thumbnail.

Anorexia Nervosa To make a diagnosis of **anorexia** several criteria must be met: a failure to maintain body weight at or above a minimally normal weight for age and height; a morbid fear of becoming fat, even though underweight; a distorted body image; and amenorrhea, in postpubertal females. Criteria for describing weight loss in anorexia include either 85% below expected weight for size or a Body Mass Index (BMI), the weight in kilograms/height in meters squared, less than or equal to 17.5 kg/m². Those that restrict their food intake may develop the signs and symptoms of starvation, whereas those who vomit or abuse laxatives may show different symptoms (see Thumbnail). In the long term, increased rates of osteoporosis, impaired fertility, and increased perinatal mortality have been reported.

Many of these individuals have increased rates of depression, obsessions, and compulsions. Those with the binging

type are more likely to have substance abuse problems and other impulse-control problems than those with the restricting type.

The prevalence of anorexia is 1% or less of the general population. It may affect males (10% of cases) and females, and seems to peak at both 14 and 18 years of age. It remains controversial as to whether this disorder is increasing in prevalence or is diagnosed more often. Higher rates are reported among certain groups, such as ballet dancers and gymnasts. First-degree relatives seem to be at increased risk of developing the disorder, and monozygotic twins show increased concordance. Abnormalities in serotonin, cholecystokinin (CCK), and the hypothalamic-pituitary-gonadal axis have been suggested. Care should be taken to rule out any possible underlying medical illness, such as a tumor or AIDS. The prognosis is generally poor, with a high dropout rate from treatment and mortality rates of 15% reported.

Bulimia Individuals with **bulimia** tend to **binge-eat** and try to **compensate** for this by purging (with vomiting or laxatives), fasting, or exercising. During these binges excessive amounts of food may be eaten in a short period of time and cannot be controlled. Often these are high-calorie and sweet foods. Typical binges may contain over 20,000 calories. This pattern of binging and compensating behaviors happens at least **twice a week for a 3-month period.** These individuals also are unduly influenced by their weight and shape but tend to be in the normal weight range. They may also have depression, anxiety, and personality disorders (borderline). Approximately one-third have substance abuse/dependence. They often have low self-esteem. The prevalence of bulimia is between approximately 1% and 3% of young women, with occasional binging reported in as many as 40% of college students. It occurs more rarely in males. Its peak age of onset is later than that for anorexia nervosa. Approximately a third of those with bulimia have a history of anorexia. The etiology is multifactorial as with anorexia, but abnormalities in serotonin have been more extensively studied in bulimia. The course may be episodic or chronic. The prognosis for individuals with bulimia is better than that of those with anorexia, but they continue to have high rates of relapse and impaired functioning.

Treatment of these disorders includes attention to any comorbid conditions, such as depression, anxiety, or substance abuse. Treatment may also require hospitalization if these individuals are suicidal or medically compromised. In anorexics a regular diet should be used to achieve an ideal body weight (e.g., a BMI of 20 to 25). Depression in bulimic patients should not be treated with selective serotonergic reuptake inhibitors (SSRIs), which may cause seizures. However, fluoxetine may help those with anorexia. Psychotherapies play an important role in the treatment of eating disorders and may involve individual, group, or family therapy. Individual therapy may be cognitive behavioral or interpersonal in type.

Family Systems Theory and Family Therapy General systems theory is used particularly in family therapy and is based on the idea of concentric and overlapping systems with various subsystems formed by individuals. There are fundamental principles of a system and they include the following:

1. Homeostasis is maintained if possible.
2. Systems operate according to rules.
3. External problems may cause a crisis.
4. Crises may cause exploration of the problem.
5. This may lead to a reorganization and thus a new homeostasis.

The family therapist can have several roles: He or she can analyze the family system and provide feedback without involvement, get involved in conflicts, or act as an authority figure to change the system. Medical decisions can be made in the context of multidisciplinary groups, so doctors need to be aware about the dynamics of a group.

There are three main schools of family therapy:

1. **Behavioral-psychoeducational:** The aim is to identify the dysfunctional behaviors and improve them.

2. **Structural-strategic:** The aim is to identify the family structure and to fix faulty alliances.

3. **Intergenerational-experiential:** The focus is to identify transgenerational patterns using genograms and to improve communication.

Group Therapy Group therapy provides the forum in which individuals can learn new and more appropriate behaviors. So the group functions as a microcosm of the individual's own world. Groups may be supportive (self-help) or psychodynamic. Analysis may be of the group as a whole or of individuals within the group. Groups can help members deal with the stressors of daily life. The therapist's responsibility is to provide support and to encourage an atmosphere in which change can occur.

Groups have several characteristics that may interfere with the group process. Groups may blame a particular individual (a "scapegoat") for difficulties that arise. Members may form alliances to protect their interests should a new leader arise. Members may also become dependent on the leader. Fight-or-flight responses may be provoked by perceived threats to the group.

Groups may generally influence behavior in several different ways through social facilitation (enhancement of task performance), social inhibition (inhibition of performance of a task as a result of the presence of others), social loafing (an individual's efforts are not evaluated, which leads to a lower work effort), identity functions, conformity, and minority influences. Some aspects of group activities may vary across different cultures (e.g., in some Asian communities group participation enhances the individual's functioning).

An individual's sense of identity is affected by the groups (e.g., social/family) he or she belongs to in society. We may try to validate our own groups compared with others, which is called social identity theory. A member can feel less like an individual within a group when there is anonymity, high levels of cohesiveness, collective action, and an external focus of attention. Groups may be more effective at making decisions than individuals. Cooperative, not competitive, atmospheres enhance such activities. Bad decisions can be made when there is polarization (may make too risky or overly conservative choices) or too much cohesion (no influence from groups within the group or outsiders).

Case Conclusion After meeting with CF and her mother you decide to refer her to a psychiatrist who specializes in eating disorders. At this consultation CF agrees to have individual psychotherapy and to participate in family therapy. A year later CF has decided that she does not want to become a professional dancer after all and has reached a more normal weight for her size. The family therapy was very beneficial.

Thumbnail: Behavioral Science—Features of Eating Disorders

	Anorexia Nervosa	Bulimia Nervosa
Physical signs and symptoms	Emaciation, hypotension, hypothermia, bradycardia, may have yellowed skin due to hypercarotenemia, dry skin and lanugo hair, edema or petechiae (due to a bleeding diathesis). Vomiters may have erosions on the inside of their teeth, calluses on their fingers, and swollen salivary glands.	Individuals may have normal weight, and the medical complications are similar to anorexia but occur less frequently and are often less severe. Binging may cause acute dilatation of the stomach. Vomiters may have enlarged parotid glands, elevated amylase levels, esophagitis, or esophageal tears. Electrolyte abnormalities are common, particularly low potassium, which may lead to renal impairment and cardiac arrhythmias. Seizures may also occur. Generally, TFTs are normal but between 30% and 50% have menstrual abnormalities. Abuse of laxatives may lead to damage of the myenteric plexus.
Investigations/labs	Leukopenia, anemia, thrombocytopenia. Elevated BUN, cholesterol, cortisol, amylase, and liver function tests. Decreased levels of phosphate, magnesium, zinc; decreased levels of LH and FSH with low serum estrogen (females), low serum testosterone (males). T4 in low normal range and T3 decreased. Vomiters may have a hypochloremic hypokalemic metabolic alkalosis, and those who abuse laxatives may have a metabolic acidosis. **Sinus bradycardia and arrhythmias diffuse abnormalities on EKG. CAT scans of the brain may reveal reversible cortical atrophy.**	Low potassium, sodium, chloride, magnesium, phosphate, and calcium. Metabolic alkalosis in vomiters, and metabolic acidosis in laxative abusers. EKG as for anorexia. Leukopenia or lymphocytosis.

Key Points

- The prevalence of anorexia is 1% or less of the general population, with males accounting for approximately 10% of the cases.
- The mortality rate for anorexia is approximately 10%.
- The prevalence of bulimia is between approximately 1% and 3 % of young women.

- Both anorexics and bulimics tend to suffer from depression and substance abuse.
- Group systems generally have rules, keep home-ostasis, and have boundaries and feedback loops.
- The three schools of family therapy include behavioral-psychoeducational, structural strategic, and intergenerational-experiential approaches.

Questions

1. CF tells you that she is not concerned that losing weight would affect her in the long term. Which of the following are considered to be more long-term complications of anorexia?
   A. Impaired fertility, osteoporosis, and seizure disorder
   B. Impaired fertility, osteoporosis, and renal stones
   C. Cardiac abnormalities, renal and cognitive impairments
   D. Cardiac abnormalities, renal and auditory impairments
   E. A mortality rate of more than 50%

2. Which of the following is a characteristic physical finding in bulimia?
   A. Excess weight
   B. Calluses on the fingers
   C. Lanugo hair
   D. Hyperchloremic, hyponatremic alkalosis
   E. Alopecia

3. Which of the following models of family therapy is correctly paired with its own theory?
   A. Structural strategic approaches: Behavior is caused by family developmental fixation.
   B. Behavioral-psychoeducational: Behavior is caused by dysfunctional attempts to adapt.
   C. Intergenerational-experiential: Behavior is caused by family developmental fixation.
   D. Structural strategic approaches: Behavior is shaped by current environmental events.
   E. Behavioral-psychoeducational: Behavior is caused by family developmental fixation.

4. Which of the following is considered a curative factor in group therapy?
   A. Scapegoating
   B. Triangulation
   C. Instillation of hope
   D. Humor
   E. Group-think

HPI: LC is a 66-year-old man with hypertension presenting to a new clinic for his regular care. He has exercised four times a week for 30 minutes for about a year but reports difficulty in maintaining a strict low-fat diet. He notes that he has struggled with his weight, trying several diet and exercise regimens without success. His highest weight was 280 pounds.

PMH: Non-Q-wave myocardial infarction 10 years ago.

Meds: metoprolol, aspirin, atorvastatin

ROS: snoring, chronic daytime fatigue, knee pain when walking for long periods. Denies having colicky abdominal pain, polyuria or polydipsia, depression, or anxiety.

PE: T 36.5°C   BP 130/90   HR 75   RR 20   Height 5' 7"   Weight 240 lbs (weight 4 months ago was 245 lbs)
He is obese with apparent truncal obesity and a waist-to-hip ratio of 1.6, and body-mass index (BMI) of 34. His head, neck, lung, and cardiac exams are unremarkable. His abdomen is obese, soft, and nontender. His knees exhibit no apparent erythema or tenderness on exam. He has no peripheral edema or abnormal skin or hair texture.

Labs/Studies: Glucose 120   TG 205   TC 210   LDL 145   HDL 29   TSH 5.2
X-rays of both knees show mild narrowing of joint space without osteophytes, cysts, or subchondral bony sclerosis.

Thought Questions

- How is obesity defined? What are the main characteristics of obesity?

- What are the main physiologic considerations and the medical consequences of obesity?

- Why are the psychological components of obesity?

- What treatment options are available for obesity?

Basic Science Review and Discussion

Obesity has many meanings in different cultural contexts and results from a complex interplay of physiology, genetics, and environment. Along with its complex pathogenesis, the medical and social consequences to the individual are equally complex, making the treatment of obesity particularly challenging, mostly for the patient. In the medical context, one defines overweight as the threshold weight associated with increased morbidity and mortality. That defines obesity as having a **body-mass index (BMI)** of *30 or above* (BMI = weight in kilograms divided by height in meters squared). However, clinically significant consequences result from BMIs as low as 25. Those patients *between 25 and 30* are considered **"overweight"** and also deserve clinical attention. It is important to note, however, that BMI does not accurately predict risk for those who have increased lean body mass. In addition to overall weight, **central obesity,** a typically android pattern of obesity marked by increased intra-abdominal fat, is higher risk than **gluteal** or **subcutaneous obesity,** a typically gynecoid pattern. This is quantified by the **waist-to-hip ratio (WHR).** Truncal obesity is defined by a WHR of more than 0.9 for women and more than 1.0 for men.

From 1976 to 1998, the prevalence of obesity (BMI > 30) in the United States has increased from 15% to 23%. Between 1991 and 1998, 50% of adults more than 20 years old were overweight (BMI > 25). Women and the poor are particularly at risk. Childhood obesity has more than doubled since 1976.

Etiology   At the most basic level, obesity is caused by a consistent intake of calories in excess of one's metabolic requirements. Body weight is regulated homeostatically through endocrine and neural signals that influence either *energy expenditure* or *intake.* Seventy percent of our energy expenditure is from the **basal metabolic rate (BMR),** the energy required to run the basic bodily functions at rest. Another 20% of our energy expenditure comes from the metabolism and storage of food as well as adaptive thermogenesis. Only 5% to 10% comes from physical activity, that which we can modify in the form of exercise. Therefore exercise alone is insufficient for weight loss; limiting food intake is the most important component of any weight reduction program.

Food intake is determined by appetite, which is influenced by several hormonal and metabolic signals (e.g., leptin, insulin, cortisol, cholecystokinin, serotonin, glucose, and ketone) as well as neural signals (e.g., those that come from the vagus nerve as a result of gut distention). **Leptin** is an important modulator of appetite, metabolism, and neuroendocrine function. It is released from adipocytes in the fed state and influences the hypothalamus by decreasing appetite, increasing energy expenditure, and influencing peripheral targets such as pancreatic beta cells. In those with typical obesity, leptin levels are found to be high, suggesting the presence of a "leptin-resistant" state. Along with psychological and cultural influences, all these factors are integrated in the hypothalamus and determine the subjective experience of hunger or satiety.

Although there are rare cases of well-defined familial obesity and secondary obesity from other medical conditions, the pathogenesis of common obesity is poorly defined and is thought to be a result of a complex interplay of genetic and environmental influences on food intake and energy expenditure. Obesity commonly runs in families, though it may be difficult to separate the environmental influence from the genetic influence. Family and twin studies support the strong influence of genetics in obesity. Strong environmental influences include the availability of food, particularly those rich in fat and simple sugars, as well as increasingly sedentary lifestyles common in industrialized societies. For instance, the high-fat content of food readily available in poor neighborhoods contributes to the high prevalence of obesity in such communities. Cultural concepts of food and body image also contribute to the accepted patterns of food intake and adiposity. Childhood obesity has been linked to decreased physical activity and increased television watching.

Disease Associated with Obesity The pathophysiologic consequences of obesity are manifold and increase mortality up to twelve times for morbidly obese individuals (>200% of ideal body weight). The cardiovascular diseases associated with obesity include **type II diabetes mellitus, hypertension,** and **hyperlipidemia.** Together these are thought to contribute to the associated increased risk of developing **coronary artery disease, stroke,** and **congestive heart failure.** Other medical conditions include **male hypogonadism, polycystic ovarian syndrome, chronic hypoventilation, sleep apnea, cholelithiasis, osteoarthritis,** and **gout.**

Although these medical conditions are significant and dangerous, perhaps the most difficult and easily ignored consequences of obesity are the social and psychological challenges. Many with obesity suffer from depression, anxiety, and poor self-esteem. Many cycles of failed dieting and exercising can lead to eating disorders such as food obsession, compulsive eating, and patterns of binging and purging. Food addiction has been described in which food is used as self-medication to relieve depression or anxiety. People with obesity suffer from social ostracism and occupational discrimination, further compounding poor self-image. Obesity has been ascribed to poor discipline and moral failure, a false assumption that is internalized by many obese individuals, making every failed attempt at weight reduction a personal failure as well. Often these psychological effects are the greatest barriers to successful weight reduction and maintenance. For others, obesity has

been accepted as a way of life, not just at the individual level but also at a larger, social and cultural level. Therefore any physician attempting to evaluate and treat obesity needs to be sensitive to the complex and varied experiences and perspectives patients have about their weight and body image. It is particularly important to not judge a patient by suggesting that they are weak or undisciplined because of their inability to lose weight. It is also important to not stigmatize a patient's body habitus, as this may compromise the doctor-patient relationship necessary for successful treatment. However, a physician can offer objective information on the consequences associated with an individual's body-mass index and offer alternatives to current eating habits and sedentary lifestyles.

Diagnosis and Treatment of Obesity To evaluate obesity, one must assess not only the objective indices of BMI and WHR, but also the comorbid conditions that increase a person's risk of developing adverse clinical consequences. This includes measuring blood pressure, triglycerides, total cholesterol, LDL, HDL, and serum glucose. Obesity secondary to other medical conditions such as Cushing's syndrome, hypothyroidism, insulinoma, and tumors involving the hypothalamus may be investigated if there is clinical suspicion from the history and physical exam. Familial obesity may be suspected in those with strong family histories, but with the exception of those with leptin deficiencies, further testing will unlikely result in changes in management. A patient's eating habits, stressors that lead to increased eating, level of physical activity, and most important, motivation to lose weight must be evaluated.

Treatment Successful weight reduction and maintenance in obesity are difficult and, sadly, uncommon. The cornerstone of treatment is reduction in food intake to below that required to maintain current body weight. A 500-kcal/day deficit will result in a weight loss of 1 pound per week. There are several long-term community programs that focus on behavioral modification, such as helping an individual to maintain a low-fat, high-fiber diet; to change eating patterns; to identify and manage stressors that lead to overeating; and to provide long-term counseling and group support. Although exercise alone will not lead to significant weight reduction, it has been shown to improve long-term maintenance of reduced weight. There are several mildly efficacious drugs available for those with BMIs of $\geq$ 30, or BMIs $\geq$ 27 with concurrent obesity-related conditions. These include **sympathomimetic and serotonergic drugs** that decrease appetite and increase energy expenditure (e.g., phentermine, sibutramine, diethylproprion); these are contraindicated in those with uncontrolled hypertension and other cardiac diseases. The other class of drugs includes the **lipase inhibitor** orlistat, which suppresses the conversion of triglycerides into free fatty acids in the gut lumen, preventing absorption. However, the most dramatic results come from surgical treatment of obesity. **Bariatric surgery** is available to those with morbid obesity (BMI > 40) who have failed all other weight loss strategies. The procedures most commonly performed to maximize weight loss benefit and minimize adverse effects like short-gut syndrome are **Roux-en-Y gastric bypass** and **duodenal switch,** both of which can be done laparoscopically, thus minimizing postoperative morbidity associated with obesity.

Case Conclusion   LC's BMI of 34 and central obesity places him at significant risk of adverse and perhaps life-threatening clinical consequences. You note that he already has several risk factors, including hypertension, hyperlipidemia, and coronary artery disease with a previous history of myocardial infarction (MI). He is also exhibiting other obesity-related conditions, such as osteoarthritis and sleep apnea. You also ruled-out several associated conditions, such as type II diabetes mellitus, and hypothyroidism. It is apparent that LC is highly motivated to lose weight but that, despite this, he is failing to limit his food intake, reflected by his minimal weight reduction in the last year and abnormal lipid profile despite medication. You therefore refer him to a community weight loss program, adjust his atorvastatin, offer nonsteroidal anti-inflammatory drugs (NSAIDs) for his mild arthritis pain, and suggest otolaryngology consultation for his sleep apnea.

Thumbnail: Behavioral Science—Obesity-Associated Medical Conditions

Condition	Description	Treatment
Hypertension	Increased peripheral resistance, cardiac output, sympathetic nervous tone, salt sensitivity, insulin-mediated salt retention	Diet, exercise, sodium restriction, beta-blockers, diuretics, ACE-inhibitors
Hypercholesterolemia	Increased LDL, VLDL, and triglycerides Decreased HDL, especially with abdominal obesity; leads to atherosclerosis and all subsequent clinical risks	Diet, statins, niacin, fibrates, resins
Sleep apnea, obesity, hypoventilation syndrome	Reduced chest wall compliance; increased intra-abdominal pressure, especially in supine position; increased minute ventilation due to increased metabolic rate; decreased total lung capacity; airway obstruction causing snoring and sleep apnea	Weight reduction, continuous positive airway pressure, surgical intervention with an ENT specialist
Type II diabetes mellitus (DM)	Hyperinsulinemia and insulin resistance; 80% of patients with type II DM are obese, especially associated with the presence of intra-abdominal fat	Metformin has efficacy in both weight reduction and glucose control
Polycystic ovary syndrome	Increased androgen production and peripheral conversion of androgen to estrogen, decreased sex hormone-binding globulin (SHBG) lead to anovulation, ovarian hyperandrogenism, oligomenorrhea, and fertility problems	Weight reduction, metformin, oral contraception
Male hypogonadism	Increased adipose tissue causes increased peripheral conversion of androgens to estrogens, reduced testosterone and SHBG leading to gynecomastia	Weight reduction
Cholelithiasis	Increased cholesterol levels promote the development of cholesterol gallstones that could become symptomatic	Weight loss, low-cholesterol diets, cholecystectomy
Cancer	In men: higher mortality in colon, rectal, prostate cancer In women: higher mortality in gallbladder, biliary, breast, endometrial, cervical, and ovarian cancer	Surgery, depending on cancer type
Osteoarthritis	Chronic added weight bearing causes gradual deterioration of weight-bearing joints (knees, hips)	Weight reduction, NSAIDs, joint replacement
Gout	Exacerbated by dietary excess and alcohol consumption	Allopurinol, colchicine

Key Points

▶ Obesity is a multifactorial disease and results from the complex interplay of genetics and environment, causing a chronic intake of calories in excess of energy expended.

▶ Obesity is associated with a large variety of medical conditions as well as several-fold increases in overall morbidity and mortality.

▶ Addressing issues of weight, body image, and obesity requires not only clinical knowledge of the problems but also cultural and emotional sensitivity to the patients that face this problem.

Questions

1. BI is a 36-year-old woman with a height of 5 feet, 4 inches and weight of 170 pounds, giving her a BMI of 29. She also has hypertension and hyperlipidemia. What weight reduction strategy is included in the appropriate management of her obesity?
   A. Fasting
   B. Low-fat, high-fiber diet
   C. Strenuous exercise
   D. Laparoscopic duodenal switch
   E. Roux-en-Y gastric bypass

2. GL is an 11-year-old boy brought to his pediatrician for an annual physical exam. He is noted to be at the 98th percentile for weight. On further inquiry, you discover that the boy spends 8 hours a day watching TV or playing video games, participates in no sports or physical activity at school, loves to drink soda, and eat potato chips and candy bars. You note that the mother is also obese. Which is the *most* appropriate in the evaluation and treatment for this patient?
   A. Inquiring about family history of obesity with subsequent serum leptin testing
   B. Leptin replacement
   C. Family counseling on proper diet and exercise
   D. Sibutramine
   E. Roux-en-Y gastric bypass

3. LC (from the case presentation) returns 4 years later complaining of gradually worsening shortness of breath and dyspnea on exertion for 1 year. He came in because he was suddenly awakened from sleep the night before and was gasping for air, after which he got up and walked around to feel better. He notes having difficulty lying down flat because of difficulty breathing and now uses three pillows to sleep at night. He previously could walk 1 mile on flat ground to work but now cannot walk 1 block without getting short of breath. He also notes worsened knee pain, which limits his activity. In addition, he continues to have daytime fatigue. On exam, he is comfortable and in no respiratory distress, with a blood pressure of 165/89, pulse 83, RR of 20, and an oxygen saturation of 97%. His BMI is now 41. His lungs are clear and he has normal heart sounds, but all other parts of his cardiac exam are difficult to assess due to his body habitus. He has bilateral pitting edema to both lower extremities. He has an EKG significant only for left ventricular hypertrophy. He has two negative tests for troponin I. Given this clinical picture, what is the *most* likely cause of his shortness of breath?
   A. Hypoventilation syndrome
   B. Coronary artery disease
   C. Restrictive lung disease due to his large body habitus
   D. Congestive heart failure
   E. Acute myocardial infarction

4. LC (from the above question) returns after having undergone all appropriate testing. He is shown to have a decreased ejection fraction of 40%. Having learned that his obesity may have something to do with his current medical condition, he would like you to help him lose weight. Which treatment is contraindicated for LC?
   A. Very-low-calorie diet
   B. Orlistat
   C. Phentermine
   D. Moderate exercise 3 times a week
   E. Roux-en-Y gastric bypass

Answer Key—Part I: Behavioral Science

Case 1
1. B
2. C
3. C
4. B

Case 2
1. B
2. C
3. E
4. B

Case 3
1. A
2. C
3. E
4. E

Case 4
1. C
2. B
3. C
4. D

Case 5
1. D
2. D
3. C
4. C

Case 6
1. E
2. E
3. D
4. D

Case 7
1. B
2. B
3. E
4. B

Case 8
1. E
2. D
3. C
4. C

Case 9
1. C
2. E
3. D
4. C

Case 10
1. D
2. A
3. A
4. B

Case 11
1. B
2. E
3. C
4. B

Case 12
1. D
2. C
3. C
4. C

Case 13
1. D
2. D
3. B
4. C

Case 14
1. E
2. D
3. C
4. B

Case 15
1. B
2. D
3. D
4. C

Case 16
1. A
2. C
3. C
4. B

Case 17
1. B
2. C
3. D
4. E

Case 18
1. B
2. B
3. C
4. C

Case 19
1. B
2. C
3. D
4. C

Part II

Neuroscience, Psychiatry, Psychopharmacology, and Psychopathology

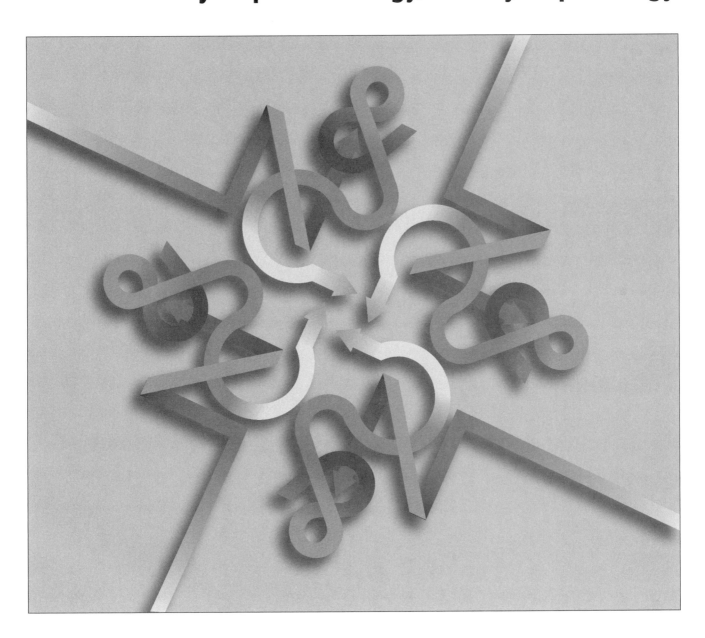

HPI: MB is a 30-year-old mother of two who comes to your clinic complaining of depressed mood. She has noticed a gradual change in her mood over the past couple of months, but things have been particularly difficult for the past 2 weeks. She has difficulty sleeping, poor appetite, low energy, and low mood with tearful episodes. Her husband, who accompanies her, confirms these changes and says her libido has decreased and that things that she used to enjoy do not seem to lift her mood anymore. There have been no recent stressors, and MB has never had a problem like this before. She has never had an episode of mania or hypomania. No previous psychiatric history. No significant medical history apart from an allergy to beestings.

In her family history, one maternal aunt has a history of recurrent depressions; otherwise, noncontributory. MB is the eldest of three daughters. Her parents are both well and live nearby. She graduated with a master's degree in art history and works as a curator in a local museum. Her husband is an accountant; they own their own home. They have two children, a son aged 4 and a daughter aged 2; both are healthy. She denies any illicit substance use, drinks alcohol rarely, and does not smoke. Lab tests were all normal.

MSE: A thin, well-dressed woman who appears her stated age; eye contact, limited; rapport, good. Affect dysphoric and tearful at times. Mood described as "down." Thought processes are logical and goal directed. Thought content includes expression of concern and guilt that she is not being a good mother or wife. She denies feelings of hopelessness or suicidal ideation. There is no evidence of psychosis. Her insight and judgment are good, and her cognitive functions are intact.

Thought Questions

- Does this woman meet the criteria for major depressive disorder?

- What other mood disorders would you consider?

- How will you treat her?

- Which agents would you consider and why?

Basic Science Review and Discussion

Depressive symptoms are commonly reported by between 13% and 20% of the general population, but the lifetime prevalence for major depressive disorder is between 10% and 25% for females and between 5% and 12% of males (see *Diagnostic and Statistical Manual of Mental Disorders*, 4th edition [*DSM-IV*] criteria in Box 20-1). Those who report depressive symptoms have been shown to have higher rates of mortality, greater disability, and lower levels of social functioning. Approximately 15% of those suffering from major depression commit suicide. Major depression is reported to be higher among primary care patients than in the general population. Risk factors include female gender, younger age, early parental loss, disruptive childhood environment, lower socioeconomic status, family history of major depression, marital separation or divorce, chronic stress, residence in an urban area, and lack of a confidante.

Various medical disorders may cause depressive symptoms, including endocrine abnormalities (hypothyroidism, hyperparathyroidism, Addison's disease, and Cushing's syndrome), central nervous system (CNS) disorders such as Parkinson's disease, multiple sclerosis, epilepsy, Huntington's disease, and cerebrovascular disease (particularly strokes with left anterior lesions), infections (HIV, brucellosis, infectious mononucleosis, hepatitis, and post influenza) and various metabolic disorders (vitamin B_{12}/folate and iron-deficient anemias, hypercalcemia, and hypomagnesia. Various

---

Box 20-1. Criteria for Major Depression

A. At least five of the following symptoms that are reported for most days for at least 2 weeks and that are a change from the usual level of functioning. [At least one of the symptoms is (i) depressed mood or (ii) loss of interest or pleasure (anhedonia).]

1. Depressed mood most of the day, nearly every day (this can be irritability in children or adolescents)
2. Significant decrease in interest or pleasure in almost all or all the activities of the day
3. Significant change in weight (either gain or loss, more than 5% of body weight in a month; in children this can be a failure to reach expected gains in weight)
4. Insomnia or hypersomnia
5. Psychomotor agitation or slowing
6. Fatigue or loss of energy
7. Feelings of guilt or worthlessness that may be delusional
8. Decreased concentration or indecisiveness
9. Recurrent thoughts of death, which may include suicidal ideation with or without a specific plan or a suicide attempt

B. These symptoms cause significant distress and impairment in normal functioning.

C. These symptoms are not due to the effects of a substance or a general medical condition.

D. These symptoms are not better accounted for by bereavement.

Adapted from *DSM-IV* published by the American Psychiatric Association.

Table 20-1. Other Mood Disorders to Consider When Taking the History and Mental State Examination

Disorder	Major Depression	Mild Depression	Mania	Hypomania
Major depressive disorder	+	±	−	−
Dysthymia	−	+	−	−
Cyclothymia	−	+	−	+
Bipolar I disorder	±	±	+	±
Bipolar II disorder	+	±	−	+

medications have also been implicated and include reserpine, L-dopa, steroids, barbiturates, nonsteroidal anti-inflammatory drugs [NSAIDs], thiazides, digoxin, and prolonged use of amphetamines).

Major depression is the most common type of mood disorder and may occur as a single episode or recur throughout the life cycle. Major depressive episodes may also occur in bipolar disorder (also called manic depression).

A mnemonic to easily remember the essential features of major depression is SIGECAPS, or "prescribe energy capsules":

S-Sleep

I-Interest

G-Guilt

E-Energy

C-Concentration

A-Appetite

P-Psychomotor agitation or retardation

S-Suicidality

Episodes of major depression may also have several specifiers, such as chronic, with catatonic features, with melancholic features (mood worse in the morning, early-morning wakening, marked psychomotor agitation or slowing, and excessive or inappropriate guilt) or with atypical features (Table 20-1).

Psychopharmacology of Major Depression   There are four main classes of antidepressants. The choice of agent depends on an individual's symptoms, presentation, history of response to a particular type of agent (or a family history of response), and potential for adverse reactions to these agents. All antidepressants have a delayed therapeutic onset of action, although their effects on amine concentrations are relatively immediate. Antidepressant effects may be seen between 2 and 8 weeks after starting treatment.

The main classes of antidepressants are outlined in Table 20-2.

Table 20-2. Main Classes of Antidepressants

Monoamine reuptake inhibitors	1. **Tricyclics:** These are further subdivided into tertiary amines (amitryptiline and imipramine), secondary amines (desimipramine and nortryptiline), and others (doxepin, clomipramine, protriptyline, and trimipramine). Tertiary and secondary amines have reuptake inhibition effects at both serotonin and norephinephrine neurons. All tricyclics affect 5HT2 receptors as well as histamine, M muscarinic, and α_1- and α_2-adrenergic receptors. 2. **Heterocyclics:** Maprotiline (a tetracyclic) and amoxepine (a dibenzoxazepine). Tetracyclics cause reuptake inhibition of norephinephrine only but may have effects at D2 dopamine receptors. Amoxepine causes reuptake inhibition of both serotonin and norepinephrine. 3. **Triazolopyridines:** Trazadone and nefazodone. These agents cause reuptake inhibition of serotonin. 4. **Propiophenone:** Bupropion. This agent causes reuptake inhibition of dopamine, serotonin, and norepinephrine.
Monoamine Oxidase inhibitors	These agents inhibit monoamine oxidase A. 1. **Hydrazine compounds:** phenelzine and isocarboxazid 2. **Nonhydrazine compound:** tranylcypromine
Selective serotonin reuptake inhibitors	These include fluoxetine, sertraline, paroxetine, fluvoxamine, and citalopram. These agents cause reuptake inhibition of serotonin, but some may also affect dopamine.
Serotonin-norepinephrine reuptake inhibitors	Venlafaxine. This affects both norepinephrine and serotonin as well as having a small effect on the reuptake of dopamine.

Case Conclusion MB indeed meets the criteria for major depressive disorder. After review of her history and discussion of the treatment options with the patient and her husband she is started on a trial of sertraline, a selective serotonergic reuptake inhibitor (SSRI) that is titrated up to 50 mg per day without adverse reaction. You also arrange for her to receive weekly psychotherapy sessions. When she returns to your clinic 1 month later she reports feeling better; 6 months later her symptoms have completely resolved.

Thumbnail: Behavioral Science—Abnormalities Reported in Depression

Neurotransmitters	**Serotonin:** Decreased plasma tryptophan, CSF, 5-HIAA (particularly in suicides), platelet 5-HT uptake and prolactin response to challenge tests with tryptophan and fenfluramine (this normalizes after treatment with antidepressants). Increased 5-HT2 receptor binding in platelets and the limbic cortex.
	Noradrenaline: Decreased growth hormone response to challenge tests with amphetamine and clonidine, cAMP turnover in platelets when stimulated by clonidine. Increased platelet alpha-2 receptor binding and beta-receptors in suicides.
	Acetylcholine: Agonists exacerbate depressive symptoms.
	GABA: Decreased plasma, CSF, and brain levels.
Neuroendocrine	**Hypercortisolemia:** Seen in up to 40% of depressed outpatients and up to 60% of depressed inpatients. Hallmark of the stress response. Failure of suppression in the dexamethasone suppression test in up to 60% of depressed patients (also seen in anorexia, schizophrenia, and alcohol dependence).
	Thyroid dysfunction: 5% to 10% of depressed patients reported to have hypothyroidism. Blunted TSH responses with TRH challenge tests.
	Growth hormone: Blunted response to clonidine.
	Somatostatin: Lower CSF levels reported.
	Prolactin: Blunted response to serotonin agonists.
Neuropathology/neuroimaging	**MRI** studies have reported decreases in caudate nucleus size. Subcortical frontal and basal ganglia cerebrovascular lesions reported in late life depression.
	Positron emission tomography (PET) studies reported decreased metabolism in the anterior brain, reduced blood flow, and metabolism in the mesocortical and mesolimbic tracts. Increased glucose metabolism reported in limbic region. Asymmetry of phosphorus metabolism in basal ganglia and left frontal lobe.
Neuropsychoimmunology	Decreased natural killer cells, T-cell replication, and interleukin-2. Increased monocyte activity.

Key Points

▶ Between 13% and 20% of the general population report depressive symptoms.

▶ The lifetime prevalence for major depressive disorder is between 10% and 25% for females and between 5% and 12% of males.

▶ Approximately 15% of those suffering from major depression commit suicide.

▶ Risk factors include female gender, younger age, early parental loss, a disruptive childhood environment, lower socioeconomic status, family history of major depression, marital separation or divorce, chronic stress, residence in an urban area, and a lack of a confidante.

▶ Medical disorders may cause depressive symptoms.

▶ There are four main classes of antidepressants: monoamine reuptake inhibitors, monoamine oxidase inhibitors, selective serotonin reuptake inhibitors, and serotonin-norepinephrine reuptake inhibitors.

Questions

1. When discussing the side effects of SSRIs with the above patient and her husband you mention the possibility of which of the following?
   A. Agranulocytosis
   B. Sexual dysfunction
   C. Dietary considerations
   D. Orthostatic hypotension
   E. Cardiac toxicity

2. Which of the following agents is incorrectly paired with other possible uses?
   A. SSRIs and OCD
   B. Tricyclics and enuresis
   C. MAOIs and narcolepsy
   D. SNRIs and bulimia
   E. Tricyclics and trichotillomania

3. A patient presents for treatment of depression. He is started on a tricyclic antidepressant medication. You counsel him that which of the following are all possible side effects?
   A. Arrhythmias, cholestatic jaundice, dry mouth, blurry vision
   B. Arrhythmias, cholestatic jaundice, priapism, constipation
   C. Dry mouth, arrhythmias, blurry vision, and constipation
   D. Dry mouth, priapism, constipation, and microcytic anemia
   E. Priapism, constipation, arrhythmias, and microcytic anemia

4. A patient presents with a depression with **atypical** features of hypersomnia and weight gain. You decide to give him a trial of an MAOI. Which of the following is a concern?
   A. Reversible binding to the enzyme MAO, hypertensive crisis with tyramine-containing foods and drinks
   B. Hypotensive crisis with tyramine-containing foods and drinks
   C. Little interaction with other CNS active agents, anticholinergic effects
   D. Little interaction with other CNS active agents, anticholinergic side effects, and postural hypotension
   E. Significant interaction with other CNS active agents, anticholinergic side effects, and postural hypotension

HPI: AD is a 32-year-old housewife who was brought to the emergency room by her husband, who was concerned that his wife "was going crazy."

Apparently, AD had not been sleeping for the past few nights, had been cleaning the house from top to bottom, and then would start all over again. Her husband became most concerned when he came home to find her emptying the woodshed of logs for the fire and cleaning it because she claimed it was dirty. She had no psychiatric history and no significant medical history. Her family history was significant for a male cousin who had been diagnosed as having bipolar disorder. She grew up the youngest of three daughters; her parents are well and live close by. She graduated from college and works as a primary school teacher. She has been married for 5 years and has no children. Her husband works as a software engineer. She denied any illicit substance abuse and drinks one or two glasses of wine a week socially. She has no legal history.

PE: Within normal limits.

MSE: AD appeared her stated age, wearing appropriate clothing with good hygiene. Eye contact tended to be intense and staring. Her speech was pressured and loud at times, particularly when she made jokes. She was very agitated at times, saying that she had to go home to finish cleaning up and accusing you of trying to conspire against her with the headmaster of the school where she worked. She said her mood was "fantastic" and her affect was labile. Thought processes were positive for flight of ideas and some loosening of associations. She denied suicidal or homicidal ideation. She denied auditory or visual hallucinations but did admit that she had "received a message" from the radio telling her to start preparing for her "next phase." She was oriented to time, person, and place. She had no insight into her condition and her judgment was impaired.

Labs: CBC, electrolytes, and thyroid function tests were normal. Utox was negative.

Thought Questions

- What is the most likely diagnosis?
- What are the characteristics of this type of disorder? What is the etiology?

Basic Science Review and Discussion

Bipolar disorder may also be referred to as manic depression and is characterized by episodes of depression and mania (Box 21-1). Only one episode of mania is needed to meet *Diagnostic and Statistical Manual of Mental Disorders,* 4th edition (*DSM-IV*) criteria. The episodes of depression in bipolar disorder have the same symptoms as in major depression but may differ in the following ways: The episodes of depression are less likely to have a specific triggering event, develop more gradually, usually do not last as long, and may be more atypical in presentation, with hypersomnia, increase in weight, and labile mood.

The *DSM-IV* criteria for mania include the following:

1. Abnormally **elevated or irritable mood for 1 week** (or less if hospitalized)
2. Three or more of these symptoms: grandiosity, decreased need for sleep, pressured speech, racing thoughts/flight of ideas, distractibility, increased goal-directed activity/

psychomotor agitation, and involvement in potentially harmful activities, such as unsafe sex, gambling, or spending sprees.

These episodes are not caused by substance abuse or a general medical condition and cause **marked impairment in functioning.**

Box 21-1. Subtypes of Bipolar Disorders

Bipolar I disorder involves at least one episode of **mania,** with or without a history of depression.

Bipolar II disorder is characterized by at least one episode of **hypomania** and at least one of **depression.** In hypomania the symptoms are milder and last at least 4 days but do not cause such interference in functioning (and generally do not require hospitalization). Insight is lost in manic episodes but is retained in hypomania.

Mixed episodes occur when there is a **combination of both manic and depressed** symptoms.

Rapid cycling occurs when there are at least **four distinct episodes** of mood disturbance within 12 months. They happen in approximately 15% of patients with bipolar I and II disorders. Rapid cycling may be triggered by antidepressants. Those with this disorder must be symptom-free for at least 2 months between episodes of mood disturbance.

Cyclothymic disorder is a chronic disorder lasting at least 2 years, with **milder episodes** of depression and elevation of mood that lasts more than 2 months. It may be chronic or may develop into a bipolar disorder.

Epidemiology The lifetime risk of bipolar I disorder is between 1% and 1.5%, whereas that for bipolar II is 0.5%. Bipolar I affects both sexes equally, but women appear to have a higher incidence of rapid cycling and mixed states, whereas bipolar II is more common in women. It tends also to present earlier in men (late teens) with a manic episode, whereas women tend to experience depression first. There is another peak of onset for women aged 40. It may start in childhood and be misdiagnosed as attention deficit disorder, but it can also occur with attention deficit disorder (ADD). Studies have reported that a high percentage of adolescents with bipolar disorder also meet criteria for ADD. It can also start in later life in those with a history of previous depressions or in conjunction with neurologic conditions such as stroke. Other risk factors reported include winter births and birth complications.

Etiology The exact etiology of bipolar disorder is unknown. Genetics accounts for only 60% of cases, so other biological and environmental factors must contribute to the development of this disorder. Increased rates have been reported in higher socioeconomic groups. It may share similar factors with schizophrenia or other psychotic disorders. These include deficiencies in reelin (a brain protein important for information processing) or an elevation in the level of VMAT2 (a brain protein that regulates the transport of neurotransmitters) in the brainstem. However, brain imaging studies have reported differences in hippocampal structures, with a significant increase in volume on the left (compared to the right) in bipolar patients, whereas a decrease in volume was reported in patients with schizophrenia. Bipolar disorder may also share similar biological mechanisms with epilepsy, including abnormalities in both of the neurotransmitters gamma aminobutyric acid and norepinephrine. This disorder may also be linked genetically to diabetes, as this condition has been reported to occur three times more commonly in those with bipolar disorder than in the general population.

Course and Prognosis If untreated, manic episodes may last up to 6 months and depressed episodes may last up to 12 months. Manic episodes tend to occur in the summer and depressive episodes to occur from autumn through the late spring. As patients with bipolar disorder become older their episodes can become more frequent and more difficult to treat. A person with bipolar disorder tends to experience an average of eight to 10 depressed or manic episodes in a lifetime. In most cases the number of depressed episodes is more than that of manic ones. Those who have early-onset bipolar disorder tend to have more complications (e.g., substance abuse, behavioral problems, and paranoid features) and a more severe form of the disorder. Between 15% and 20% of untreated bipolar patients may commit suicide, and it has been reported that up to 50% of bipolar patients may have attempted suicide at some stage during their illness. Periods of increased risk include depressed and mixed episodes. Studies have also reported that bipolar II patients may be at higher risk of suicide than those with either bipolar I disorder or depression.

Up to 60% of patients with bipolar disorder also have substance abuse problems during their illness. The most common substance abused is alcohol, followed by marijuana and cocaine. Males and those with mixed episodes appear to be at higher risk for developing substance abuse.

Other complications of this disorder may include high rates of divorce, legal problems due to impulsive manic behaviors, and high economic cost to the country. Direct costs include those due to patient care and suicide. Indirect costs include losses in productivity and costs to the justice system. Both have been reported to cost $45 billion.

Case Conclusion AD was admitted to the hospital and started on valproate and an atypical antipsychotic. Benzodiazepines were used as needed for anxiety, agitation, and insomnia. Her valproate was titrated with good effect (serum level of 85µg/mL. A week later she was no longer manic, was sleeping normally, and was discharged to the care of her husband with close follow-up.

Thumbnail: Behavioral Science—Genetics of Mood Disorders

Data from twin, adoption, and family studies have provided support for the genetic contributions to bipolar disorder.

	Lifetime Risk in the General Population	Lifetime Risk in First-Degree Relatives	Twin Concordance
Bipolar disorder	1%	Bipolar 7.8% (1.5% to 17.9%) Unipolar 11.4% (0.5% to 22.4%)	MZ, 79% DZ, 19%
Unipolar depression	2% to 5%	Bipolar, 0.6% (0.3% to 2.1%) Unipolar, 9.1% (5.9% to 18.4%)	MZ, 58% DZ, 23%

MZ, monozygotic; DZ, dizygotic

Key Points

▶ In bipolar I disorder there is at least one episode of mania with or without a history of depression. Bipolar II disorder is characterized by at least one episode of hypomania and at least one of depression.

▶ The lifetime risk is between 1% and 1.5% for bipolar I and is 0.5% for bipolar II.

▶ Bipolar I affects both sexes equally. Bipolar II is more common in women. Genetics accounts for only 60% of cases.

▶ Females have a higher incidence of rapid cycling and mixed states.

▶ Bipolar patients may experience eight to 10 depressed or manic episodes in a lifetime.

▶ Between 15% and 20% of untreated bipolar patients may commit suicide. Up to 60% of patients with bipolar disorder also have substance abuse problems.

Questions

1. When this patient's husband asks you about risk factors for developing bipolar disorder, you tell him that which of the following may be risk factors?
   A. Age > 65
   B. Substance abuse
   C. A family history
   D. Female gender
   E. Male gender

2. He is concerned about any future children they might have. What other conditions have a higher incidence rate in the families of persons with bipolar?
   A. Schizophrenia
   B. Eating disorders
   C. Kleptomania
   D. Depression
   E. Mental retardation

3. Which of the following statements concerning the genetics of psychiatric disease is correct?
   A. If twin concordance rates are higher in dizygotic twins than in monozygotic twins, then genetic factors are implicated.
   B. Simple Mendelian modes of transmission explain the mechanisms of genetic transmission in psychiatric disorders.
   C. There is no evidence of trinucleotide repeat expansions in bipolar disorder.
   D. Linkage studies in bipolar disorder have been well replicated.
   E. Chromosome 18 may be linked to bipolar disorder.

4. Which of the following medical conditions may present with manic symptoms?
   A. Addison's disease
   B. Hypothyroidism
   C. Cushing's syndrome
   D. Turner's syndrome
   E. Pancreatitis

HPI: BT is a 50-year-old married housewife who has carried a diagnosis of bipolar disorder since she was 26 years old. BT has just been hospitalized with a mixed episode. She has been experiencing symptoms of both mania and depression over the previous 3 days prior to admission. These symptoms included hypersomnia, dysphoria, and labile mood with tearfulness, extreme irritability, and short-lived spells of euphoria. Her husband confirms that she has been taking her medications as prescribed and mentions that their youngest son has just left home to start college in another state. Her initial presentation at the age of 26 was with an episode of severe depression for which she was hospitalized and treated with lithium and thiothixene (Navane). She has been maintained on lithium since that time as prophylaxis with two more episodes of depression and one of mania. There has been no history of suicide attempts or assaultive behavior. She has been taking a slow-release preparation of lithium (Eskalith-CR) 450 mg twice daily.
BT has two older brothers and her parents live in a retirement community in another state. She graduated from high school, trained as a paralegal, and worked until she got married at the age of 25. Her husband is a lawyer and they have two grown sons 21 and 18 years of age. She does not drink alcohol, smoke, or abuse substances.

PE: Within normal limits excluding the tremor mentioned above.

MSE: BT was disheveled with poor hygiene. Eye contact was poor and rapport was limited. Her affect was irritable and she described her mood as "just fine." A fine tremor was evident in both hands. Her thought processes were tangential, and there was flight of ideas. She denied SI/HI but admitted to command auditory hallucinations telling her to visit her son and "organize his dorm properly."
She has no insight into her current condition and her judgment is impaired.

Labs: CBC reveals a mild leukocytosis; Chem 20 and TFTs were within normal limits. Utox is negative and her serum level of lithium on admission is 0.8 mmol/L.

Thought Questions

■ How should bipolar disorder be treated?

■ Are mixed episodes treated differently?

■ Describe the pharmacology of mood stabilizers?

Basic Science Review and Discussion

The treatment of bipolar disorder includes mood-stabilizing medications, antipsychotic agents, antianxiety agents, antidepressants, electroconvulsive therapy (ECT), and psychotherapy. Different phases of the illness may require different interventions.

Mania   Usually, patients with mania require hospitalization, particularly if they are psychotic, suicidal, or homicidal. Pharmacologic control of acute mania usually involves a combination of a mood stabilizer and an antipsychotic agent. Mood stabilizers used include lithium, valproate, or carbamazepine (see Thumbnail). It has been reported that olanzepine (Zyprexa), an atypical antipsychotic, may be effective as a single agent. Other neuroleptics include other atypical agents [clozapine (Clozaril), risperidone (Risperidal), quetiapine (Seroquel), zisprasidone (Geodon), and aripiprazole (Abilify) or older typical agents such as haloperidol (Haldol). Antianxiety agents include clonazepam (Klonopin)

and lorazepam (Ativan). If a patient does not respond to medications or cannot take these medications (e.g., pregnant patients), then ECT may be useful.

Depression   Here mood-stabilizing agents may be helpful, particularly lamotrigine (Lamictal). If there is no improvement in depressive symptoms, then an antidepressant may be tried, but with care, as these agents may precipitate a manic episode. Agents that are reported to be less likely to cause mania include bupropion (Wellbutrin), venlafaxine (Effexor), paroxetine (Paxil), and sertraline (Zoloft). ECT may also be used. Antipsychotics may be used if there is severe depression or psychotic symptoms.

Patients with **mixed episodes or rapid cycling** may not respond to lithium, and valproate or carbamazepine is preferred. Other medications that may be useful in patients with rapid cycling include lamotrigine, levothyroxine (synthetic T4), and nimodipine (calcium channel blocker).

Lifelong **maintenance therapy** is considered for patients who are thought to be at high risk of recurring episodes and involves treatment with a mood stabilizer and even perhaps in combination with an atypical antipsychotic agent. Maintenance ECT may also be helpful. Other interventions include maintaining a good sleep pattern and avoiding stimulants, caffeine, alcohol, or illicit substances. It is very important that patients with bipolar disorder obtain good sleep, as insomnia may precipitate a manic episode.

Psychological treatments include psychoeducation and psychological and supportive therapies, which can enhance medication compliance (a serious problem in some patients who like to be manic or hypomanic). Traditional analytic psychotherapy has not been found to be effective in these disorders. Cognitive behavioral therapy (CBT) can improve outcomes in combination with medication. Interpersonal therapy can also help with difficulties in relationships, which may be precipitating stressors. Family therapy can help the patient comply with treatment and support a stressed spouse or family unit. Families should be encouraged to attend support groups. The treatment of bipolar II disorder is along the same guidelines as that for bipolar I, with mood stabilizers.

Case Conclusion As BT was experiencing a breakthrough of mixed symptoms while taking lithium it was decided to convert her to valproate. She was given olanzepine 15 mg every night for her psychotic symptoms. Her lithium was tapered and discontinued, and the valproate was added and titrated to a serum level of 78 mmol/L with good clinical effect and no adverse effects reported apart from some mild sedation initially. After about 1 week on the valproate her mood was euthymic and she was discharged home with follow-up on valproate 1000 mg twice daily and olanzepine 10 mg every night.

Thumbnail: Behavioral Science—Pharmacology of Mood Stabilizers

Lithium (Eskalith, Lithobid)	**Early side effects:** Nausea, vomiting, and diarrhea, fine tremor, **dry mouth, fatigue, drowsiness, nasal congestion, and metallic taste.** Long term: Nephrogenic **diabetes insipidus** with polyuria and polydipsia due to distal tubule becoming resistant to ADH in approximately 9% to 20% of users. **Hypothyroidism** in approximately 5% of users, females. Edema and weight gain. Cardiac effects include T-wave flattening and arrhythmias. Neurologic disorders include choreoathetosis, ataxia, dysarthria, tardive dyskinesia, and memory impairment. Acne and alopecia. Increased risk of **Ebstein's anomaly** in fetuses. Reported hypotonicity and cyanosis in infants. Thiazides decrease lithium clearance by 30% to 50%. Low-salt diets, pregnancy, and diarrhea/vomiting/dehydration may increase levels. NSAIDs may also increase levels. Levels and risk of neurotoxicity may be increased by neuroleptics and carbamazepine. Levels of lithium are decreased by theophylline, caffeine, antacids, acetazolamide, and osmotic diuretics.
Valproate/valproic acid /divalproex (Depakote)	Side effects: **GI upset** (nausea, vomiting, heartburn can occur in up to 50% of patients), headaches, tremor, agitation, tinnitus, hair loss, **weight gain,** sedation, visual disturbances, and menstrual abnormalities. More serious side effects include hepatitis, thrombocytopenia, seizures, coma, and possibly fatal pancreatitis. Long-term treatment may be associated with reversible cognitive impairment and parkinsonian symptoms. Teratogenic effects include **neural tube defects** in 1% to 1.5%. Should be avoided in breast-feeding and liver disease. Aspirin and cytochrome P450 inhibitors increase levels. Baseline liver function tests and drug levels with follow-up every 6 months are recommended.
Carbamazepine (Epitol, Tegretol)	Side effects: **Dizziness,** diplopia, weight gain, ataxia, sedation, dry mouth, **rash (rarely, Stevens-Johnson syndrome),** leucopenia, agranulocytosis, and hyponatremia. Avoid in acute intermittent porphyria, with MAOIs, with oral contraceptives, and in pregnancy. **Teratogenic effects** include spina bifida, craniofacial abnormalities, finger and nasal hypoplasia. It is metabolized in the liver and excreted by the kidneys. It induces its own metabolism, so dosages may need to be increased.
Oxcarbazepine (Trileptal)	Side effects: Skin rash and hematologic disorders may occur less frequently than with carbamazepine, but **hyponatremia** may occur more often. There may be cross sensitivity in those allergic to carbamazepine. Caution in renal impairment and pregnancy.
Lamotrigine (Lamictal)	May be used as add-on therapy but not with valproate, as this increases the risk of a rare but potentially fatal rash called **Stevens-Johnson syndrome.** Metabolized by the liver and excreted by the kidneys. Metabolism induced by carbamazepine. Other adverse reactions include **aplastic anemia,** hemolytic anemia, thrombocytopenia, pancytopenia, and liver failure. Other side effects include fatigue, dizziness, confusion, impaired memory, diplopia, blurred vision, nystagmus, headache, aphasia, rash, nausea, and vomiting. Contraindicated in breast-feeding
Topiramate (Topamax)	It is the only mood-stabilizing agent associated with **weight loss.** It may be used as an adjunctive agent or to reduce weight gain caused by other mood stabilizers. Reduce dose if there is renal impairment. Do not use in hepatic impairment, with oral contraceptives, or in young children. Serious reactions include **nephrolithiasis,** myopia, and acute-angle **glaucoma.** More common side effects include fatigue, dizziness, somnolence, impaired concentration, confusion, language difficulties, psychomotor slowing, mood disturbances, depression, nystagmus, diplopia, tremor, and abdominal pain. Excreted primarily in the urine.

Key Points

- The treatment of bipolar disorder includes mood-stabilizing medications, antipsychotic agents, antianxiety agents, antidepressants, ECT, and psychotherapy.

- Mania is treated with a combination of a mood stabilizer and an antipsychotic agent.

- Depressive episodes are treated with mood stabilizers but may require careful use of an antidepressant or ECT.

- Mood stabilizers include lithium, valproate, carbamazepine, lamotrigine, and topirimate.

- Mixed episodes are usually treated with valproate or carbamazepine.

- Rapid cyclers may respond to valproate, carbamazepine, lamotrigine, or augmentation with levothyroxine.

- Lamotrigine may cause a potentially fatal rash called Stevens-Johnson syndrome.

Questions

1. When starting a young female patient on a mood stabilizer which of the following would you caution her about?
   A. Avoiding oral contraceptives
   B. Not to be concerned about getting pregnant
   C. Avoiding sun exposure
   D. Avoiding ranitidine
   E. Avoiding selenium and zinc

2. MQ is a 24-year-old male with bipolar disorder. He has been taking lithium for approximately 2 weeks, since he was first diagnosed with bipolar disorder. He arrives at the clinic telling you that he feels "something isn't right." Which of the following would be an early side effect of lithium?
   A. Edema
   B. EEG changes
   C. Alopecia
   D. Diarrhea
   E. Ataxia

3. Which of the following medications is correctly paired with its mode of action?
   A. Carbamazepine   ⇓ Glutamate
   B. Valproate   ⇓ Calcium
   C. Lithium   ⇑ GABA
   D. Gabapentin   ⇓ G proteins
   E. Topiramate   ⇓ Glutamate

4. CD is a 32-year-old male with a history of bipolar disorder first diagnosed at the age of 26. Since then he has had one manic episode and two depressed episodes. He has just been promoted and is very concerned about having another episode. What can you advise him about prophylaxis?
   A. Lithium has an effectiveness rate of approximately 80%.
   B. Lithium levels should be maintained between 1 and 2 meq/L.
   C. Carbamazepine is more effective than lithium in preventing mania and depressive episodes.
   D. Rapid cycling may respond to thyroid augmentation.
   E. Extended periods of wakefulness can prevent mania.

HPI: You are going to colead a psychotherapy group for patients with anxiety disorders. Before the first group you review the descriptions of the group participants.

AG is a 30-year-old woman who works in the filing department of an accounting firm. She joined the group because of extreme shyness, an inability to participate in social activities for fear of people watching her and making a fool of herself.

RP is a 23-year-old man who has a new job in an advertising firm. He finds that when he has to make a presentation he becomes extremely anxious, tachycardic, and diaphoretic, with a dry mouth. He has been turning down projects or allowing his coworkers to get the accolades for his work, for fear of having to speak in public.

DB is a 20-year-old college student with a morbid fear of rats. He joined the group after realizing that his summer job in a prestigious laboratory included the responsibility of feeding and caring for the rats. He decided to address this fear rather than avoid the situation and find another summer job.

ET is a 47-year-old woman who describes a 20-year history of anxiety. "It's all of the time." It isn't related to any specific situation and it causes her a great deal of distress. Her sleep is often interrupted, she feels "wound up" and tense, is often irritable, and finds it hard to concentrate because of her anxiety.

Thought Questions

- What disorders do these people have?

- What is known about their biology? Treatment?

Basic Science Review and Discussion

AG has social phobia, generalized type. RP has social phobia, specifically related to performance. DB has a specific phobia. ET has generalized anxiety disorder.

Social and Specific Phobias A phobia is defined as an irrational fear that results in a compelling desire to avoid the phobic stimulus. This can be a specific object, activity, or situation. The person realizes that the fear is excessive or out of proportion to any danger.

Specific Phobia A specific phobia relates to a persistent excessive fear of a specific thing (e.g., dogs, blood) or situation (e.g., flying, getting an injection, elevators). Exposure causes significant anxiety or distress, even a cued panic attack. The person realizes that the fear is excessive, and it causes significant distress or interferes with social or occupational functioning. Phobias are among the most common psychiatric disorders. Findings based on large community samples yielded lifetime prevalence estimates of approximately 11%. Most specific phobias are more common in women than in men. The mean age at onset differs, depending on the type of phobia. In childhood, phobias of animals, blood, storms, and water tend to begin, whereas phobias of heights tend to begin in the teens, and situational phobias (e.g., claustrophobia) have mean ages at onset in late teens to mid 20s.

Blood-injection-injury phobias tend to cluster together, as do animal phobias, natural environment phobias, and situational phobias. Up to 30% of patients with an anxiety disorder have a comorbid specific phobia.

There is a higher risk of specific phobias in first-degree relatives of people with specific phobias than in controls (approximately 30% vs 10%). Unfortunately, there are no good adoption studies of specific phobias, and in general there is a dearth of biologic research on specific phobias.

Social Phobia In social phobia, the individual's central fear is that he or she will act in such a way as to humiliate or embarrass him- or herself in front of others. Socially phobic individuals fear and/or avoid a variety of situations in which they would be required to interact with or perform a task in front of other people. There are two subtypes of social phobias. One is generalized, in which the social fear encompasses most social situations. This causes more morbidity than the other type, in which the social phobia is circumscribed to one or two specific activities. Common phobias are of speaking or eating in public, using public lavatories, and attending parties or interviews. A common fear of socially phobic individuals is that other people will detect and ridicule their anxiety in social situations.

In social phobias the anxiety is stimulus-bound. When confronted with the phobic situation, the individual experiences profound anxiety accompanied by a variety of somatic symptoms, such as sweating, blushing, and dry mouth. Actual panic attacks may also occur in response to feared social situations.

Individuals who have only circumscribed social fears may function well overall and be relatively asymptomatic unless confronted with their phobic situation. When faced with this, they are often subject to intense anticipatory anxiety. Generalized social phobia can lead to chronic demoralization, social isolation, and disabling vocational and interpersonal impairment.

Epidemiology Social phobia may be slightly more prevalent in women. The median age of onset is in the mid teens. The lifetime prevalence is between 3% and 13%. Interestingly, in a large epidemiologic study, despite significant functional impairment only a minority had sought professional help. Generalized social phobia usually has an earlier age of onset than more circumscribed social phobias, and affected patients are more often single and have more comorbidity with depression and alcoholism.

Genetics A strong familial risk for social phobia has been identified and is believed to be partly heritable and partly environmental. First-degree relatives of persons with generalized social phobia have an approximately tenfold higher risk for generalized social phobia or avoidant personality disorder. Environmental factors also play a significant role. Prospectively, the personality trait of behavioral inhibition, assessed in toddlerhood, has been found to be a strong predictor of social anxiety in adolescence.

Neurochemistry and Neuroimaging The biology of social phobia has not been well documented. Despite the documented efficacy of serotonin reuptake inhibitors in treating social phobia, little is directly known about serotonergic involvement in the disorder. The neuroimaging of social phobia is also poorly elaborated, and studies are small and often not replicated. Provocation paradigms that evoke social anxiety symptoms during imaging suggest an increase in activity in areas involved in emotional processing, and possibly in the amygdala. (See discussion of fear response in Case 26.)

Course and Prognosis Social phobia has its mean age of onset in late adolescence and early adulthood, and the course is chronic, often lasting decades or longer. The onset of symptoms is usually insidious over months or years and without a clear-cut precipitant. Occasionally, the onset is triggered by a humiliating social experience. Predictors of good outcome in social phobia are onset after age 11, absence of psychiatric comorbidity, and higher educational status.

Generalized Anxiety Disorder Generalized anxiety disorder **(GAD)** is defined in the *Diagnostic and Statistical Manual of Mental Disorders,* 4th edition (text revision) (*DSM IV-TR*), as excessive anxiety or apprehension occurring more days than not, about a number of things, and lasting at least 6 months. There are three or more associated symptoms, such as feeling restless or keyed up, having difficulty concentrating, feeling easily fatigued or irritable, having muscle tension, and/or experiencing sleep disturbance (including difficulty falling or staying asleep). The anxiety must cause significant distress or impairment of functioning and should not be due to substance use, a medical problem, or another

Axis I diagnosis (e.g., worry about dirt and contamination in someone with obsessive compulsive disorder).

GAD is seen more frequently in women and often starts in the 20s. The lifetime prevalence is approximately 5%. The course may be chronic, with many people reporting years of symptoms before presentation for help. The literature on the course of GAD is sparse. Twin studies suggest that there does seem to be some heritable susceptibility to GAD, with a higher proportion of monozygotic twins being concordant.

There is some evidence that serotonin is involved in GAD. This is partially related to the data from pharmacologic intervention trials that demonstrate efficacy of 5-HT_{1A} partial agonists and 5-HT_2 antagonists in the treatment of GAD symptoms. Challenge studies provoking symptoms in GAD patients have been consistent with this. A great deal of exploration is still needed to elaborate this system.

Treatment Cognitive behavioral therapy has been used in treatment of all anxiety disorders. The cognitive therapy is based on finding disordered cognitions (e.g., the expectation of failure or of anxiety), making it explicit, and then helping to find a way to replace it with a different cognition. The basic principle of the behavioral component to the therapy is that anything that triggers is avoided and thus becomes more frightening over time. If it is repeatedly confronted without leading to the anticipated bad or dangerous outcome, it becomes less frightening.

In social phobia, the cognitive work focuses on distorted expectations of negative social outcomes and hypercritical self-evaluations. The behavioral component is based on graded exposure (or systematic desensitization) to increasingly challenging situations to allow desensitization to occur. Groups are quite useful to practice exposure exercises and to help observe and correct other distorted self-assessments, which may lead to improved self-awareness as well. Specific phobias are treated with graded exposure as well. The patient must participate in creating a set of appropriate graded exposures and then practice them through imaging as well as "in the field." The treatment of GAD is less well defined but may respond to similar cognitive work in evaluating distorted expectations, using cognitive restructuring to reinterpret the physical symptoms of anxiety. In addition, relaxation training may be useful.

Pharmacology Generalized anxiety disorder is often treated with buspirone, antidepressants (e.g., selective serotonergic reuptake inhibitors [SSRIs] or tricyclics) and/or benzodiazepines. Generalized social phobia may also respond, in part, to antidepressants (e.g., SSRIs, tricyclics, or monoamine oxidase inhibitors [MAOIs] and/or benzodiazepines). In social phobia limited to performance situations beta-blockers such as propranolol are often employed at low doses before the performance.

Case Conclusion You and your coleader decide that the group will use a cognitive behavioral model. In the context of the group each participant will help the others find cognitive distortions and work out plans for graded exposures. In addition, AG, who had a generalized social phobia, started an SSRI; RP, who had a fear of public speaking, was given a prescription for propranolol, to use adjunctively with his graded exposure plan; DB, who had the specific phobia of rats was not prescribed anything, although when he begins work he may have a short course of benzodiazepines; and ET, who had generalized anxiety disorder, had extra "homework" with relaxation exercises and was prescribed an SSRI.

Thumbnail: Behavioral Science—Antianxiety Agents

Medication	Mechanism of Action	Metabolism	Side Effects
Buspirone	Serotonin (5-HT$_{1A}$) agonist. Suppresses neuronal firing in the dorsal raphe	Primarily by oxidation to hydroxylated derivatives and an active metabolite	Dizziness, light-headedness, headache, little sedation, no tolerance or physical dependence
Benzodiazepines	Allosterically enhance GABA binding, causing increased influx of Cl$^-$ with GABA binding	Most are both demethylated and glucuronidated. Lorazepam and oxazepam are only glucuronidated.	Dizziness, ataxia, drowsiness, tolerance, physical dependence, confusion, amnesia. Those with longer half-lives and active metabolites increase risk of falling among the elderly. Withdrawal can lead to seizures.
Barbiturates	Allosterically enhances GABA binding (different site than BZDs)	Hepatic, induces P450 enzymes	Tolerance (including cross-tolerance to all CNS depressants), withdrawal, life-threatening respiratory depression in overdose

Key Points

Specific Phobia

▶ Inappropriate persistent, excessive fear of a specific thing or situation

▶ Cognitive-behavioral therapy (CBT), systematic desensitization, sometimes benzodiazepines

Generalized Social Phobia

▶ Fear of humiliating oneself in a variety of social situations, with social avoidance

▶ Antidepressants, CBT

Limited Social Phobia

▶ Fear of humiliating oneself in a particular social situation (e.g., public speaking), with resultant dysfunction

▶ Beta-blockers, benzodiazepines, CBT

Generalized Anxiety Disorder

▶ Excessive anxiety occurring more days than not, about a number of things, lasting at least 6 months with associated physical symptoms

▶ Buspirone, antidepressants, benzodiazepines, relaxation therapy, CBT

Questions

Questions 1 and 2 relate to the following clinical scenario:

GZ is a 45-year-old woman who comes in to your office complaining of anxiety. She has restricted her activities, has taken a job where she can work from home, and sees only one long-standing friend and her siblings. She has a pervasive fear of humiliating herself and being ridiculed.

1. Which of the following is her likely diagnosis and what is the probable course?
   A. Social phobia—chronic, long-standing
   B. Social phobia—episodic, long-standing
   C. Generalized anxiety disorder—chronic, long-standing
   D. Generalized anxiety disorder—episodic, long-standing
   E. Generalized anxiety disorder—brief episodes followed by long remissions

2. What can be said about the treatment of this disorder?
   A. Propranolol is an efficacious medication.
   B. Selective serotonin reuptake inhibitors are efficacious medications.
   C. Cognitive behavioral therapy is not effective.
   D. Long-standing high-dose benzodiazepines are the treatment of choice.
   E. Buspirone is the treatment of choice.

Questions 3 and 4 refer to the following scenario:

When JP is confronted with a social situation, especially a large party or a speaking engagement, he becomes extremely anxious and at times will have palpitations, diaphoresis, nausea, and tremulousness.

3. If he takes a lorazepam prior to the stressful event, he can circumvent these feelings. Which of the following is true about the pharmacology of lorazepam?
   A. It allosterically modulates the serotonin receptor.
   B. It allows an increase in the net efflux of calcium ions from the cell.
   C. It has multiple active metabolites and a half-life of 56 hours.
   D. It will not directly open the gamma aminobutyric acid receptor.
   E. It is an agonist at the 5-HT$_{1A}$ receptor.

4. His sister gives him some of her benzodiazepine prescription to take prior to her daughter's college graduation party. He is able to tolerate the experience with minimal anxiety. He decides that he wants to take this "all the time" and convinces his doctor to give him enough so he can take it four times a day. Which of the following is a likely adverse effect of this class of medication?
   A. Weight loss
   B. Weight gain
   C. Constipation
   D. Withdrawal seizures
   E. Headaches

HPI: TR is a married 37-year-old woman with no significant medical history who presents to her physician complaining of fatigue. In reviewing her symptoms, she admits to having disrupted sleep, with multiple awakenings in the night. She states that she used to be a sound sleeper, but at this point a dog barking on the street is enough to awaken her. She also admits to anxiety, difficulty concentrating during the day, irritability, and nightmares. She dates this to some time in late September 2001. She describes that she is an administrative assistant who worked in an office in the World Trade Center in New York. She saw the plane hit the first tower and ran down 47 floors to safety. In addition, she describes avoiding tall buildings, elevators, and the media barrage of the event. She has found a job in New Jersey, where she lives, which pays 50% of what she made at the financial institution but "is on the first floor, and it's a small building in a small town." She denies other constitutional symptoms, and her physical exam and lab work are all normal.

Thought Questions

■ What psychiatric disorder might account for her symptoms?

■ What is the known biology of this disorder?

Basic Science Review and Discussion

Posttraumatic stress disorder (PTSD) is a pathologic response to trauma that occurs in only a fraction of people exposed to a traumatic event. Overall, 20% of those exposed to a severe trauma will develop PTSD. Different traumas are more or less likely to result in the development of PTSD, and PTSD can occur even if the trauma happens to someone else. The severity and duration of the trauma influence the incidence of PTSD. Characteristics of the individual that influence the risk of developing PTSD include having a pre-existing depression or anxiety, or an early history of trauma.

Four factors are necessary for a *Diagnostic and Statistical Manual of Mental Disorders,* 4th edition (text revision) (*DSM-IV-TR*) diagnosis of PTSD—a trauma, reexperiencing phenomena, avoidance, and hyperarousal. These symptoms must last for at least 1 month and cause significant distress or impairment in functioning.

A trauma is defined as experiencing or witnessing an event that involved actual or threatened death or serious injury or a threat to the physical integrity of oneself or others. In response, the individual must have experienced fear, help-lessness, or horror. Reexperiencing refers to intrusive recollections, recurrent nightmares, and acting or feeling as if the traumatic event were reoccurring ("flashbacks"). Avoidance may include avoiding anything associated with the trauma; attempts to avoid thoughts, feelings, places, or people associated with the trauma; inability to recall important aspects of the event; feelings of detachment; a restricted range of affect; or a sense of a foreshortened future. Symptoms of increased arousal include difficulty falling or staying asleep, irritability or outbursts of anger, difficulty concentrating, hypervigilance, or exaggerated startle response.

This woman clearly meets criteria for PTSD. She experienced a trauma and has reexperiencing phenomena (nightmares), avoidance (avoiding tall office buildings, elevators, any media coverage of 9/11), and hyperarousal (disrupted, light sleep, irritability, difficulty concentrating).

It is important to contrast this with acute stress disorder, which lasts between 2 days and 4 weeks and occurs within a month of the trauma. The criteria for acute stress disorder are having experienced a trauma, having dissociative symptoms during or after the event (e.g., a sense of numbing or detachment, being in a daze, derealization, or depersonalization). In addition, there are reexperiencing phenomena, hyperarousal, and avoidance, as in PTSD. Of course, the symptoms must cause clinically significant distress or dysfunction.

The Biology of PTSD The biology of PTSD has been most studied in terms of the sympathetic nervous system (SNS), along with the locus coeruleus and amygdala, and the hypothalamic-pituitary-adrenal (HPA) axis.

The SNS is implicated in the pathophysiology of PTSD, particularly in the symptoms of hyperarousal. The SNS is involved in the fight-or-flight response. Blood flow to muscles and organs increases, the pupils are dilated, and the peripheral vasculature is clamped down. In general, PTSD subjects have significantly elevated levels of dopamine, epinephrine, and norepinephrine metabolites (HVA, 5-HIAA) in 24-hour urine collection studies, and fewer α_2-adrenergic receptors on the surface of platelets as compared with normal controls. This may be the result of down-regulation secondary to high circulating levels of catecholamines. Functional neuroimaging has shown increased reactivity of the amygdala. These areas of the brain are involved in fear responses.

Briefly, the neurocircuitry of fear involves the amygdala with inputs from the thalamus and prefrontal cortex, and outputs to various areas, including the locus coeruleus (which is the primary noradrenergic nucleus in the brain and mediates arousal), areas of the brainstem that mediate respiratory activation, the HPA axis (discussed later) and again the cortex, which then is involved in the cognitive interpretations of the information.

The HPA axis is stimulated via the fear response, and cortisol can be thought of as a break on the system, reversing the SNS activation after the stressful event has passed. Human studies of cortisol levels in the acute aftermath of trauma (e.g., rape, motor vehicle accidents) suggest that people with lower levels of cortisol are more likely to

develop PTSD. In patients with chronic PTSD there may be down-regulation of pituitary corticotropin releasing factor (CRF) receptors, due to chronic hypersecretion of CRF, yet overall levels of cortisol are low. There appears to be increased negative feedback sensitivity of the HPA axis.

Hippocampal volume is decreased in PTSD. Animal models show that elevated glucocorticoid levels cause dendritic pruning or neuronal death in the hippocampus. Hippocampal volume is negatively correlated with trauma severity.

Case Conclusion TR meets criteria for PTSD. She experienced a trauma, has a reexperiencing phenomenon, avoidance, and hyperarousal. She was offered a selective serotonin reuptake inhibitor but decided to opt for a trial of cognitive behavioral therapy and group therapy for survivors of 9/11. The therapy focused on helping her to restore a sense of safety and control, to mourn and reintegrate her memories of the trauma, and gradually to face her avoidance. It also integrated relaxation training to help her control her anxiety by reducing physiologic arousal and reactivity. Over time her symptoms diminished, although she decided to remain in her job in New Jersey.

Thumbnail: Behavioral Science—Feedback Pathways in PTSD

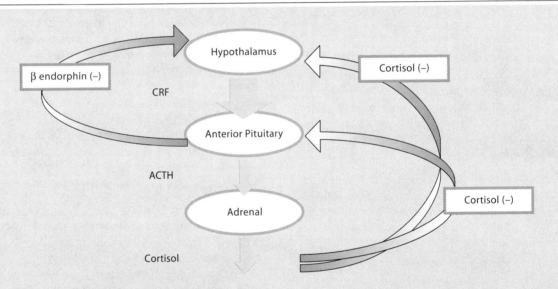

In patients with PTSD, CRF is high but cortisol is low. In fact, there is hyperresponsivity to the negative feedback mechanism. This can be demonstrated using exogenous steroids (such as dexamethasone), which causes exaggerated suppression of cortisol. This is probably related to an increase in receptor sensitivity because of the low levels of circulating cortisol.

Key Points

- PTSD symptoms must last more than 1 month. If the symptoms appear more than 6 months after the trauma, it is considered to have a delayed onset.

- Acute stress disorder lasts 2 days to 4 weeks and occurs within 4 weeks of a trauma.

- In PTSD the locus coeruleus and amygdala are hyperreactive, and there is an increase in circulating catecholamines. The negative feedback of the HPA axis is hyperreactive, cortisol levels are low, and CRF is high.

- PTSD is treated pharmacologically with antidepressants (selective serotonin reuptake inhibitors, tricyclics, and monoamine oxidase inhibitors) as well as occasionally with clonidine (an α_2-agonist) and benzodiazepines. Psychotherapy, group therapy, and support groups may all be helpful.

Questions

Questions 1 and 2 refer to the following case:

GR is a 73-year-old widowed white male whose wife died 1 year ago. Since that time he has been experiencing more difficulty sleeping and has had nightmares. Upon questioning it becomes clear that his nightmares relate to his experiences in the Holocaust, when he saw his parents taken away to be killed and his younger sister shot as she tried to go after them. He was in a concentration camp for 3 years before it was liberated. He has never slept well, has had occasional nightmares, and has always been irritable as well as "extra-protective" of his family. He has never been able to remember large periods of his experiences in the camps. His energy, appetite, and concentration are unchanged. He is not suicidal.

1. What is the most likely diagnosis for this gentleman?
   A. Bereavement
   B. Major depression
   C. Sleep terror disorder
   D. Posttraumatic stress disorder
   E. Hypnopompic hallucinations

2. If this man were given a dose of dexamethasone (a steroid) in the evening, what would you expect his cortisol to be the next morning?
   A. It would fail to suppress it because the receptors in the hypothalamus are less sensitive than normal.
   B. It would fail to suppress it because the receptors in the hypothalamus are normal.
   C. It would be strongly suppressed because the receptors in the hypothalamus are more sensitive than normal.
   D. It would be strongly suppressed because the receptors in the hypothalamus are less sensitive than normal.
   E. It would fail to suppress it because the receptors in the hypothalamus are more sensitive than normal.

Questions 3 and 4 refer to the following case:

BA is a 52-year-old Vietnam veteran who was in heavy combat, lost most of his unit on three different occasions, and finally was sent home after stepping on a mine and having to have a great deal of shrapnel removed from his leg. He describes "freaking" every time a car backfires and has thrown himself to the ground when hearing a helicopter overhead. On two occasions he said that for a few minutes it was as if he were "back in the jungle." He is constantly on edge, will never sit with his back to an open door or room, has nightmares, and "prowls" his house at night, checking the doors and the windows and looking in on his stepchildren. He never goes into crowds, generally feels "detached" from everyone, and has very few friends outside of his wife and one participant in the group he attends at the Veterans Administration. He describes having a "very short fuse," especially during the 20 years that he was a heavy substance abuser (benzodiazepines, occasional intranasal heroin, alcohol, marijuana) after leaving the service. "I don't hit people any more, but I get really angry." Since he's been "sober" he has been coming to the Veterans Administration for treatment.

3. Which of the following is a criterion for PTSD?
   A. Worthlessness
   B. Hypervigilance
   C. Paranoid delusions
   D. Substance abuse
   E. Night terrors

4. Which neurobiological correlates would you expect to see in this gentleman, compared with a normal control?
   A. Increased urinary cortisol
   B. Increased urinary HVA and 5-HIAA
   C. Increased hippocampal size
   D. Marked temporal and parietal atrophy on CT scan
   E. Decreased amygdala activity seen on functional imaging after a stressor

HPI: RG is a recently married woman who comes to your office at the urging of her husband. She says that before their marriage she was always extremely neat and orderly, but since they are living together she is miserable because of his habits, and he is "going nuts" because of hers. She describes needing to have things "just so," with all of the CDs, books, and canned foods, organized by size and color. She spends at least 2 hours each morning reorganizing these items. In addition, all the picture frames, shades, blinds, rugs, and incidentals (vases, decorative boxes, etc.) must be precisely in the correct place and orientation. This adds at least another hour to her day. She is always vigilant about dirt, allows no shoes or coats into the house, and washes her hands either 14 or 21 times a day, for 7 minutes each time. She worries that the dirt on the coats, bags, or shoes will somehow get into the house and make them sick. She works as an executive secretary and is extremely organized. Her boss, who is also "a bit compulsive," lets her keep the place "however she wants to."

Since her marriage, having her husband come in and move things, put his coat on the couch, inadvertently change the order of the CDs or books, or move things around the apartment makes her intolerably anxious, and she spends most of her evenings following him around "undoing his mess." He has tried to change his habits, but there is no way he can meet her "standards." Before her marriage she always thought of herself as "a little too neat," but now she realizes that her inability to "relax a bit" and allow some variability in her surroundings is excessive and might actually cost her her marriage.

Thought Questions

- What is the likely etiology of her symptoms?
- What is known about the diagnosis, biology, and treatment of this illness?

Basic Science Review and Discussion

The essential features of obsessive-compulsive disorder (OCD) are obsessions and/or compulsions. In *Diagnostic and Statistical Manual of Mental Disorders,* 4th edition (text revision) (*DSM-IV*-TR), OCD is classified among the anxiety disorders because anxiety is often associated with obsessions. Resistance to compulsions causes anxiety or tension and is often immediately relieved by yielding to compulsions. Common presentations include obsessions about dirt and contamination, with rituals that include compulsive washing and avoidance of contaminated objects; pathologic counting and compulsive checking; obsessions but no compulsions; hoarding for fear of someday needing something discarded; and so on.

An obsession is an intrusive, unwanted mental event usually evoking anxiety or discomfort. Obsessions may be thoughts, ideas, images, or impulses, and are often aggressive, sexual, or religious. Much obsessive thinking involves horrific ideas of an aggressive or sexual nature (e.g., rape, murder, child molestation). Obsessional fears often involve dirt or contamination, harm coming to oneself or to others as a consequence of one's misdoings (e.g., failure to check the door and a killer getting into the house, or running over a pedestrian because of careless driving). Obsessional think-

ing may also involve persistent doubting. Patients variably try to resist these thoughts, causing significant anxiety or distress. Obsessions are usually accompanied by compulsions but may also occur as the main or only symptom. Approximately 10% to 25% of OCD patients are purely or predominantly obsessional.

Compulsions usually arise to try to control or decrease obsessional thoughts. For instance, excessive washing may arise to address obsessions about contamination, and repeated checking may arise because of persistent doubting. A compulsion usually reduces discomfort but is carried out in a rigid fashion. Compulsions include rituals involving washing, checking, repeating, avoiding, and being meticulous. The most common compulsion is washing, which represents about 25% to 50% of OCD cases. These individuals may spend many hours a day washing their hands, showering, or avoiding germs or bodily wastes. The second most common compulsion is checking. Checkers have pathologic doubt and compulsively check to see if they have run over someone with their car or left the ignition on. Not all compulsions are physically acted out. Mental compulsions include counting or mentally replaying conversations over and over. A rare and disabling form of OCD is called primary obsessional slowness. In this form of the illness it may take many hours to get dressed or get out of the house.

Epidemiology OCD usually begins in adolescence or early adulthood. Almost one-third of cases begin between ages 10 and 15, with 75% developing by age 30. The course is most often chronic. OCD was previously considered one of the rarest mental disorders. Current data suggest that OCD is actually fairly common, with a lifetime prevalence rate of 2.5%. The ratio of males to females is about 1:1, although in childhood-onset OCD, about 70% of patients are male.

Twin and family studies have found a greater degree of concordance for OCD among monozygotic twins compared with dizygotic twins, although there are no studies of OCD in adopted children or monozygotic twins raised apart. Studies of families and first-degree relatives of OCD patients show an increased incidence of anxiety disorders and obsessive-compulsive symptoms. It appears that OCD which begins before age 18 is associated with much higher rates of familial OCD. Family studies also suggest a genetic link between OCD and Tourette's syndrome. No candidate serotonin-related genes have reliably emerged in familial studies.

Biological Theories   It is important to note that there is a subset of patients whose symptoms result from a neurologic insult, including abnormal birth events, head injury and seizures, or association with the encephalitis epidemic in 1916–18 (von Economo's encephalitis). In addition, OCD may be associated with a number of subtle neurologic findings, including the presence of neurologic soft signs and abnormalities on electroencephalogram and auditory evoked potentials.

Recent neuroimaging techniques suggest that orbitofrontal-limbic-basal ganglia circuits are involved in the pathophysiology of OCD. Interestingly, after effective treatment of OCD with serotonin reuptake inhibitors or with behavior therapy, functional imaging studies have shown a normalization of hyperactivity in areas such as the caudate, orbitofrontal lobes, and cingulate cortex. One hypothesis is that the basal ganglia act as a gating station, filtering input from orbitofrontal and cingulate cortex and mediating motor patterns. Another theory is that OCD behaviors such as excessive washing or saving may be dysregulated manifestations of normal grooming or hoarding behaviors. The neurotransmitter serotonin has been implicated in the pathophysiology of the illness, particularly because of the therapeutic success of potent serotonin reuptake inhibitors.

Course and Prognosis   Approximately 5% to 10% have periods of remission or even sustained remissions; 5% to 10% may have a progressive, deteriorating course; 30% have a fluctuating course; and more than 50% have a continuous course. Before the use of current modalities, OCD had a poor prognosis. With the use of serotonin reuptake inhibitors and/or behavioral therapy, the prognosis is improved, although up to 30% to 60% may not have a significant clinical response, depending on how response is defined. Untreated, the disorder has a major impact on daily functioning, with some patients spending many waking hours consumed with their obsessions and rituals. This may lead to social isolation, marrying at an older age,

and in males, high celibacy rates. Depression and anxiety are common comorbid disorders with OCD.

Treatment   The principal pharmacologic agents used to treat OCD are the selective serotonergic reuptake inhibitors (SSRIs), which include, for example, fluoxetine, fluvoxamine and sertraline, and the tricyclic antidepressant clomipramine. In general, patients may require higher doses of SSRIs to treat OCD than to treat depression. If a patient fails to respond to an SSRI, an antipsychotic medication may serve as an augmenting strategy.

Either alone or in combination with pharmacotherapy, behavioral therapy has been shown to be effective in the treatment of OCD. Overall, 50% to 70% of patients are helped by behavioral therapy. About 20% refuse or cannot tolerate the anxiety that is induced, and another 25% fail to improve for other reasons. Behavioral therapy may have more long-term effects than pharmacology alone, with studies suggesting that up to 75% of people who respond to behavior therapy continue to do well, although often not symptom-free, after the therapy has ended.

Behavioral therapy is based on the principle of exposure and response prevention. Briefly, the patient is asked to endure the anxiety that an obsession provokes while refraining from acting on the compulsion. For example, the patient with obsessions about contamination would choose a series of graded exposures (e.g., touching a doorknob, touching the floor, touching something in a bathroom) and not wash. By learning to tolerate the anxiety, it will eventually decrease on its own (i.e., habituation will occur), and the need to perform the ritual will eventually disappear. The behavioral therapy therefore helps the patient habituate to the anxiety and extinguish the compulsions by breaking the cycle of obsessions temporarily relieved by compulsions. This principle is applied to many types of behavioral therapy and is referred to as *systematic desensitization*. For instance, in the treatment of phobias patients are asked to create a hierarchy of anxiety-provoking experiences. Through imaging (i.e., imagining the experience) and through actually confronting the experience, the anxiety is tolerated and finally extinguished. This is done in a graduated manner, starting with the least threatening and gradually working up to the most anxiety-provoking exposure.

Occasionally, even with adequate pharmacotherapy and/or behavioral therapy, patients still experience intractable incapacitating symptoms, and neurosurgery may be considered. Obviously, the symptoms must be very severe, and the patient must have proven resistant to multiple psychological and somatic therapies over the course of many years. The success rate is about 50% to 70%. In general, the surgical procedures used (anterior capsulotomy, cingulotomy, and limbic leukotomy) aim to interrupt the connection between the cortex and the basal ganglia and related structures.

Case Conclusion   RG decided to opt for a combination of pharmacotherapy and behavior therapy. She was treated with an SSRI, and with her therapist, devised a series of graded exposures first in the office and then at home. With the combination of these treatment modalities, she was able to significantly decrease her time spent on her OCD symptoms, and learned how to accept her husband (and his "mess"). Although in times of stress she had some recurrence of her symptoms, she was able to function well with only minimal disruption by her OCD.

Thumbnail: Behavioral Science—Obsessive-Compulsive Disorder vs Obsessive-Compulsive Personality Disorder

Obsessive-Compulsive Disorder	Obsessive-Compulsive Personality Disorder
Obsessions	No obsessions
Compulsions	No compulsions
Ego dystonic (incompatible with the individual's self-concept)	Ego syntonic (compatible with the individual's self-concept)
Obsessions and compulsions are time consuming and interfere with daily functioning	Personality style that is inflexible, perfectionistic, and detail oriented

Key Points

▶ **Obsessions:** Recurrent and persistent thoughts, impulses, or images cause marked anxiety or distress. They are not excessive worries about real-life problems. The person either attempts to ignore or suppress them, or to neutralize them with some other thoughts or actions.

▶ **Compulsions:** Repetitive behaviors or mental acts that the person feels driven to perform in response to an obsession, or according to rigid rules. The acts are aimed at preventing or reducing distress or neutralizing or preventing the obsessions and are clearly excessive.

▶ In the **diagnosis** of OCD, the obsessions or compulsions cause marked distress, are time-consuming (e.g., take more than 1 hour per day), or interfere significantly with the person's normal routine, social, occupational, or academic functioning.

▶ The orbitofrontal-limbic-basal ganglia circuits are implicated in OCD, and serotonin is thought to be the major neurotransmitter affected.

▶ The pharmacologic treatment of OCD is with SSRIs. Antipsychotics occasionally may be used as augmentation. Behavioral therapy is also effective. In rare cases of resistant, incapacitating OCD, psychosurgery is used.

Questions

1. PJ presented to the dermatologist for a cream for a rash on his hands. Upon examination his hands were red, irritated, and dry. He had no other manifestations on other parts of his body. In reviewing his habits, he admitted to washing his hands 50 or more times per day. His work in a hospital made him acutely aware of and concerned about germs and contamination. He is worried that if he does not continually wash, he will make his family or himself sick. He avoids touching most surfaces with his hands (e.g., doorknobs), and if he does he has to wash. Each time he washes he spends 10 minutes. If he is prevented from washing he becomes very anxious and upset. Which of the following would probably be the most beneficial treatment of his condition.

   A. Recommend that he not wash so frequently.
   B. Explain that he is causing the condition by his excessive washing.
   C. Educate him about universal precautions and when to wear latex gloves.
   D. Set up a structured program of exposure and response prevention.
   E. Encourage him to take a microbiology course to better understand which pathogens are harmful.

2. FD is a 22-year-old student who comes for an evaluation because of increased difficulty completing his work. He explains that when he reads he becomes overwhelmed with the idea that he has missed a paragraph or a page and thus reads everything six times. He has recently found it harder to get out to class in the morning because he needs to check that the hot plate is off, the door is locked, his books are in a certain order, and his shoes are lined up in a particular way. He admits that he has an irrational fear that if things aren't perfect his dorm room will catch on fire or that something terrible will happen to his parents or brother. Which of the following neurotransmitter systems has been most consistently implicated in this disorder?

   A. Serotonin
   B. Norepinephrine
   C. Acetylcholine
   D. GABA
   E. Dopamine

Questions 3 and 4 refer to the following case:

SD is plagued with the notion that she has run over a child in her car or has inadvertently killed a baby. She stopped driving 5 years ago, but before that she would need to stop every block and get out to reassure herself that she had not hurt anyone. Whenever she saw a child in the street she would stare at him or her to convince herself that the child was well and unharmed. She has two grown children who are well, and she has never hurt anyone, child or adult, in her life. She has suffered from intrusive thoughts on and off throughout her adult life, but now, in her 40s, she spends hours every day plagued with these thoughts and horrific images of mutilated children or children crushed under the wheel of a car. This has been significantly interfering with her life and ability to function at work or socially over the past few years. She has had multiple psychiatric admissions because of her distress.

3. Which of the following is an appropriate treatment strategy?

   A. Decreasing her current SSRI medication (fluvoxamine)
   B. Adding lithium to her therapy
   C. Adding methylphenidate to her treatment
   D. High-dose clozapine therapy
   E. Adding behavioral therapy to her treatment

4. Assuming that she has failed multiple adequate treatment regimens and augmentation strategies, what is a possible treatment option for refractory OCD?

   A. Occipital lobe ablation
   B. Surgery on the cingulate cortex
   C. Frontal lobotomy
   D. High-dose desipramine therapy
   E. Augmentation of fluoxetine with an acetylcholinesterase inhibitor

HPI: SA is a 25-year-old accountant living in a small city. She has no significant medical history. She describes that abruptly when she was taking the subway home from work, she developed acute shortness of breath, felt as if her throat was closing, became quite frightened, was fearful of dying, and broke out in a cold sweat. She was sure that she was having a heart attack. She got out at the next station and sat for 10 minutes and began to gradually recover. Within 20 minutes all symptoms were gone. She went to her internist, who performed a physical exam; EKG; and some blood work, including thyroid function tests. Everything was unremarkable. She stopped taking the subway because of fear of further attacks, but over the next month, she experienced several more episodes, usually when she would go out shopping or was on the bus. Over the next few weeks, she began to avoid going out alone; was tense, nervous, and fearful throughout the day; and had difficulty falling asleep. She began to do more and more of her work from home, "the only place I feel safe." She would only go out with her mother or her best friend. She went to her internist, who reviewed her symptoms, and after convincing her that there was no organic etiology to her symptoms, sent her for a psychiatric evaluation.

Thought Questions

- What psychiatric disorder explains these symptoms?
- What medical conditions need to be evaluated?

Basic Science Review and Discussion

Panic disorder is defined by four or more symptoms (Box 26-1) that occur spontaneously, peak in about 10 minutes, and are associated with significant worry about additional attacks or of "losing control" or dying. Because there are numerous medical illnesses and substances that can cause symptoms similar to panic disorder, it is important to take a careful history and do a complete physical exam. Examples include hyperthyroidism, hypoglycemia, neuroendocrine tumors (e.g., carcinoid, pheochromocytoma), cardiac conditions (e.g., ischemia, arrhythmias, possibly mitral valve prolapse), stimulant use, or depressant (e.g., alcohol) withdrawal.

Box 26-1. Symptoms of Panic

Palpitations or tachycardia
Nausea, abdominal distress
Derealization or depersonalization
Sweating
Chest pain/discomfort
Chills or hot flashes
Trembling or shaking
Dizzy, light-headed, unsteady
Paresthesias (numbness, tingling)
Fear of dying
Shortness of breath, smothering
Fear of losing control or going crazy
Sensation of choking

Adapted from *DSM-IV.*

Many people experience an occasional unexpected attack of panic, but the diagnosis of panic disorder is only made when the attacks occur with some regularity and frequency, and are associated with anticipatory anxiety. The patient comes to dread the attacks and starts worrying in the between attacks. This can progress until the fearfulness and autonomic hyperactivity between panic attacks becomes debilitating. In addition, many patients with panic disorder develop agoraphobia, the fear of going out because of a fear of having a panic attack and being unsafe or out of control.

Epidemiology The lifetime prevalence rate for panic disorder is approximately 1.5%. Women have almost double the rate of that found among men. It most commonly begins in the third decade.

Genetics Several family and twin studies of panic disorder have consistently supported the presence of a moderate genetic influence in the expression of panic disorder. Panic attacks have been found to be five times more frequent in monozygotic than in dizygotic twins. However, the absolute concordance rate in monozygotic twins is only 31%, suggesting that nongenetic factors also play an important role in the development of the illness.

Biological Theories The locus ceruleus (LC), located in the pons, contains more than 50% of all noradrenergic neurons in the entire central nervous system. It sends afferent projections to a wide area of the brain, including the hippocampus, amygdala, limbic lobe, and cerebral cortex. In animals, electrical stimulation of the LC produces fear and anxiety. Ablation renders an animal less susceptible to fear in the face of danger. In humans, drugs that are known to increase LC firing are anxiogenic (e.g., yohimbine, an $\alpha2$-antagonist), whereas many drugs that decrease LC firing and central noradrenergic turnover (e.g., benzodiazepines, clonidine, tricyclics, antidepressants) tend to decrease anxiety.

In patients with panic attacks but not normal controls, sodium lactate infusion can provoke panic attacks. The mechanism is unclear, but theories have included induction of metabolic alkalosis and transient intracerebral hypercapnia, among others. Similarly, sodium bicarbonate infusion or breathing 5% carbon dioxide mixed with room air also provokes panic attacks in patients. In control subjects, hyperventilation and respiratory alkalosis do not routinely provoke panic attacks. One theory is that panic disorder patients may have hypersensitive brainstem CO_2 chemoreceptors in the medulla. Infused lactate is metabolized to bicarbonate, which is then converted in the periphery to CO_2. Thus, CO_2 constitutes the common metabolic product of both lactate and bicarbonate. CO_2 then crosses the blood-brain barrier and produces transient cerebral hypercapnia. The hypercapnia sets off the brainstem CO_2 chemoreceptors, leading to hyperventilation and panic. This is described as a "false suffocation alarm" theory of panic. Of note, hyperventilation causes a decrease in serum calcium, which may account for some of the paresthesias.

Other neurochemical circuits have been implicated in the pathophysiology of panic disorder. Benzodiazepines are very effective anxiolytics, and interestingly, decreased benzodiazepine receptor binding has been seen on SPECT and PET in brain areas that may be involved in the "fear circuit"

described later. Selective serotonin reuptake inhibitors are also used in the treatment of panic. Serotonergic medications may act by desensitizing the brain's fear network via projections from the raphe nuclei to the LC inhibiting noradrenergic activation, and from the raphe nuclei to the hypothalamus inhibiting the release of corticotropin-releasing factor (CRF). They may also act directly at the level of the amygdala, inhibiting excitatory pathways from the cortex and the thalamus.

An important concept in understanding anxiety and panic disorder is that of the "fear circuit." The model proposes that panic attacks may be manifestations of dysregulation of the brain circuits underlying conditioned fear responses. Panic is speculated to originate in an abnormally sensitive fear network, centered in the amygdala. Input into the amygdala is modulated by both thalamic input and prefrontal cortical projections. There are amygdalar projections to several areas involved in various aspects of the fear response, such as the LC and arousal, the brainstem and respiratory activation, the hypothalamus and activation of the hypothalamic-pituitary-adrenal (HPA) stress axis, and the cortex and cognitive interpretations. This model is thought to explain why biologically diverse agents have panicogenic properties: they act at different pathways in the circuit. This is a very comprehensive and theoretically exciting biological model of panic and needs further empirical validation.

Case Conclusion   SA was diagnosed with panic disorder after a negative work-up of other possible causative factors. She was treated with a selective serotonin reuptake inhibitor and cognitive behavioral therapy. Her panic attacks stopped, and she learned to understand that her body's reaction was not related to any real threat. Through the therapy she was able to understand that her phobic avoidance of going outside was purely related to her panic disorder, and over time she was able to resume her previous activities.

Thumbnail: Behavioral Science—The Fear Circuit

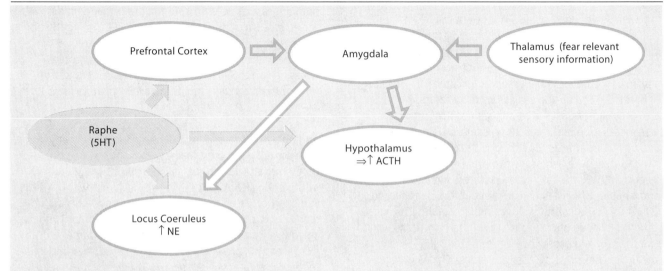

The fear circuit is an important concept in conceptualizing the mechanism of a number of psychiatric disorders, including PTSD and panic disorder, as well as other anxiety disorders. Interestingly, serotonin projections from the raphe nucleus inhibit the LC, as well as the hypothalamus and prefrontal cortex. This diagram is a simplified representation.

Input into the amygdala is modulated by both thalamic input and prefrontal cortical projections, and there are amygdalar projections to several areas involved in various aspects of the fear response, such as the LC and arousal, the brainstem and respiratory activation, the hypothalamus and activation of the HPA stress axis, and the cortex and cognitive interpretations.

Key Points

▶ Panic disorder is associated with episodic panic attacks and is often associated with agoraphobia.

▶ Attacks can be induced by CO_2, lactate, and bicarbonate.

▶ Mitral valve prolapse may be more common in patients with panic disorder.

▶ There does seem to be a genetic component.

▶ The treatment of panic disorder with or without agoraphobia includes antidepressants (tricyclics and selective serotonin reuptake inhibitors) and cognitive behavioral therapy.

Questions

Questions 1, 2, and 3 relate to the following case:

DS, a 21-year-old mechanic, presents to the emergency room complaining of light–headedness, tingling in his fingers, overwhelming anxiety, palpitations, tachypnea, and mild nausea. He says that these symptoms came out of the blue when he was fixing an ambulance in the hospital lot. He reports that he had similar symptoms once before 4 years ago, right before an exam in school.

1. Which of the following etiology—symptom pairs is correct?
   A. Peptic ulcer disease—palpitations
   B. Six cups of coffee that morning—paresthesias
   C. Alcohol withdrawal—hypotension
   D. Hyperthyroidism—palpitations
   E. Hypercalcemia—paresthesias

2. Assuming that this constellation of symptoms stems from a panic attack, what is the most likely etiology of the tingling in his fingers?
   A. Hyperventilation-induced alkalosis and hypocalcemia
   B. Hyperventilation-induced alkalosis and hypercalcemia
   C. Hyperventilation-induced acidosis and hypocalcemia
   D. Hyperventilation-induced hypercapnia and acidosis
   E. Hyperventilation-induced hypercapnia and hypercalcemia

3. Which of the following would be most likely to cause a panic attack in this patient?
   A. Sodium bicarbonate po
   B. An α_2-agonist
   C. Sodium lactate infusion
   D. A beta antagonist
   E. Breathing 100% CO for 30 minutes

4. PT is a 45-year-old female with a 20-year history of recurrent episodes of panic disorder. She last had a panic attack 3 years ago and has been off medication for a year. She comes in to your office for a consultation stating that she is having a recurrence of her symptoms. She describes episodes of feeling suddenly panicked, with a sensation of choking, nausea, trembling, shaking, pain in her chest that radiates to her jaw, hot flashes, auditory hallucinations, and the sensation of being outside herself watching the scene. Which of her symptoms is least consistent with a panic attack?
   A. Nausea
   B. The sensation of choking
   C. Auditory hallucinations
   D. Depersonalization
   E. Hot flashes

HPI: EC is a 68-year-old woman who was brought to her doctor because of increasing confusion. The family described that she was doing well living in an assisted-living apartment until yesterday, when she started to "act strangely" and called her daughters from her home, asking them about the family cat who had died years ago and wondering when she was going to go home. She has no significant medical history. When she presented to the emergency room she was at times agitated, disoriented, and confused; at other times she was more lucid.

PE: She has decreased breath sounds on the right. Her chest x-ray revealed an infiltrate on the right, and her labs are all normal except for a white blood cell count of 15.

Thought Questions

- What is wrong with this woman?
- What is the likely etiology of her cognitive problems?

Basic Science Review and Discussion

EC has pneumonia. Her change in mental status is probably due to delirium. Delirium is characterized by an acute, fluctuating change in mental status. Delirious patients exhibit reduced awareness of the environment, altered levels of consciousness, and reduced ability to focus attention. Delirium may be associated with perceptual disturbances in any modality (frequently tactile or visual) and with delusions, which are often disorganized and paranoid. The patient may be agitated, or psychomotorically retarded, may have a disturbance in the sleep-wake cycle, and may be emotionally labile. Symptom severity can fluctuate significantly.

Delirium generally presents in an acute or subacute manner (i.e., over hours or days) that may help differentiate it from dementia, which (except in the case of poststroke dementia) usually has an insidious gradual onset over months to years. Delirium is often undetected. As many as 70% of cases may go undiagnosed or untreated by physicians.

Epidemiology of Delirium Risk factors for delirium include advancing age, dementia, drug/alcohol use, brain damage, chronic or severe physical illness, sensory impairment, and medications. Children may also be at greater risk. The prevalence of delirium in older persons living in the community is approximately 1%. In hospitalized inpatients the prevalence of delirium is approximately 10% to 25%. In hospitalized patients with dementia it may be up to 40%. In general, delirium is more frequent in post coronary artery bypass graft (CABG) and patients who have had hip surgery, burn patients, and people with low serum albumin (which can lead to increased free fractions of drugs). Of course, it is also frequently seen in people intoxicated with or withdrawing from various substances, most commonly alcohol or benzodiazepines. Delirium can last from less than a week to more than a month. It is often more protracted in the elderly.

Delirium is associated with increased mortality rates during hospitalization and after discharge. It also is associated with increased hospital length of stay, increased health care expenditures, poor function, caregiver burden, persistent cognitive impairment, and increased costs for rehabilitation, institutionalization, and home care. In elderly patients, estimates of the risk of death during the incident hospitalization are 22% to 75%. Studies have also found a link between in-hospital delirium and functional decline, need for nursing home placement, increased length of stay, and so on. Given this, it is of concern that delirium is often underrecognized. Thus it is very important to recognize a delirium and treat the underlying cause.

Pathophysiology and Etiology The pathophysiology of delirium is unclear. Dysfunction of the reticular activating system has been implicated, as has a reduction in central nervous system oxidative metabolism leading to neurotransmitter abnormalities, increased cerebral cytokines that impair neurotransmitter system function, neuronal signal transduction, and second messenger systems. In addition, older persons are at increased risk of delirium due to age-related changes in brain neurochemistry and pharmacodynamic and pharmacokinetic alterations in the metabolism and excretion of medications.

The etiologies of delirium are diverse. The following list provides a sample. The etiology of delirium is most often multifactorial but frequently involves medications.

- *Medications, drugs, pesticides, solvents.*
  - Many medications are associated with delirium and psychotic symptoms, including nonsteroidal anti-inflammatory drugs (NSAIDs), quinolones, and H2 blockers.
  - Many medications have anticholinergic side effects that may be cumulative. Medications that are not traditionally thought of as anticholinergic, such as cimetidine, meperidine, and prednisolone, do have some anticholinergic activity.

- Drug-drug interactions (e.g., change of free fraction of drugs by protein-binding interactions, or alterations in P450 metabolism) may cause a delirium.
- *Cardiovascular*—Hypertensive encephalopathy, hypoperfusion
- *Intracranial bleeding*—especially with focal neurologic signs
- *Infections*—Meningitis/encephalitis, sepsis, pneumonia, and in patients with dementia, even a urinary tract infection
- *Withdrawal* from various substances including alcohol, benzodiazepines, and barbiturates
  - Alcohol withdrawal is usually seen 24 to 96 hours after the last drink and is associated with autonomic hyperactivity (tachycardia, diaphoresis, hypertension).
  - Delirium tremens often has associated prominent visual or tactile hallucinations and seizures. The mortality of delirium tremens, if untreated, is about 20%. This is usually due to medical complications, such as pneumonia, renal or hepatic disease, or cardiac disease.

- The time required for symptoms of benzodiazepine withdrawal to develop depends on the half-life of the specific benzodiazepine.
- *Wernicke's encephalopathy* (confusion, ataxia, lateral gaze paralysis)
  - Most commonly seen in alcoholics
  - Due to thiamine deficiency
  - If not immediately treated with IV thiamine it can progress to irreversible Korsakoff's dementia (confusion, retrograde and anterograde amnesia)
- *Metabolic*—acid-base disturbances, electrolyte abnormalities, liver or kidney failure, hypoglycemia
- *Paraneoplastic syndromes* (sometimes called limbic encephalopathy) secondary to a number of neoplasms, including ovarian, small cell, thymoma, seminoma, testicular cancer
- *Miscellaneous:* sleep deprivation, overstimulation in an intensive care unit

---

Case Conclusion EC was diagnosed with delirium secondary to pneumonia. After a course of IV antibiotics her mental status improved. She was able to concentrate, was oriented to time and place, and had no more ruminations or confusion about the cat. She was able to return to her assisted-living situation with the same minimal level of care that she had before admission.

Thumbnail: Behavioral Science—Differentiating Delirium from Dementia

Delirium	Dementia
Impaired level of consciousness	Level of consciousness not impaired
Acute or subacute onset	Usually insidious onset over months to years
Marked fluctuation in symptoms	Symptoms more stable over time
Frequently reversible	Rarely reversible (~5%)
May have marked autonomic dysfunction	No autonomic dysfunction

Key Points

- ▶ **Delirium**
  - ▶ *Risk factors:* age (young children or elderly), dementia, drug/alcohol use, brain damage, chronic or severe physical illness, sensory impairment, and medications
  - ▶ *Prevalence:* Hospitalized inpatients—10% to 25%. Hospitalized patients with dementia, 40%.

- ▶ *Course:* days to greater than a month. More protracted in the elderly.
- ▶ Delirium is associated with increased morbidity and mortality rates during hospitalization and after discharge.
- ▶ Delirium is often underrecognized.

Questions

1. LS is a 75-year-old woman who was brought to her internist by her son. He notes that over the past week she has been more confused, at times hallucinating about a man coming into her apartment at night. On exam she is noted to be flushed, have a dry mouth, and to complain of constipation and blurry vision. She started a new medication within the past 2 weeks. Which of the following medications is most likely responsible for her symptoms?
   A. Atenolol
   B. Warfarin
   C. Diphenhydramine
   D. Diazepam
   E. Ranitidine

2. A 56-year-old man is brought into the emergency room by the police after he was found staggering and incoherent in the train station. On exam he is ataxic, is confused, and has lateral gaze paralysis. What treatment should be instituted immediately?
   A. IV folic acid
   B. IV thiamine
   C. IV glucose
   D. Oxygen
   E. IV diazepam

3. A 45-year-old woman is admitted to the hospital for a broken leg. Two days after admission she becomes confused and begins to complain that groups of children are coming into her room and laughing at her. Later she tells you that she needs to pull her car out of the parking space and that you are blocking her way. She also is markedly tremulous, hypertensive, and tachycardic. What is the most likely etiology of her symptoms?
   A. New-onset schizophrenia
   B. Mania brought on by general anesthesia
   C. An adverse reaction to antibiotics
   D. Cocaine intoxication
   E. Alcohol withdrawal

4. An 83-year-old man has been admitted to the hospital for a urinary tract infection. On admission he is confused, disoriented, and disheveled. On exam, he is febrile and is intermittently irritable and falling asleep. He is treated for his infection with IV antibiotics and is rehydrated and discharged. At a follow-up visit 1 month later with his internist, he is able to sustain his attention, is able to groom himself but remains disorientated to time and the name of the street where his doctor is located; in addition, he cannot remember three words in 5 minutes. Otherwise his neurologic exam is normal. In talking to the son, what is the most likely history? He was
   A. Cognitively normal, working as a lawyer, and had a sudden onset of symptoms prior to hospitalization.
   B. A retired lawyer, has impaired short-term memory, has been unable to pay his bills for the last year, but has been living independently; he experienced acute worsening of symptoms before hospitalization.
   C. A retired lawyer and needed to move to a nursing home 4 years ago; there was no appreciable change in his cognition and behavior on admission.
   D. A boxer who was knocked unconscious multiple times, with an acute worsening of cognitive symptoms before admission.
   E. A man with a large middle cerebral artery stroke 1 year ago; he experienced acute worsening of his symptoms on admission.

HPI: JD is a 79-year-old retired lawyer who was brought in by his wife for an evaluation of his memory. They note that he has been having difficulty with short-term memory, often forgetting what his wife told him hours before. He often asks her the same questions repeatedly; for instance, about social engagements or family concerns. He also describes that his desk and financial affairs, which were always immaculately organized, have become less so, to the point that last month he forgot to pay the electric bill and his broker had to call him three times to decide what to do with the money from a bond that was coming due. He was an avid bird-watcher and notes that for the last 6 months he has been having problems naming the birds that he sees. He has no significant medical problems, his physical exam and laboratory work-up, including thyroid, vitamin levels, hepatic function, renal function, and blood counts, are all unremarkable.

Thought Questions

- What is wrong with this gentleman?

- Given his normal physical, history, and lab results, what is the likely etiology of his problems?

Basic Science Review and Discussion

This gentleman meets criteria for dementia (see below) with deficits in short-term memory and difficulties with executive functioning and language. Given his history and work-up, he most likely has Alzheimer's disease (AD).

Diagnosis and Epidemiology of Dementia Dementia is defined as the presence of consistent deficits in short-term memory, coupled with a decline in another area of cognitive function–aphasia (impaired or absent comprehension or production of, speech, writing, or signs), apraxia (difficulty in carrying out familiar purposeful movements not due to physical limitations [e.g., severe arthritis]), agnosia (impairment of ability to recognize or comprehend the meaning of various sensory stimuli) or disturbance of executive function (e.g., planning, organizing, sequencing, abstracting). Such cognitive deficits must cause marked impairment in social or occupational function, and must represent a significant decline from a previous level of functioning. These deficits may not occur exclusively during the course of a delirium.

Dementia may be due to a medical condition (e.g., stroke, Alzheimer's disease, Parkinson's disease), the enduring effects of substance use (e.g., alcohol, toxins), or a combination of etiologies. The prevalence of moderate to severe dementia in different population groups is approximately 5% in the general population over age 65; 20% to 40% in the general population over 85 years of age; 15% to 20% in outpatient general medical practices; and 50% in chronic care facilities.

The course of dementia varies according to the etiology, but most dementias are progressive. The following descriptions discuss general syndromes, although the actual presentation of diseases can vary enormously. Diseases that affect the cortical areas (such as Alzheimer's or Pick's disease) usually present with significant memory symptoms and difficulties in language, praxis, and executive functioning. Diseases that are primarily subcortical, such as Parkinson's disease and Binswanger's disease, often have prominent apathy, movement disorders, and less severe memory difficulties. Disorders affecting the frontal lobes, such as Pick's disease, often have marked disinhibition, other personality changes, and slowed movement and thought. Dementias may be complicated by behavioral disturbances (e.g., wandering, hallucinations, paranoia, and aggression). These are more prevalent in the moderate and severe stages of disease. In the terminal stage patients may be contracted, immobile, incontinent, unable to swallow properly, unable to clear their secretions, and prone to pressure ulcers. Infections are usually the proximal cause of death (e.g., pneumonias, urosepsis, infected ulcers).

Etiology The most common causes of dementia in individuals more than 65 years of age are Alzheimer's disease (which accounts for approximately 60%), vascular dementia (15%), and mixed vascular and Alzheimer's dementia (15%). Other illnesses account for approximately 10%, including Pick's disease, normal-pressure hydrocephalus, alcoholic dementia, infectious dementia such as HIV or neurosyphilis, prion diseases such as Creutzfeldt-Jakob disease, tumors, and Parkinson's disease (see Thumbnail). Some sources suggest that up to 5% of dementias evaluated in clinical settings may be attributable to reversible causes, such as metabolic abnormalities (e.g., hypothyroidism), nutritional deficiencies (e.g., vitamin B_{12} or folate deficiencies), or dementia syndrome due to depression. The dementia syndrome due to depression was previously referred to as pseudodementia.

The diagnosis of dementia is made by taking a careful history and using selected diagnostic tests. The clinical history should always be corroborated with a family member or other knowledgeable informant, as patients with memory disorders are often poor historians. The history and physical serve to evaluate various exposures, risk factors, potentially reversible etiologies, and neurologic findings (e.g., focal neurologic signs). A family history of dementia is particularly important in early-onset Alzheimer's disease or other known genetically transmitted diseases such as Huntington's chorea.

Genetic Causes Various etiologies of dementia are thought to have a genetic basis. Certainly this is clear in diseases caused by known mutations, such as Huntington's disease. The genetics of Alzheimer's disease is more complicated. There are known mutations on chromosomes 1, 14, and 21, which account for approximately 2% of all AD cases. These mutations are seen primarily in early-onset patients with strong family histories of AD, and they tend to be transmitted in an autosomal dominant pattern. The gene for Alzheimer's precursor protein (APP) is coded on chromosome 21, and people with Down syndrome (trisomy-21) universally exhibit the microscopic pathology of AD as they age. The other two genes, on chromosomes 1 and 14, code for presinillins, which are thought to be involved in APP processing.

Late-onset AD is also thought to have a genetic component. The precise genetic contributions have not been defined, but part of this is attributable to the effects of polymorphisms in the APO E gene coded on chromosome 19. ApoE plays a role in redistribution of lipids associated with neurodegeneration, and promotes $A\beta$ deposition into plaque (see possible etiologies below). The gene has three major alleles, $\epsilon2$, $\epsilon3$, and $\epsilon4$, which code for the apo E2, E3, and E4 isoforms, respectively. The $\epsilon4$ allele has been found in up to 50% of AD patients, versus 16% of controls, and the rare $\epsilon2$ allele may be protective against illness development. A gene dosage effect exists, strengthening the association. Homozygosity for $\epsilon4$ conferred an eightfold increased risk over $\epsilon3/\epsilon3$, and a sixteenfold increased risk over $\epsilon2/\epsilon3$.

Alzheimer's Disease-Possible Etiologies Overproduction or decreased clearance of $A\beta$ (also called β-amyloid) is implicated as a central process in the pathophysiology of AD. $A\beta$ is formed by processing of APP via the β- and γ-secretase enzymes. $A\beta$ easily aggregates into β pleated sheets, which aggregate to form insoluble extracellular amyloid plaque. All the known familial mutations (discussed earlier) are associated with an increase in $A\beta$ production. APP can also be cleaved by the nonamyloidogenic α-secretase, which does not form toxic $A\beta$, and releases soluble APP into circulation.

The other neuropathologic hallmark of Alzheimer's disease is paired helical filaments of hyperphosphorylated τ (tau) seen in intracellular neurofibrillary tangles. τ is a central nervous system (CNS) protein that is involved in microtubular assembly. Microtubules are vital to normal neurotransport, and the abnormal τ interferes with that process.

Many neurochemical deficits are observed in AD, but abnormalities in the cholinergic system are most consistently described. Choline acetyltransferase activity is substantially reduced in patients with AD, and this has been confirmed on autopsy of patients with at least a moderate stage of the illness, but not in patients with mild illness.

Macroscopically, the brains of early AD patients may appear grossly normal. As the disease progresses, widened sulci and increased ventricular size are seen. Atrophy in the temporal, parietal, and frontal lobes is often most prominent. The atrophy is due to neuronal loss, with up to 10% of the large neocortical neurons lost, primarily in the frontal and temporal lobes.

Microscopically, the characteristic lesions of AD are amyloid plaques and neurofibrillary tangles. The early stages begin with relatively selective involvement of the entorhinal cortex and hippocampus. Later stages involve other areas of the limbic lobes and finally the neocortex. Plaque contains an amyloid core that is composed of β pleated sheets of the peptide $A\beta$. The central core is surrounded by dystrophic neuritis, microglial cells, and reactive astrocytes. Neurofibrillary tangles are intracellular inclusion bodies, containing paired helical filaments composed of abnormally phosphorylated tau. Plaques and tangles are not unique to AD and are observed in other illnesses, but the presence of the two together in abnormally high density is pathognomonic for AD.

Alzheimer's Disease-Management The two strategies that are currently used in the management of the cognitive decline in AD are replacement and neuroprotection. Replacement strategies focus on the neurochemical deficits in AD (such as acetylcholine), whereas neuroprotective strategies aim to retard the progression of the illness by slowing further neuronal injury or loss.

The only class of drugs currently FDA approved for the treatment of AD are the acetylcholinesterase inhibitors (AChEIs). These agents exemplify the replacement strategy because they decrease the breakdown of acetylcholine in the synapse, increasing the effective amount of acetylcholine (ACh) available. These medications are generally associated with a clinical improvement of approximately 6 to 12 months' duration. After this the patient continues to decline at a rate similar to that of untreated patients. The agents currently available are tacrine, donepezil, rivastigmine, and galantamine. Tacrine, the first medication approved by the FDA, is rarely used today because of its side effect profile (marked gastrointestinal (GI) disturbance, frequent liver function abnormalities). The common side effects of this class of medications include nausea and diarrhea, although with gradual titration they are usually mild.

The most commonly used agent for neuroprotective effect is vitamin E, probably for its antioxidant properties. Vitamin

E was shown in one double-blind randomized clinical trial to increase the time for moderate-stage patients to reach a poor outcome (i.e., loss of two or more activities of daily living, nursing home placement, or death), suggesting a slowing of illness progression.

Other Dementias   **Vascular dementia** is the second most common cause of dementia after AD. The symptomatology depends on the areas of infarction. Vascular dementia may be distinguished from AD by its relatively sudden onset, its focal neurologic signs, its history of stroke, and the likely presence of multiple risk factors for cerebrovascular disease.

Binswanger's disease, a vascular dementia, is characterized by microinfarctions of white matter with sparing of the cortex. It is a subcortical dementia with executive dysfunction, inattention, memory loss, slowed motor function, ataxia, incontinence, and loss of verbal fluency. Apathy, behavioral disturbance, and parkinsonian symptoms are also common findings.

Dementia with Lewy bodies (DLB) is a progressive dementia with parkinsonian symptoms, fluctuation in the level of attention and the severity of cognitive deficits and visual hallucinations. Delusions and sensitivity to the side effects of neuroleptic medications are common. The exact prevalence is unknown, but it may be the third most prevalent dementia. Lewy bodies are eosinophilic intracytoplasmic structures and are composed of ubiquitin or alpha-synuclein. The presence of Lewy bodies in AD portends a more malignant course.

Frontotemporal dementia includes a heterogeneous group of sporadic and familial diseases that result in personality and behavioral changes, with variable degrees of language and cognitive impairment, including Pick's disease, primary progressive aphasia, semantic dementia, and corticobasal degeneration. Frontotemporal dementias account for 5% to 20% of degenerative dementias. The age of onset ranges from 35 to 75 years. Pick's disease is characterized by Pick cells, which appear swollen and stain pink with hematoxylin-eosin.

AIDS dementia complex (ADC) is seen in patients with advanced AIDS and is associated with high viral load. Before the introduction of highly active antiretroviral therapies (HAART) ADC developed in 60% of patients. Now the incidence is less than 10% of AIDS patients. ADC is probably related to neuronal loss. The neuropathologic findings include diffuse inflammatory changes with microscopic foamy macrophages and multinucleated giant cells that invade subcortical white matter. ADC is characterized by cognitive decline and motor slowing, HIV is also associated with many CNS opportunistic infections.

Dementia due to Parkinson's disease occurs in 20% to 30% of patients. The typical age of onset of Parkinson's disease is 50 to 60 years. This dementia affects executive functioning and memory. Pathology reveals Lewy bodies in the cytoplasm of neurons in the substantia nigra.

Dementia due to Huntington's disease typically begins between the ages of 25 and 50 years. More trinucleotide repeats are correlated with earlier age of onset. Huntington's disease is transmitted in an autosomal dominant pattern with complete penetrance and results from an unstable trinucleotide repeat sequence (CAG) on chromosome 4. Damage occurs through neuronal loss in the caudate nucleus and putamen by an unknown mechanism.

Huntington's disease is characterized by psychiatric symptoms and cognitive impairment followed by the classic choreoathetoid movements. Psychopathology may include depression, psychosis, anxiety, and personality changes. Cognitive impairment is gradual and progressive. Initial symptoms may include mild memory deficits with subtle difficulty in executive functioning. Complex task performance worsens as the disease progresses, as do learning and verbal and visuospatial abilities.

Dementia due to Creutzfeldt-Jakob disease (CJD) occurs as a result of one of a group of rare but fatal neurodegenerative diseases. Transmissible spongiform encephalopathy results from CJD, Gerstmann-Straussler-Scheinker disease, fatal familial insomnia, bovine spongiform encephalopathy, and kuru. These diseases are caused by a *proteinaceous infectious particle,* or prion. Prions may incubate for decades before symptoms emerge. Transmission is through invasive body contact, such as corneal transplants, contaminated surgical instruments, cannibalism, or the ingestion of infected animal products. The infection produces a diffuse neurodegenerative process characterized by dementia, hypertonicity, and electroencephalographic changes. The progression is rapid, and death typically ensues within a year. Histopathology is diagnostic and shows neuronal loss, astrocyte proliferation, and a resultant spongiform appearance to the gray matter of the cortex, striatum, and thalamus. Creutzfeldt-Jakob disease is extremely rare.

Case Conclusion JD clearly has a dementia because he has difficulty with short-term memory, executive functioning, and mild difficulty with language. Given his negative work-up for other causes and his gradual and progressive course, his most likely diagnosis is Alzheimer's disease. He was treated with a cholinesterase inhibitor and vitamin E, which had a modest effect in improving his cognitive functioning. He and his family were encouraged to discuss health care proxy and advanced directives with their internist, and were referred to the Alzheimer's Association for more information about financial planning and support groups available in the community.

Thumbnail: Behavioral Science—Possible Etiologies of Dementia

Degenerative dementias	Alzheimer's disease Frontotemporal dementias (e.g., Pick's disease) Parkinson's disease Lewy body dementia Progressive supranuclear palsy
Cardiac/vascular/anoxia	Infarction Binswanger's disease Hemodynamic insufficiency (e.g., hypoxia, hypoperfusion)
Tumor	Primary or metastatic (e.g., meningioma, metastatic breast or lung cancer)
Trauma	For example, dementia pugilistica, subdural hematoma
Metabolic/nutritional	Vitamin deficiencies (e.g., vitamin B_{12}, folate) Endocrinopathies (e.g., hypothyroidism) Chronic metabolic disturbances (e.g., uremia)
Infection	Acquired immunodeficiency syndrome Neurosyphilis Prion diseases (e.g., Creutzfeldt-Jakob, bovine spongiform encephalitis)
Drugs/toxins	Alcohol Heavy metals Irradiation Pseudodementia due to medications

Key Points

Neuropathologic and neurochemical hallmarks of AD

▶ Plaque–extracellular, made primarily of Aβ, seen very early in the disease in the hippocampus.

▶ Tangles–intracellular dystrophic neuritis with paired helical filaments of hyperphosphorylated τ protein.

▶ As the disease progresses, atrophy and ventricular enlargement are seen.

▶ In moderate-stage disease or more advanced, a loss of cholinergic neurons and a decrease in choline acetyltransferase are seen on autopsy.

Genetics of AD

▶ Known mutations, usually associated with early-onset disease (<65) are on chromosomes 1, 14, and 21.

▶ The APO E gene has polymorphisms (ε2, ε3, ε4), which seem to modify risk of developing AD.

▶ The APO E–ε4 gene confers the greatest risk, whereas the ε2 gene may be protective.

Questions

Questions 1 and 2 relate to the following case:

WS is a 75-year-old woman who was brought in by her daughter for evaluation of her memory. She noted that her mother has been more forgetful over the past year but until recently had been paying her bills. Three months ago the daughter had gone to her house instead of meeting at a restaurant and was appalled at the stacks of papers, memberships, bills, and solicitations for contributions that were piled up on the desk. Since that time she has taken over financial management. She also noticed that her mother would repeat questions, forget conversations, and could no longer do the crossword puzzle.

1. Which of the following would be appropriate diagnostic tests?
   A. RPR, total body CT scan, TSH levels, vitamin K
   B. Vitamin C levels, RPR, MRI of the brain, TSH
   C. Vitamin B_{12} levels, RPR, MRI of the brain, TSH
   D. Total body CT scan, TSH, RPR, vitamin B_{12}
   E. Ceruloplasmin, RPR, MRI of the brain

2. She underwent all the appropriate testing above, as well as renal and hepatic function tests, a complete blood count, a physical and a neurologic exam, which were all unremarkable. Having ruled out other etiologies of dementia, she is presumed to have Alzheimer's disease. Which of the following statements is most likely true?
   A. She has a mutation on chromosome 1.
   B. She has a mutation on chromosome 21.
   C. She has an APOE-ε4 allele.
   D. She has an APOE-ε2 allele.
   E. She has trinucleotide repeats on chromosome 4.

3. An 85-year-old woman died of pneumonia. Her sons requested an autopsy because they wanted a definitive diagnosis of her 8-year history of memory loss. At the time of her death she was incontinent, needed assistance in all of her activities of daily living, often did not recognize her sons. Which of the following neuropathologic findings would confirm a diagnosis of Alzheimer's disease?
   A. Alpha-synuclein containing intracellular inclusion bodies
   B. Astrogliosis, neuronal loss, and spongiform change
   C. Ischemic periventricular leukoencephalopathy
   D. Increased choline acetyltransferase
   E. Intracellular paired helical filaments of hyperphosphorylated tau protein

4. An 83-year-old man has had a stroke. His symptoms include irritability, impulsivity with poor executive functioning, and a marked change in his personality. Which area of the brain does the stroke most likely affect?
   A. Frontal
   B. Temporal
   C. Occipital
   D. Parietal
   E. Brainstem

HPI: KR is a 22-year-old female college junior who is brought in to the student health service by her roommates because they found her superficially cutting her arms with a razor blade when they came home from a dinner. She told them that she was "fine," but they insisted on bringing her into urgent care. Upon questioning you find that she felt "lonely and empty" when her roommates went out together to a dinner and that cutting herself made her feel more "real." She denied current suicidal ideation, although she admitted to feeling suicidal in the past, with two overdoses at the time relationships were nearing an end. She took a leave of absence from college after the second suicide attempt. She returned to school 7 months ago. She admits that her relationships with friends and boyfriends are usually volatile, sometimes extremely close, sometimes with angry fights. She explains that it has been difficult because she has terrible troubles with self-image, can "never figure out who [she is]," and has had multiple problems with binge alcohol use, impulsive promiscuous sex, and binge eating and vomiting. She denies current bulimic behaviors. She has engaged in these self-mutilatory "cutting" behaviors since age 14. She was only in therapy once, briefly after the second suicide attempt.

Thought Questions

- What is the likely diagnosis of this woman?

- Does she meet criteria for a personality disorder?

Basic Science Review and Discussion

This woman meets criteria for borderline personality disorder. *Diagnostic and Statistical Manual of Mental Disorders,* 4th edition (text revision) (*DSM-IV*-TR), defines borderline personality disorder (BPD) as a pervasive pattern, beginning in early adulthood, of instability of interpersonal relationships, self-image, and affect, associated with marked impulsivity. It must be present in a variety of contexts and may include frantic efforts to avoid real or imagined abandonment, unstable self-image, reckless impulsivity (e.g., sex, substance abuse, binging), mood instability, recurrent suicidal or self-mutilatory behavior, chronic feelings of emptiness, inappropriate intense anger, marked swings in interpersonal relationships that swing from idealizing to devaluing, and transient stress-related paranoia or severe dissociation.

Personality disorders are by definition a pervasive maladaptive pattern of behaviors that begin in early adulthood and affect functioning. People with personality disorders do not necessarily see these symptoms/behaviors as an illness, or as alien to themselves, and therefore often do not seek treatment. Clearly, in the example above, the amount of pathology associated with some personality disorders brings the patient into contact with mental health care providers. In *DSM-IV* they are coded on Axis II.

In general there are three clusters of personality disorders as defined by the *DSM-IV*. Cluster A, the "odd" cluster, is comprised of paranoid, schizoid, and schizotypal personality disorders. This cluster is characterized by disturbance of interpersonal relatedness and cognitive function. Cluster B, the "dramatic" cluster, consists of histrionic, narcissistic, borderline, and antisocial personality disorders. It is characterized by disturbance of affective stability and impulsivity, with dramatic emotional expressiveness. Cluster C, the "anxious" cluster, is avoidant, dependent, and obsessive-compulsive personality disorders. It is characterized by the constriction of assertiveness and sociability in the service of avoiding anxiety.

Borderline Personality Disorder The cluster B disorders are associated with the greatest morbidity and mortality. There are various theories about the pathogenesis of personality disorders and various theories by which to understand them. (Adapted from Kaplan and Sadock 2001 Ch 24.) Psychoanalytic theory (especially Otto Kernberg) describes borderline personality structure as characterized by ego weakness (lack of impulse control, lack of anxiety tolerance, blurred self—other boundaries, occasional distorted reality testing), problematic object relations (seeing the same "object" as all good or all bad), immature defense mechanisms (e.g., splitting), and a fragmentary self-concept. These are seen at various immature phases of normal development, but in personality disorders they persist. The psychobiological approach sees personality disorders as an interaction of temperament (which has a strong genetic component) with character (which is formed more by family and other environmental influences). Family life and other environmental influences help form character, which allows the person, with his or her own unique temperament, to interact with the world. Thus a person who is quite impulsive and novelty seeking could either be self-directed and cooperative and become a successful entrepreneur or be goal-less, undisciplined, and uncooperative, and end up with a personality disorder. Studies show that maturation increases self-directedness and cooperation, leading to a decline in impulsivity and "acting out" with age.

Impulsive Aggression A common component of many of the cluster B personality disorders is impulsive aggression. It is important to understand that impulsive aggression, whether self- or other-directed, is associated with decreased serotonergic activity, as reflected in reduced cerebrospinal fluid (CSF) 5-hydroxy indoleacetic acid (5-HIAA), and reduced prefrontal metabolic activity in response to serotonergic agents. The prefrontal cortex is implicated in aggression, as was seen by the famous case of Phineas Gage, who was a calm, capable, and efficient person who became irascible and impulsive following injury to the orbital frontal cortex (in a freak accident on a railroad construction site that left him with a tamping iron blown through his head).

Epidemiology/Course Borderline personality disorder occurs in 2% to 3% of the general population. The M:F ratio is 1:3. It is five times more common in first-degree relatives than in the general population. The mortality is approximately 10%. The course often shows greatest instability and impulsivity in early adult years, often improving in the 30s and 40s. It is also associated with physical or sexual abuse in childhood. The morbidity of this disorder is high, because of associated behaviors and disorders, such as impulsive promiscuity, reckless behaviors, substance use, depression, bulimia, other self-destructive or self-mutilatory behaviors, suicidality, and suicidal attempts.

Treatment Medications may be useful in borderline or other personality disorders. In general, they are used to treat some of the comorbid Axis I disorders. Some core symptoms of disorders may respond to medication. For instance, the impulsive aggression in borderline and antisocial personalities may respond to selective serotonergic reuptake inhibitors (SSRIs). In general, cognitive and behavioral approaches are often useful, as is group therapy. Since these are personality constructs, the support, reflection, and confrontation by other group members may be particularly useful. In borderline personality disorders various individual and group methods have been used to help patients find alternative ways to deal with feelings of emptiness, abandonment, depression, or anger rather than substance use or self-mutilation.

Case Conclusion KR meets criteria for borderline personality disorder. She denies current Axis I symptoms of major depression or an eating disorder. Because of her history of binging and vomiting, you check her electrolytes, which are within normal limits; she has no other stigmata of bulimia (e.g., parotid enlargement) and is of normal weight. Her cuts are superficial and do not require suturing. While she is in the emergency room, she is labeled as a "difficult patient," as she is somewhat seductive and idealizing of the medical student who examined her wrist and hostile and devaluing to the nurse and the emergency room resident. You note this behavior, evaluate her, and talk to her about her experiences and behaviors but decide not to admit her. She agrees to come in the following day to begin outpatient cognitive behavioral therapy.

Thumbnail: Behavioral Science—Review of Personality Disorders

Cluster	Disorder	Features	Epidemiology	Comments
Cluster A	Paranoid	Suspiciousness over interpreting others' motivations or actions	0.5% to 2.5% of the population M> F	Experience of their paranoid symptoms as ego syntonic (part of who they are), thus rarely seek treatment
	Schizoid	Detached, restricted range of affect; disinterest in social relationships	0.5% to 7% of the population Possibly M > F Possible family association with schizophrenia	Experience of their symptoms as ego syntonic
	Schizotypal	Discomfort with and reduced capacity for close relationships, cognitive and perceptual aberrations, behavioral eccentricities	General population: approximately 3% Possibly M > F Increased in families of schizophrenics, and increased risk of schizophrenia in families with schizotypal personality disorder (PD)	Correlates of central nervous system dysfunction in schizophrenia seen in schizotypal PD, including tests of visual and auditory attention and smooth pursuit eye movement
Cluster B	Histrionic	Excessive emotionality; attention seeking; sometimes seductive, shallow, theatrical, speech may be vague or impressionistic	2% to 3% of the general population, much higher in psychological and medical samples Diagnosed in F > M	May have a higher rate of somatic complaints, depression, and substance abuse
	Narcissistic	Grandiosity; need for admiration; lack of empathy; interpersonally exploitative, envious, arrogant	<1% of the general population; 2% to 16% of psychiatric clinical populations. M > F.	Associated with devaluing parenting. Sense of worth contingent upon accomplishment. Increased risk of depression, rage, or paranoia with injury to self-image.
	Borderline	Instability of interpersonal relationships, self-image, and affect; associated with marked impulsivity	General population: 2% to 3% M:F = 1:3	Associated with physical or sexual abuse. Associated with substance use, suicide (approximately 9%), depression, eating disorders.
	Antisocial	Disregard for and violation of rights of others. Lying, illegal behavior, impulsivity, aggressive, remorseless.	Rate in prison 20% to 50%. General population: 3% of men, 1% of women. Possible genetic predisposition.	Childhood: physical or sexual abuse or neglect, empathy and warmth discouraged or punished. Associated with substance abuse, depression.
Cluster C	Avoidant	Social inhibition, feeling inadequate, hypersensitive to criticism. Avoiding people or occupational pursuits because of feeling inadequate.	0.5% to 1% of the population M:F = 1:1	Intense desire for acceptance. Overlap with social phobia.
	Dependent	Need to be taken care of, clingy, fear of separation, need for constant reassurance, helpless	Two percent to 3% of the population. Seen frequently in psychology medical settings because seeking help and support. Possibly F > M	Intense need for relationships and social approval. Treatment to help assertiveness. Associated with depression and anxiety disorders.
	Obsessive-compulsive	Preoccupation with orderliness, perfectionism, inflexibility, control	1% in the general population M> F Not significantly associated with OCD	May view their symptoms as positive. No intrusive obsessions or ego dystonic compulsions. May be self-critical and lack social closeness and therefore may have increased depression.

Key Points

- The cluster A disorders may have the strongest genetic components, and schizoptypal PD may have the greatest genetic relationship to an Axis I disorder (schizophrenia).
- The cluster B disorders are associated with the greatest morbidity and mortality, especially borderline and antisocial personality disorders.
- Some personality disorders are significantly associated with childhood trauma or neglect (e.g., borderline and antisocial).

- Borderline and histrionic PD are diagnosed in more women than men.
- Narcissistic, antisocial, and probably paranoid and obsessive-compulsive personality disorders are seen more frequently in men.

Questions

1. DP is a 33-year-old man who is seen for an initial appointment for routine health maintenance. He comes in with a large folder in which his daily activities and diet are catalogued, along with his immunization history and record of all doctors appointments that he has had since college. He reports that he has always been organized and it is one of the things he likes most about himself. He is self-employed as a computer programmer and cites the disorder and lack of rational structure in offices as the reason he works on his own. He admits that the environment in the office at his last job made him anxious. He has few relationships and he admits to being "a bit controlling." His most likely diagnosis is
   A. Avoidant personality disorder
   B. Antisocial personality disorder
   C. Obsessive-compulsive personality disorder
   D. Schizoid personality disorder
   E. Obsessive-compulsive disorder

2. GR is a 39-year-old single female who comes in for a routine checkup because her astrologer told her that there was an excess of gamma and microwaves that she should be concerned about. She has few close social contacts or friends. She spends some time with a group of people with whom she discusses numerology and astrology. Her work history is somewhat checkered, because after working in a place for a while she usually has some conflict with the other staff or management and feels singled out. She often feels that things are indirectly giving her messages (e.g., hearing a specific song while on a bus and knowing that it is a sign she should look for a job in the neighborhood of the next stop). She has no significant medical history, complaints, physical or lab findings. Which of the following is probably true?
   A. She is no more likely to have a family member with schizophrenia than the general population.
   B. She may have abnormalities in smooth pursuit eye tracking.
   C. She has more than a 50% chance of developing schizophrenia.
   D. She probably sees her beliefs as being odd and not compatible with her self-image.
   E. This disorder is seen predominantly in women.

3. ZC is a 56-year-old businessman who comes in for treatment of depression after being downsized from his company. Before seeing you he tells you that he was referred by the chairman of another department and plays golf with a vice president of the hospital. He also confirms your academic rank and membership on the board of a local philanthropic organization. In your evaluation you find that he has been downsized because his division did not weather the recession and that it was probably due to some poor management decisions on his part. He is furious and is convinced that it is their fault and that they will call him back. He seems to lack empathy and in many of his stories comes across as being arrogant and exploitative. Which of the following is probably true?
   A. This disorder is seen in women more frequently than men.
   B. This man probably has histrionic personality disorder.
   C. This man probably has no difficulty accepting feedback.
   D. This man probably has no difficulty in sustaining long-term intimate relationships.
   E. His feelings of insecurity may be masked by arrogance.

4. NF is a 45-year-old man who has been running a prostitution and drug ring from his suburban home, where his wife and two young children also live. As a younger man he abused substances, was expelled from high school for selling homework answers and marijuana, and tried to put the responsibility on his friend, who was actually uninvolved. He also had stolen various things as a child, and although he wasn't caught, he "borrowed" cars frequently and actually crashed two or three of them. He also frequently got into physical fights and at times had hit his wife. He laughs when he tells you about some of his exploits and how various people got hurt in the process. His wife apparently thought he was doing direct marketing and called the police when she found a crate of semiautomatic weapons in the basement. Which of the following is true?
   A. This disorder is seen in 90% of prison inmates.
   B. This disorder is seen in 3% of men.
   C. This disorder has no association with childhood abuse or neglect.
   D. This disorder is more common in women than men.
   E. This disorder has diagnostic EEG findings.

HPI: FS is a 39-year-old single female who is trained as an LPN but is currently working as an office clerk. She has had multiple hospitalizations for infections in her left foot and has been delirious on a number of occasions with bacteremia. She has had some odd pathogens colonize her foot, including *Enterobacter.* She has been to a number of hospitals in the area. Because her course has been so difficult to manage, you mention this patient to an infectious disease colleague, who says that she saw her at another hospital and was convinced that she was either retarding the healing process or actively infecting the wound. The patient has no reason (i.e., financial or legal) to be producing her symptoms.

Thought Questions

- What is this woman's likely disorder?
- What is the difference between malingering and factitious disorder?

Basic Science Review and Discussion

Some patients exaggerate or produce physical or psychiatric symptoms. This may be for a number of reasons, including financial gain (feigning a back injury to collect workers' compensation), avoiding legal responsibilities (feigning suicidality or psychosis to avoid prison time), getting drugs (feigning severe pain to get narcotics), and so on. When there is a clear secondary gain, this behavior comes under the diagnostic heading of malingering.

There is another, more psychologically complex reason that people exaggerate or produce physical or psychiatric symptoms, and this is to assume the sick role. Someone might do this for a number of theoretical reasons. People who are sick are excused from many of society's obligations. Illness may get others to nurture. People with a poorly defined sense of self may feel more in control in the well-defined role of a patient. Abusive inadequate parenting may lead to associating nurturing with pain and feeling deserving of abuse.

Many presentations exist, ranging from misrepresenting medical history, exercising or drinking hot beverages to affect vital signs, producing infections (e.g., by injecting or rubbing feces on a wound or into a line), taking medications to produce laboratory abnormalities (e.g., insulin, diuretics), and so on.

The prevalence of factitious disorder is approximately 1% of psychological consultations and 4% to 10% of fevers of unknown origin. It is most prevalent in single, unemployed, estranged middle-aged men and women in their 20s to 40s who have some medical experience (e.g., nursing). Comorbid personality disorders are common and are usually in cluster B (most frequently borderline personality disorder).

Münchausen's by proxy (in which symptoms are caused in another, usually a child) tends to be seen in women with young children who have engaged in factitious behaviors before. There is obviously a significant morbidity and mortality in those children associated with the behaviors. Approximately 10% die before reaching adulthood. Symptoms may be produced by the surreptitious administration of laxatives or diuretics, apnea due to smothering, and so on. The perpetrators are usually extremely involved in the hospital care and are happy to sign consent for multiple invasive procedures. Mysteriously, the children do better when the mother is absent. In the last few years, videotapes were made of women smothering their children with pillows in the hospital to simulate apneic events. Because of the risk to the child and to other children in the family, these cases must be referred to social services, and the children should be placed outside the home.

Treatment Of course the first step in treatment is to investigate and treat any underlying physical disorder. Often people with factitious disorders do have real medical concerns as well. There may also be comorbid psychiatric disorders, including mood or psychotic disorders. These must be evaluated and treated as well.

There is no proven treatment for factitious disorder. Medication is not useful in factitious disorder itself. Cognitive behavioral therapy has not been studied. Supportive therapy to address issues in day-to-day life, without colluding in the factitious disorder may help. A team approach may decrease splitting and foster open discussion of the emotional, ethical, and legal issues associated with taking care of these complex patients.

Case Conclusion   You find yourself angry at the patient for having induced the symptoms. Therefore the following day you confront her with the evidence. She becomes very guarded and the following day leaves the hospital against medical advice. You decide to hold an interdisciplinary case conference to think through alternate ways of managing a patient like this, and managing the attendant frustrations and anger that she evoked. She certainly is someone at risk for considerable morbidity and even mortality. In the conference your consensus recommendations include that she should have been treated by a team, in a supportive, nonconfrontational environment while the medical condition is under treatment. A patient like this should be offered ways to save face (i.e., ways to relinquish the symptoms without having to admit to it directly) and some supportive psychotherapy. If she were felt to be a significant danger to herself, she might well require an inpatient psychiatric hospitalization, where these symptoms and behaviors could be further evaluated.

Thumbnail: Behavioral Science—Sick Role

Disorder	Description
Somatization	Multiple physical complaints in multiple body areas requiring medical evaluation, tests, and interventions. Symptoms are not deliberately produced.
Somatiform pain	Pain in one or more sites that warrants clinical attention, and significant distress, but psychological factors are thought to have a significant role in the onset, severity, or maintenance of the symptoms. But the symptom is not intentionally caused or feigned.
Hypochondriasis	Preoccupation with health concerns, belief that one has a serious illness, despite appropriate evaluation and work-up, but with no delusions.
Body dysmorphic	Preoccupation that some aspect of one's bodily appearance is grossly abnormal.
Conversion	Symptoms affecting motor or sensory function, not caused by a neurologic or medical problem, and not created intentionally. Psychological concerns are judged to be important in the onset or maintenance of the symptom.
Factitious	Relating to the intentional production of symptoms or signs for the purpose of assuming the sick role
Münchausen's	An eponym for severe factitious disorder
Münchausen's by proxy	The feigning of symptoms in another (usually a child by a parent) for the purpose of assuming the sick role
Malingering	Intentional production of symptoms or signs for the purpose of financial gain or avoidance of legal responsibility

Key Points

▶ Physical or psychiatric symptoms can be exhibited by patients for numerous reasons.

▶ Patients frequently somatize their psychological distress, and 25% of patients in primary care are thought to have some somatization.

▶ If the symptoms are created unconsciously, they are considered in the realm of somatization disorders. These include somatization disorder, conversion disorder, somatiform pain disorder, hypochondriasis, and body dysmorphic disorder.

▶ If the symptoms are created consciously to assume the sick role, they are factitious disorders. These include factitious disorder and Münchausen's by proxy.

▶ If the symptoms are created consciously for a secondary gain (e.g., financial or legal), then they fall under the heading of malingering.

Questions

1. IJ is a 58-year-old man who presents to the emergency room late on a Saturday night complaining of a variety of odd symptoms, including intermittent fevers and diarrhea. He states that he has a rare immune disease and has recently returned from a remote tropical region and is concerned that he has been exposed to an infectious agent. He regales the staff with interesting tales of his journeys and experiences in the military. He is fairly vague about the details of his life and has no visitors. Over the following weeks he undergoes multiple diagnostic procedures, including colonoscopies and biopsies. He continues to have intermittent spiking fevers and diarrhea. One day the medical student notes that a box of laxatives is half covered by his sheets. The temperature spikes seem to coincide with meals, at which he always gets tea. Which of the following is probably true?
   A. This man probably has somatization disorder.
   B. SSRIs are the treatment of choice for him.
   C. The best course of action is to stage an "intervention" and confront him with all of your suspicions.
   D. He most likely has factitious disorder.
   E. He is most likely malingering.

Questions 2 to 4 relate to the following case:

VO is a 45-year-old woman who has had a more than 20-year history of multiple medical problems, for which she has seen multiple doctors and had many different opinions and treatments. She has had a number of different pain syndromes, including migraines, backaches, abdominal and menstrual pain, for which she has seen numerous doctors and had many laboratory tests, even including a laparoscopy to evaluate possible endometriosis. All tests were negative. She also complains of nausea and bloating, and has had tests for this condition, including a barium swallow and an endoscopy. She has irregular menses. Recently she has gone to her neurologist because she has had localized weakness and loss of sensation in one hand. She is currently scheduled for an MRI of her neck and an EMG of her arm. Because of these problems, she has had to take significant time off from work, and her career has suffered. For the most part her work-ups have been negative, although she has had some significant side effects from some of the treatments.

2. This patient has a somatizing disorder (one in which psychological distress is manifested physically). Which of the following is her likely diagnosis?
   A. Conversion disorder
   B. Factitious disorder
   C. Hypochondriasis
   D. Body dysmorphic disorder
   E. Somatization disorder

3. In general, which is the correct pairing of illness and something that might help understand someone with that disorder?
   A. Somatization disorder—Physical illness may be more stigmatizing than psychiatric illness.
   B. Factitious disorder—Directly motivated by the desire to avoid incarceration.
   C. Malingering—Illness may be unconsciously associated with being taken care of.
   D. Factitious disorder—Illness may work unconsciously to bring a socially isolated person into contact with support systems.
   E. Somatization disorder—Financial gain.

4. Given the fact that this patient has a somatizing disorder, which of the following is true about treatment?
   A. Once the diagnosis is made, no further invasive tests should be done.
   B. Once the diagnosis is made there is no need to look for comorbid psychiatric disorders.
   C. Confronting the patient by explaining that the symptoms are "in your head" is a good way to help the patient stop somatizing.
   D. Patients with this disorder are at risk for iatrogenic complications.
   E. Once the diagnosis is made, the physician should never refer the patient to a specialist.

HPI: LD is a 19-year-old single, white male, second-semester college junior who presents to the university student health clinic one evening because he is afraid that someone is trying to make him fail out of school. He describes that last spring his roommate Jim joined the chess club, and since the beginning of this year Jim and three other members are plotting to make him fail in school. He is very worried because second-semester midterms have just been returned and he did much more poorly than previously. He attributes this to two things. One is his inability to concentrate due to the constant plotting by these four boys, talking behind his back, telling the dining hall workers and the campus police about him. The other is the constant net of people watching him and reporting back to Jim. He describes that he can tell by certain gestures that people make (e.g., the way they look at their watches) whether they are looking out for him or reporting on him. He notes that this has been happening all year but has gotten worse. He tried to tell his RA a little about his concerns, but when she gently suggested that his roommate would have no reason to make him fail, he ended the conversation.

Thought Questions

- Define the types of symptoms that he is manifesting.

- What other symptoms should you look for?

- What is in the differential diagnosis of psychotic symptoms?

Basic Science Review and Discussion

LD is exhibiting a number of symptoms that are commonly seen in psychotic disorders. The most prominent ones in his presentation are delusions and ideas of reference.

- *Delusions: paranoid type.* A delusion is a fixed false belief. LD believes that people are plotting against him (and that some are "looking out" for him). Delusions may be of many types (e.g., delusions of grandeur, in which the person believes that he or she possesses exaggerated power, importance, knowledge, or ability; or erotic delusions—that someone is in love with him or her).

- *Ideas of reference.* A delusional belief that media content, gestures, or other unrelated information is about oneself. LD believes that when people check the time, they are actually sending him messages.

There are many other symptoms that are associated with psychotic illness (see Table 31-1). These include **hallucinations,** which are false sensory perceptions that can be in any sensory modality. Auditory hallucinations are the most common. Hallucinations must be differentiated from **illusions,** which are misinterpretations of a real sensory experience. **Hypnagogic hallucinations** are disorders of perception occurring in a semiconscious state while going to sleep; **hypnapompic hallucinations** are disorders of perception occurring in a semiconscious state upon awakening.

Thought disorder is another important sign associated with psychotic illness. This may come in various forms, including the following:

- **Incoherence**—thinking processes so disrupted that they do not result in a complete idea. The most severe form is *word salad,* in which words are strung together in an apparently unrelated fashion.

- **Loosening of associations**—idiosyncratic switching from topic to topic, a lack of logical relationships between contiguous thoughts or ideas.

- **Neologisms**—newly invented words.

- **Poverty of content**—decreased content of speech, which may be a negative symptom of schizophrenia.

- **Thought blocking**—sudden cessation in a train of thought that is unexplainable to a patient.

- **Thought broadcasting**—the belief that others can hear or read one's thoughts.

- **Thought insertion**—the belief that others can insert thoughts into one's mind.

Schizophrenia—Epidemiology The prevalence of schizophrenia is 1%. Schizophrenics are more commonly born in the winter months, whether in the Northern or Southern Hemisphere. This suggests that there may be an association with viral infection or other intrauterine exposure during pregnancy. One epidemiologic study in Scandinavia associated an increase in the number of births of schizophrenics in a year of an influenza epidemic. Approximately 50% of monozygotic and 15% of dizygotic twins are concordant for schizophrenia.

The peak age of onset for schizophrenia is 15 to 25 in males and 25 to 35 in females. Good prognostic signs are associated with good interpersonal functioning, acute onset, and older age at onset. People with schizophrenia are at increased risk for suicide. Approximately 25% to 50% will attempt suicide, and about 10% will die from suicide. Risk factors for suicide include previous attempts and being male, being young, being hopeless [especially in the context of lost expectations (e.g., college education and significant ambitions)], having multiple relapses, suffering from depressed mood, living alone, and engaging in substance use.

Table 31-1. Psychiatric Illnesses with Psychotic Symptoms

Delusional disorder	Nonbizarre delusions (such as being followed or deceived), lasting for at least a month, and apart from the ramification of the delusion, no marked effect on functioning.
Schizophrenia	Positive symptoms (bizarre delusions, auditory hallucinations, disorganized behavior) or negative symptoms (flat affect, avolition [lack of motivation], anhedonia [lack of enjoyment], social withdrawal, poverty of speech) lasting for more than 6 months. Associated with significant social or occupational impairment.
Brief psychotic disorder	Psychotic symptoms lasting 1 day to 1 month, often precipitated by significant life stressors.
Schizophreniform disorder	Symptoms of schizophrenia, but lasting 1 to 6 months.
Schizoaffective disorder	In this disorder major depressive, manic, or mixed episodes occur concurrently with active symptoms of schizophrenia, but there must be at least 2 weeks with delusions/hallucinations without prominent mood symptoms.
Bipolar disorder, manic with psychotic symptoms	Criteria for mania (see Case 21), including increased energy, decreased need for sleep, racing thoughts, with hallucinations and/or delusions. Delusions are usually mood congruent (e.g., delusions of omnipotence or grandeur).
Major depression with psychotic symptoms	Criteria for major depression (see Case 20), including depressed mood, decreased energy, appetite, concentration, change in sleep associated with hallucinations and/or delusions. Delusions are usually mood congruent (e.g., delusions of having a fatal illness).
Psychotic symptoms due to substance use or underlying medical condition	In this disorder major depressive, manic, or mixed episodes occur concurrently with active symptoms of schizophrenia, but there must be at least 2 weeks with delusions/hallucinations without prominent mood symptoms.

Case Conclusion On further examination, LD admits that over the past 6 months he has been hearing a male voice, which at first was just warning him about people's motivations, but recently has also been commenting on his actions. He denies substance use or abuse, and his urine toxicology is negative. His family history is significant for a maternal great uncle who had "odd beliefs," was a "loner," and was never steadily employed. His physical and neurologic examination is unremarkable, as were his laboratory tests. Given his symptoms of paranoid delusions, auditory hallucinations, and ideas of reference associated with social withdrawal and decline in his school performance, lasting for 6 months, this young man most likely is experiencing a first break of schizophrenia.

With the encouragement of the school and his family, LD takes a medical leave of absence from school. He is started on an atypical antipsychotic, which he tolerates well and which reduces his paranoid ideation and hallucinations.

Thumbnail: Behavioral Science—Differential Diagnosis of Schizophrenia

	Duration of Psychotic Symptoms	**Course**	**Comments**
Schizophrenia	> 6 months	Relapsing/chronic	Must have two or more of the following: delusions, hallucinations, disorganized speech, disorganized behavior, negative symptoms (e.g., avolition, flat affect), with significant social and/or occupational dysfunction
Schizophreniform disorder	1 to 6 months	Single episode	Clinical criteria for schizophrenia but not long enough duration.
Schizoaffective disorder	≥ 2 weeks of psychosis without mood symptoms	Relapsing	Must both have concurrent major mood disorder and meet criteria for schizophrenia, as well as have the psychotic symptoms in absence of the mood symptoms.
Delusional disorder	≥ 1 month	Usually, gradual onset, chronic	Apart from the impact of the delusions, behavior or functioning is not affected.
Brief psychotic disorder	1 day to 1 month	After the episode, return to premorbid functioning	Often in response to a significant stressor
Major depression with psychotic symptoms	> 2 weeks	Episodic	Psychotic symptoms only in context of major depression
Mania with psychotic symptoms	> 1 week	Episodic	Psychotic symptoms only in context of mania

Key Points

The *Diagnostic and Statistical Manual of Mental Disorders,* 4th edition (text revision) (*DSM-IV*-TR) criteria for schizophrenia include characteristic symptoms, such as delusions, hallucinations, disorganized speech, grossly disorganized or catatonic behavior, and negative symptoms. These symptoms must persist for at least 1 month (6 months, including prodromal or residual deficits) and lead to significant social or occupational dysfunction. These symptoms cannot be caused by a substance or underlying medical condition.

▶ Positive symptoms of schizophrenia

   ▶ Hallucinations (most frequently auditory but can be in any modality)

   ▶ Delusions (paranoid, jealous, religious, somatic, grandiose, thought broadcasting, thought insertion, etc.)

▶ Bizarre behavior (inappropriate clothing, appearance, agitated or stereotyped repetitive behaviors)

▶ Formal thought disorder (tangentiality, circumstantiality, incoherence, distractible speech, etc.)

▶ Negative symptoms of schizophrenia

   ▶ Avolition (reduction or inability in initiating and persisting in goal-directed behavior)

   ▶ Alogia (an impoverishment in thinking, poverty of content of speech)

   ▶ Affective flattening (unchanging facial expression, decreased spontaneity, poor eye contact, lack of vocal inflections)

   ▶ Anhedonia (lack of pleasure in anything, including recreational, social activities, and intimate or peer relationships)

Questions

Questions 1 and 2 refer to the following case:

SJ is an 18-year-old with a 6-month history of bizarre delusions about religious figures and rock stars. Two months ago she lost her job in a fast-food restaurant because she was chronically late and was unable to complete the tasks assigned to her. She admits to some auditory hallucinations and has become disheveled, refuses to bathe, and wears odd combinations of clothes that she has found on the street.

1. Which of the following is true about the epidemiology of schizophrenia?
   A. Schizophrenics are more commonly born during the summer months.
   B. The worldwide prevalence of schizophrenia is 1%.
   C. Eighty percent of monozygotic twins are concordant for this disease.
   D. Fifty percent of dizygotic twins are concordant for the illness.
   E. First-degree relatives have the same prevalence of schizophrenia as the general population.

2. Which of the following subtype of schizophrenia does this patient probably have?
   A. Catatonic
   B. Disorganized
   C. Grandiose
   D. Residual
   E. Paranoid

3. FR is a 21-year-old man recently diagnosed with schizophrenia, after a year of gradually increasing paranoid behavior, lining his hats with tinfoil to protect him from "rays" (i.e., ideas of reference about TV newsmen relaying messages to him from aliens) and auditory hallucinations commenting on his actions. With his permission you agree to speak to his parents about their concerns. Which of the following is consistent with the course of schizophrenia?
   A. This patient will not likely have a chronic course.
   B. Seventy-five percent of patients will have remission or very mild symptoms.
   C. About 50% of patients with schizophrenia will attempt suicide.
   D. This patient will most likely return to college and do as well as he did before the onset of his symptoms.
   E. About 75% of patients will have a severe debilitating course.

4. PD is a 45-year-old male with a 20-year history of schizophrenia. His symptoms are currently well controlled with medications. His elder sister comes with him for a medication visit and they reminisce about what he was like before his first episode. Which of the following symptoms is consistent with prodromal schizophrenia?
   A. Auditory hallucinations
   B. Grossly disorganized thought process
   C. Paranoid delusions
   D. Social withdrawal
   E. Thought broadcasting

HPI: JL is a 19-year-old single, white male, college junior whom you saw yesterday in the student health service and diagnosed with a first episode of schizophrenia, with auditory hallucination, paranoid delusions, and ideas of reference. You decided to hospitalize him, which made him feel much safer, and told him you would start him on medications in the morning. You are the attending physician on the psychiatry service, and during morning rounds you sit down with the medical students to review certain things about the etiologic theories of schizophrenia and pharmacologic options. You review these theories and then go to the nursing report, in which the night nurse describes the patients' status overnight. She tells you that JL had been quite agitated and the resident on call prescribed a dose of haloperidol and that the patient required another dose this morning. When you and the team go to see him, his neck is stiff and turned to one side. He states that he is not sure how this happened but he is quite uncomfortable. He is also having difficulty moving his eyes. His vital signs are normal, as is the rest of his physical exam.

Thought Questions

- What neurotransmitter abnormalities are thought to be associated with schizophrenia?

- What has happened to this young man?

- What kinds of medications are used for schizophrenia? What differentiates antipsychotics?

Basic Science Review and Discussion

Neurotransmitter Abnormalities in Schizophrenia   A number of hypotheses related to major neurotransmitter systems have been set forth to explain the symptoms of schizophrenia. The three major theories relate to dopamine, serotonin, and glutamate.

The Dopamine Hypothesis of Schizophrenia   Schizophrenics have too much dopamine, especially in the striatum and limbic system, and this is responsible for the positive symptoms of schizophrenia. Many of these symptoms are mimicked by giving large doses of amphetamines, which cause dopamine release. Traditional antipsychotics act by blocking dopamine receptors, particularly the D2 receptor, in the brain. This model is overly simplistic, as negative symptoms seem to be associated with a hypodopaminergic state in the prefrontal cortex.

The Serotonin Hypothesis   Because lysergic acid diethylamide (LSD), a serotonin (5-HT) postsynaptic agonist, causes hallucinations, some suggested that there is a relationship between serotonin and schizophrenia. Serotonin is implicated in many behaviors, including cognition, pain sensitivity, mood, impulsivity, aggression, and sexual drive. Alterations in serotonergic functioning affect multiple neurotransmitter systems (including dopamine, glutamate, gamma aminobutyric acid [GABA], and norepinephrine). There is now considerable evidence that the atypical antipsychotic drugs, such as clozapine, olanzapine, quetiapine, risperidone, sertindole, and ziprasidone, are more effective than the older medications, and they are all antagonists of the 5-HT$_{2A}$ receptor. In fact, although most of them have some activity as D2 antagonists, they are much more potent at the 5-HT$_{2A}$ receptor.

The Glutamate Hypothesis   The glutamate hypothesis proposes a hypofunctional glutamate system in schizophrenia. The origins of the glutamate hypothesis of schizophrenia can be traced to the observations that the dissociative anesthetic ketamine, which is similar to phencyclidine (PCP), produced psychotic symptoms in a subgroup of surgical patients. This continues to be under investigation.

Neurotransmitters in Schizophrenia, Anatomic Location, and Metabolic Pathways   *Dopamine* is a catecholamine. Dopamine cell bodies are found in the substantia nigra (SN) and the ventral tegmental area (VTA). The VTA sends its axons to the prefrontal cortex (implicated in attention and working memory) and the nucleus accumbens (associated with motivation). The SN projects to the striatum (associated with motor function) (see Figure 32-1).

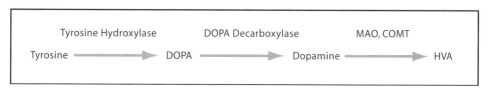

Figure 32-1: Dopamine—metabolic pathway

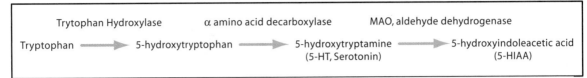

Figure 32-2: Seratonin—metabolic pathway

Serotonin is an indolamine. Serotonin cell bodies are primarily found in the raphe nuclei. Most areas of the brain receive at least some serotonergic innervation (see Figure 32-2).

Glutamate is an excitatory amino acid neurotransmitter. Glutamate is the major excitatory neurotransmitter in the central nervous system and the glutamate receptors play a vital role in the mediation of excitatory synaptic transmission. It is synthesized either from α-ketoglutarate via an aminotransferase or from glutamine via glutaminase.

Antipsychotic Medications and Their Side Effects This patient is having a dystonic reaction to haloperidol. Dystonic reactions are either spasmodic or sustained involuntary contractions of muscles in the face, neck, trunk, or extremities. They are very uncomfortable and often produce significant distress. Treatment with anticholinergic agents such as benztropine (Cogentin) or diphenhydramine (Benadryl) is extremely effective, and the symptoms resolve within minutes. The reaction is more common in young male patients and with high-potency drugs such as haloperidol. The usual etiology is nigrostriatal dopamine D2 receptor blockade leading to an increase in striatal cholinergic output. You explain this to him and give him an injection of benztropine, which results in rapid resolution of his dystonia. He asks you what kind of medication you suggest to help him feel "less upset" about the incessant voices and his anxiety related to his belief of being persecuted.

There are two broad classes of antipsychotic medications. One is the *typical,* or conventional, antipsychotic; the other is the *atypical,* or "second-generation," antipsychotic. Typical antipsychotics have their primary site of action at the D2 dopamine receptor. Examples include haloperidol, chlorpromazine, and perphenazine. They are usually classified by their potency, which reflects both the dosage used to have an effect and their side effect profile. In general, the high-potency medications (e.g., haloperidol) are less sedating and less anticholinergic but cause more extrapyramidal (parkinsonian) symptoms. The low-potency medications (e.g., chlorpromazine) are more sedating and anticholinergic but cause fewer extrapyramidal symptoms.

Atypical antipsychotics usually have antagonistic actions at a number of receptors, including 5-HT_{2A}, dopamine D4, and some D2. As a rule they are better tolerated, cause fewer extrapyramidal side effects, and are less likely to cause a dystonic reaction. They still may be associated with sedation, weight gain, orthostasis. Examples of medications in this class include risperidone, olanzapine, and clozapine.

Another common side effect of the typical antipsychotics and of risperidone is an increase in prolactin levels, caused by the dopamine blockade, which can result in galactorrhea, breast enlargement, amenorrhea, and sexual dysfunction. Many medications can also cause conduction abnormalities or QT prolongation.

Case Conclusion JL was started on an atypical antipsychotic and tolerated it well. Over the next week he had a decrease in the auditory hallucinations and paranoia and felt "calmer." He was able to be discharged to outpatient follow-up.

Thumbnail: Psychiatry—Review of Antipsychotic Medications and Their Side Effects

Typical or Conventional Antipsychotics

Potency	Example	Side Effects
High	Haloperidol (Haldol), thiothixene (Navane)	Akathisia (an internal sense of restlessness), extrapyramidal (parkinsonian) symptoms (EPS)
Mid	Perphenazine (Trilafon)	Mildly sedating, some anticholinergic effects, less EPS than with high-potency medications
Low	Thioridizine (Mellaril), chlorpromazine (Thorazine)	More sedating, significant anticholinergic effects (dry mouth, constipation, urinary retention, blurred vision), orthostatic hypotension, lowered seizure threshold. Thioridizine may cause irreversible pigmentation of the retina. Chlorpromazine may cause corneal deposits and/or photosensitivity and blue gray skin coloration.

Atypical Antipsychotic Agents

Medication	Comments/Side Effects
Risperidone	EPS in higher doses, some sedation, orthostatic hypotension, tachycardia, anticholinergic effects
Olanzapine	Sedation, weight gain, orthostatic hypotension, tachycardia, anticholinergic effects
Quetiapine	Orthostatic hypotension, tachycardia, anticholinergic effects
Clozapine	Indicated for resistant symptoms, is more effective, may improve negative symptoms, results in less tardive dyskinesia (TD), neuroleptic malignant syndrome (NMS), and EPS but is sedating, lowers the seizure threshold, causes orthostatic hypotension, and requires weekly blood work to monitor for agranulocytosis.
Aripiprazole	Insomnia, nausea/vomiting, akathisia, and anxiety

Key Points

▶ The dopamine hypothesis is the classic hypothesis for the etiology of symptoms in schizophrenia.

  ▶ Increased dopamine function in the limbic system is thought to be important in the etiology of the positive symptoms of schizophrenia.

  ▶ Decreased dopamine function in the prefrontal cortex is thought to be important in the etiology of the negative symptoms of schizophrenia.

▶ Typical antipsychotics act as antagonists at the dopamine D2 receptor.

▶ Atypical antipsychotics have antagonistic actions at a number of receptors, including 5-HT2A, dopamine D4, and some D2.

In general, the atypical agents have a more benign side effect profile and are less likely to cause extrapyramidal symptoms, dystonia, and akathisia. Clozapine is thought to confer minimal risk of tardive dyskinesia.

Questions

Questions 1 and 2 refer to the following case:

TR is a 56-year-old woman who has been maintained on the same conventional neuroleptic for the past 30 years. She comes into the emergency room with an exacerbation of her auditory hallucinations. She complains that there are too many side effects to her medications and admits to having stopped them 1 week before.

1. The medical student in the emergency room tells you that he's confused about the "typical antipsychotics" and asks which of the following is true:
   A. Their primary effect is through blockage of the muscarinic receptor.
   B. Haloperidol is a low-potency medication.
   C. Thioridizine is associated with sedation and orthostatic hypotension.
   D. Potent D2 receptor agonists are particularly effective medications.
   E. Akathisia refers to the parkinsonian rigidity associated with these medications.

2. Which of the following is true about the atypical antipsychotics?
   A. Perphenazine (Trilafon) is an example of an atypical antipsychotic.
   B. Clozapine is associated with agranulocytosis and lowered seizure threshold.
   C. Atypical agents have no effect on dopamine receptors.
   D. All atypical agents have marked agonist effects on the 5-HT receptor.
   E. Risperidone has its primary action at the nicotinic receptor.

3. BR has a 15-year history of antipsychotic use prescribed for chronic paranoid schizophrenia. He comes to your office for an initial visit and you notice that he is smacking his lips, his tongue occasionally protrudes from his mouth, and he seems to have some choreoathetoid movements in his hands. What is this syndrome called and what medication is most likely to have caused it?
   A. Tardive dyskinesia—chlorpromazine
   B. Akathisia—haloperidol
   C. Akathisia—olanzapine
   D. Tardive dyskinesia—clozapine
   E. Extrapyramidal symptoms—clozapine

4. You are called to see a 38-year-old patient in the emergency room, who was brought in because he had a high fever and had become confused, rigid, and sweaty. You check his laboratory results and find that his white blood cell count and his CPK are elevated. His other labs are pending, and his PE is otherwise unremarkable. He is on hydrochlorothiazide and perphenazine. What is the most likely etiology for his symptoms?
   A. Influenza A
   B. *Neisseria meningitidis* meningitis
   C. Neuroleptic malignant syndrome
   D. Malignant hyperthermia
   E. Enterovirus meningitis

> **HPI:** SG is a 7-year-old boy brought in by his mother at the school's recommendation. His mother describes him as disruptive and often uncooperative. In his unstructured preschool he did well, but he has had a great deal of difficulty adjusting to the structure of first grade. He has a difficult time sitting in his chair and gets up multiple times when the class is having a lesson or "quiet time." His teacher describes him as "on the go." He always fidgets or leaves his seat in class, or blurts out answers without raising his hand. She says that he is a nice child who sometimes has difficulty with his peers because he is unable to wait his turn in class, gym, or on class trips. She notes he often acts on impulse and has had a couple of playground accidents as a result.

Thought Questions

■ What psychiatric disorder might account for these symptoms?

■ What is the known biology of this disorder?

Basic Science Review and Discussion

To make a diagnosis of attention deficit hyperactivity disorder (ADHD) there must be at least 6 months of either six inattentive or six hyperactive/impulsive symptoms (see Table 33-1). In addition, the symptoms must be maladaptive and inconsistent with developmental level, must occur in more than one setting, and must cause an impairment of functioning. ADHD is not usually diagnosed until the child enters primary school, probably because of the more stringent requirements of school. In general, it is crucial to differentiate what are normal, age-appropriate exuberance and short attention span of a toddler or preschooler from developmentally inappropriate behavior. It is extremely important to get corroborative information from the school or other programs. In general, it is also very important to

rule out possible organic causes for his behavior, such as hyperthyroidism, stimulant use (e.g., caffeinated beverages), or, if he is primarily inattentive, conditions such as absence seizures. Other conditions that should be evaluated include mood disorders, mental retardation, and learning disorders.

Epidemiology The prevalence of ADHD varies by the criteria used and the threshold chosen to make the diagnosis. Currently, it is thought to affect 3% to 5% of children in the United States. In the United Kingdom the numbers are lower (approximately 1% to 2%) because of more stringent criteria. The male-to-female ratio is at least 2:1, if not higher (depending on the study). Confounding variables include the fact that boys are often more active than girls, and girls may be underdiagnosed, as they more often have the inattentive subtype.

Many disorders are seen with increased frequency in people with ADHD. Up to half of patients with ADHD have comorbid oppositional defiant disorder (ODD) or conduct disorder (CD), 25% have comorbid anxiety disorders, up to 33% have mood disorders, and 20% to 25% have a learning disorder. Tourette syndrome (TS) is seen in approximately 2% of

Table 33-1. Criteria for ADHD

Inattention	Fails to give close attention to details or makes careless errors in schoolwork
	Has difficulty sustaining attention in tasks or play
	Does not seem to listen when spoken to directly
	Does not follow through on instructions and fails to finish work (not because of opposition or failure to understand)
	Has difficulty organizing tasks and activities
	Avoids or dislikes tasks that require sustained mental effort
	Loses necessary things (toys, books, etc.)
	Is easily distracted by extraneous stimuli
	Is forgetful in daily activities
Hyperactivity	Fidgets or squirms
	Talks excessively
	Has difficulty playing quietly
	Runs or climbs excessively in inappropriate situations (in adolescents may be subjective feeling of restlessness)
	Is "on the go," as if "driven by a motor"
	Leaves seat in class or when sitting still is expected
Impulsivity	Blurts out answers before question is completed
	Has difficulty awaiting turn
	Interrupts or intrudes on others

children with ADHD. Although this number seems low, the prevalence is greatly increased as compared with the general population. Fifty percent of TS patients have ADHD.

Of note, ADHD is also associated with increased risk of accidents. Excessive activity combined with impulsivity and inattention make children accident-prone and increases the risk of motor vehicle accidents in adolescence.

The risk factors for ADHD include male sex, family history of ADHD and alcoholism, family discord, and low socioeconomic status. Many of the same risk factors are also risk factors for the common comorbid disorders, so it is difficult to sort out the factors specifically associated with ADHD.

Biology of ADHD Dysregulation of the central noradrenergic and dopaminergic network has long been hypothesized to underlie the pathophysiology of ADHD. This hypothesis is derived largely from pharmacologic data documenting that drugs that modulate noradrenergic and dopaminergic function show efficacy in treating ADHD. The noradrenergic system has been associated with the modulation of higher cortical functions, including attention, alertness, and vigilance. Changes in dopaminergic and noradrenergic function appear necessary for the clinical efficacy of the stimulants.

A number of genes have been evaluated in family studies of ADHD, including candidates associated with dopaminergic function (such as receptor or transporter polymorphisms).

None has been sufficiently replicated. In general, genetic studies show greatly increased (two to eight times) familial risk. Twin studies show a 60% to 80% concordance rate, and heritability is supported by adoption studies. The most probable mode of inheritance is polygenic.

Course As individuals get older the gross motor activity and impulsivity do decrease. But a substantial proportion may have academic and vocational difficulty as they age. For those who do not have complete remittance of symptoms, feelings of restlessness; a need to take many breaks to walk around; and impulsivity in relationships, driving, and work may all persist.

Treatment A number of medications have been evaluated in the treatment of ADHD. The first-line treatment for ADHD is the stimulants. In general, stimulants have been shown to increase attentiveness, reduce distractibility, enhance concentration, and decrease motor restlessness and hyperactivity in roughly 75% of children with ADHD. The most common side effects include headache, nausea, vomiting, anorexia, dizziness, and insomnia. Tics and growth suppression have also been reported. Various antidepressants, particularly the tricyclics and bupropion, have been used as second-line agents. These agents are discussed in depth in the context of treatment for depression.

Case Conclusion This child meets criteria for ADHD, hyperactive impulsive subtype. He has at least seven hyperactive/impulsive symptoms. He was treated with a stimulant medication and his school and family were involved in learning behavioral techniques to help manage his behavior and to help him learn to interact with peers. Over the next year he has made more friends and is doing better in school.

Thumbnail: Behavioral Science—Stimulant Medications

Medication	Mechanism of Action	Side Effects
Dextroamphetamine	Increases extracellular dopamine via acting as a false substrate for the dopamine transporter and promoting reverse transport of intracellular dopamine into the extracellular compartment.	Common: palpitations, excitability, nervousness, insomnia, tremors, pupil dilation, increased blood pressure and heart rate, nausea and vomiting, anorexia, and growth suppression. Large doses: hyperactivity, dyskinesia, seizures, insomnia, hallucinations
Methylphenidate	Blocks dopamine and possibly norepinephrine and serotonin reuptake.	As above
Pemoline	Probably via dopaminergic actions, exact mechanism unknown	As above, fewer peripheral sympathomimetic actions. Potential hepatic toxicity

Key Points

▸ ADHD is diagnosed with the presence of at least 6 months of either inattentive or hyperactive/impulsive symptoms that are maladaptive and inconsistent with developmental level, occur in more than one setting, and cause an impairment of functioning.

▸ ADHD affects approximately 3% to 5% of children, and there seem to be at least twice as many boys as girls affected.

▸ Comorbid disorders include oppositional defiant disorder, conduct disorder, anxiety disorders, mood disorders, and learning disorders. The frequency of Tourette syndrome is also increased.

▸ The standard pharmacologic treatment of ADHD is stimulant medications.

Questions

Questions 1 and 2 refer to the following case:

DB is a 10-year-old boy who has been getting into trouble at school since first grade. He has always had trouble concentrating in class, constantly loses things or does not seem to listen to assignments, does not sit still, gets up or calls out in class and is constantly interrupting others, and does not wait his turn.

1. Which of the following pharmacotherapy is not recommended in the treatment of this child?
   A. Tricyclic antidepressants
   B. Benzodiazepines
   C. Dextroamphetamine
   D. Methylphenidate
   E. Dopaminergic antidepressants (e.g., bupropion)

2. Which of the following is true?
   A. He is at no greater risk for anxiety disorders than the general population.
   B. He is at no greater risk for mood disorders than the general population.
   C. He is at no greater risk for psychotic disorders than the general population.
   D. He is at no greater risk for disruptive behavior disorders than the general population.
   E. He is at no greater risk for learning disorders than the general population.

3. KB is an 8-year-old boy with attention deficit disorder who has done well on amphetamine. He is less restless and is better able to concentrate and organize himself. How does this medication affect CNS receptors?
   A. It blocks the reuptake of dopamine into the presynaptic neuron.
   B. It blocks the breakdown of dopamine in the cytoplasm.
   C. It increases release into the extracellular compartment.
   D. It inhibits the breakdown of dopamine by acetylcholinesterase.
   E. It blocks postsynaptic dopamine D2 receptors.

4. MT is an 11-year-old boy who has moved to a new school this year. He has been having more behavior problems, is extremely active, interrupts teachers or other students, talks excessively, and has gotten into two fights. Without knowing other information about his history, which of the following should be included in the differential diagnosis of his behavior?
   A. Crohn's disease
   B. Bipolar disorder, depressed
   C. Dissociative fugue
   D. Hypothyroidism
   E. Understimulation of an extremely bright child

HPI: WK is a 65-year-old man with a history of alcoholism who is brought by ambulance to the emergency department after being found unconscious on a street corner, smelling of alcohol and vomit. He is somnolent but arousable to painful stimulus. His finger-stick blood sugar is 55. He is given oxygen, naloxone, thiamine, and vitamin B_{12}, 1 amp of $D_{50}W$, and started on IV normal saline with 5% dextrose by the paramedics, to which he responds minimally. Upon arrival to the emergency department he has the following readings

PE: T 35.9°C   BP 110/65   HR 97   RR 16   Sao$_2$ 92% room air, 98% with 100% O$_2$
He is lying in the bed, difficult to arouse, grunting with sternal pressure with a GCS of 10. His head is atraumatic and he is anicteric. He has multiple **spider angiomata** and **telangiectasia** on his chest. He has a normal lung and cardiac exam. He has a large, distended abdomen with a **positive fluid wave** and **migrating dullness to percussion** and a 5-cm liver span. He has brown heme-positive stool. He has bilateral symmetric wasting of upper and lower extremities, **palmar erythema,** diffuse ecchymoses, and 2+ pitting edema to the sacrum. His pupils are equal, with his right eye slightly deviated inwardly, 1+ deep tendon reflexes bilaterally.

Labs: WBC 6200/mL; Hgb 10 (13.5–17.5); Hct 30% (41–53%); Plt 95,000 (150,000–400,000); MCV 100 (80–100); Na 132 (136–145); K 3.5 (3.5–5.0); glucose 115 (70–110); total bilirubin 1.7 (0.1–1.0); direct bilirubin 0.6 (0.0–0.3); AST 90 (8–20); ALT 45 (8–20); alkaline phosphatase 132 (20–70), albumin 2.5 g/dL; total protein 5.5 g/dL; PT/PTT/INR 30 s/43 s/3.2; UA −3+ ketones, lipase 205; ABG-7.35/50/95/20 (pH/CO$_2$/O$_2$/HCO$_3$)

Studies: Abdominal CT–marked ascites and nodular cirrhotic liver; no evidence of acute pancreatitis; head CT–diffuse cortical atrophy with no other parenchymal abnormalities.

Thought Questions

■ What are the definitions of *alcohol abuse, tolerance,* and *dependency?*

■ What are the clinical manifestations of alcohol intoxication? Withdrawal?

■ What are the acute and chronic medical and cognitive complications of alcoholism?

■ How are alcohol intoxication, withdrawal, and alcohol-related medical diseases managed acutely and chronically?

Basic Science Review and Discussion

Alcoholism is an exceedingly common condition affecting 7% of adults and has a lifetime prevalence of 14%. While alcohol may be benign within the context of safe and responsible drinking, when taken to excess in unsafe conditions, a person may acutely fall victim to its secondary hazards, including falls, car accidents, sexual assault, and other violence. Alcohol is a pervasive element in crime, violence, and poverty, and its greatest effect may take place silently in an individual of any socioeconomic class or background. It not only affects the individual but also his or her job performance, relationships with friends and family, with rippling effects to society at large.

Mechanism of Action   Ethanol is a central nervous system (CNS) depressant and acts by enhancing the activity of the inhibitory **gamma aminobutyric acid A (GABA$_A$) receptor** and by inhibiting the excitatory **N-methyl-D-aspartate (NMDA) receptor**. Its immediate effects include sedation, disinhibition, impaired judgment and motor coordination, and in severe cases, "blackout" (or a temporary amnesia of all events surrounding the period of alcohol ingestion). A person who drinks an excessive amount over a short period of time (e.g., in hazing rituals) may induce enough CNS depression to cause respiratory depression, a common cause of alcohol-induced death. Otherwise, acute physiologic effects include some nutritional and metabolic derangements. A drink is approximately one 12-ounce can of beer, one 4-ounce glass of wine, or one shot (1.5 ounces) of liquor. One drink produces a blood alcohol level of about 30 mg/dL. "Legal intoxication" is reached at blood alcohol levels of 80 mg/dL and above (about two to three drinks, depending on a person's weight). Ethanol is metabolized to acetaldehyde by the liver primarily via the **alcohol dehydrogenase (ADH) pathway** and does so at a constant rate of approximately 30 mg/dL/hr, approximately one drink per hour.

Epidemiology   Risk factors for alcoholism include male gender, low socioeconomic status, unemployment, depression, anxiety, narcotic abuse, antisocial personality disorder, family history or dysfunction, and peer pressure. Often psy-

Table 34-1. *DSM-IV* Criteria for Alcohol Abuse vs Alcohol Dependence

Alcohol Abuse	Alcohol Dependence
Continued drinking despite repetitive problems, at least one out of four of the following: *Mnemonic: "When alcohol takes **HOLD** of you."* **H**azardous situations—(e.g., driving under the influence) **O**bligations unfulfilled—social/occupational debilitation **L**egal problems—crime, violence **D**ifficulties with interpersonal relationships	Presence of three out of seven of the following within a 12-month period *Mnemonic: "**WE** are unable **TO CUT** our drinking."* **W**ithdrawal symptoms **E**xcessive drinking (progressively increasing amounts) **T**olerance **O**ccupational/social abandonment (in order to drink) **C**ontinued use despite occupational/social consequence **U**ncontrolled use—person unable to control drinking **T**ime increasingly occupied by drinking

chological conditions such as depression and anxiety precede the substance abuse, which develops as a result of a person's attempt to self-medicate. Those susceptible to addiction may develop a habit of alcohol consumption, which can induce **tolerance.** First, a **metabolic tolerance** develops as hepatic clearance accelerates. Next, a **cellular tolerance** develops as alcohol induces neurochemical changes that make neurons dependent on alcohol for normal functioning. Finally, a person adapts to chronic intake by modifying behavior (**behavioral tolerance**). *Alcoholism* describes the interface between the physiologic event of *tolerance* and the internal and external ramifications of *behavior.* Two terms subdivide the syndrome of alcoholism, **alcohol abuse** and **dependence,** both of which predict recurrent problems with drinking and shortened life span (see Table 34-1).

There are several classic signs of chronic alcoholism (Box 34-1). Given the significant morbidity and mortality associated with alcoholism, it is important to detect and offer intervention for this disease. An established clinical screening method is the CAGE method (see Box 34-2).

Over time, physiologic and psychological dependence to alcohol can develop. Any decrease in alcohol intake can unmask the compensatory overactivity of the nervous system to alcohol and induce symptoms of withdrawal. Mild withdrawal include **tremors, agitation, mild anxiety, GI upset, headache, insomnia,** and **palpitations** 6 hours after the last drink. More severe withdrawal symptoms starting 1 to 4 days after the last drink include generalized tonic-clonic **seizures** within 48 hours, alcoholic **hallucinosis** (usually visual) within 12 to 24 hours, and **delirium tremens** 48 hours after the last drink. Delirium tremens is an uncommon but life-threatening condition without intervention. It includes unorientable delirium, hallucination, agitation, diaphoresis, and **autonomic instability** with increases in all four vital signs. **Benzodiazepines** (e.g., chlordiazepoxide, lorazepam) are GABA receptor agonists and are used to suppress withdrawal symptoms. **Thiamine** is also given to prevent Wernicke-Korsakoff syndrome, described later.

Otherwise, patients who present with acute intoxication and evidence of chronic alcoholism need to be stabilized and offered a long-term plan for rehabilitation. After discharge, those who express a desire to quit can undergo detoxification (monitoring and support for withdrawal symptoms) for several days. This can be followed by long-term rehabilitation; this includes organizations that support behavior modification like Alcoholics Anonymous. Private therapy and residential rehabilitation programs are also effective. Pharmacotherapy to supplement the rehabilitation regimen includes **naltrexone** and **acamprosate,** which reduce cravings for alcohol and reduce relapse rates.

Box 34-1. Classic Signs of Chronic Alcoholism (from Head to Toe)

Alcohol odor in breath
Scleral icterus/jaundice
Opthalmoplegia (Wernicke's)
Spider angiomata/telangiectasia
Firm, distended abdomen (ascites)
Caput medusa (portocaval shunt)
Large liver span (steatohepatitis)
Small liver span (cirrhotic liver)
Palmar erythema
Asterixis (encephalopathy)
Peripheral neuropathy/ataxia
Mental status changes (dementia)
↑ AST, ↑ ALT (AST:ALT = 2:1)
↑ Total and direct bilirubin
↓ Albumin/protein, ↑ PT/PTT

Box 34-2. CAGE Screening

Have you ever tried to **C**ut down?
Have you ever been **A**nnoyed by people telling you to stop drinking?
Have you ever felt **G**uilty about drinking?
Have you ever needed an **E**ye-opener?
≥ 2 positive answers makes alcoholism likely

Case Conclusion   WK is stabilized and given lorazepam for withdrawal prophylaxis. He is also given a multivitamin and vitamin K injection for his coagulopathy. He is diagnosed with having had an episode of acute alcohol intoxication with combined respiratory and metabolic acidosis from respiratory depression and alcoholic ketoacidosis, respectively. He is subsequently admitted. During his stay it is established that he has cirrhotic liver disease that is causing ascites. This hepatic insufficiency is thought to be responsible for his hypoproteinemia and edema, hyperbilirubinemia, and coagulopathy from insufficient coagulation factor production. In addition to the direct toxic effects of alcohol, poor nutrition, liver insufficiency, and occult GI bleeding may be responsible for his anemia, leukopenia, and thrombocytopenia. His moderately elevated lipase suggests that he has a chronic pancreatitis. Paracentesis is performed to relieve him of some of the abdominal pressure from his ascites. He is given supportive therapy and discharged to a medical detoxification program, after which he enters a residential rehabilitation program. He is currently taking naltrexone and has been abstinent for 2 months.

Thumbnail: Behavioral Science—Common Medical Complications of Chronic Alcohol Abuse

	Acute Conditions	Chronic Conditions

Neurologic	Acute alcohol intoxication
	Alcoholic withdrawal syndromes
	  Tremors-"shakes"
	  Seizures
	  Alcoholic hallucinosis
	  Delirium tremens
	Hemorrhagic stroke
	Subdural/epidural hematoma
		Alcohol tolerance/dependency
		Peripheral neuropathy (B_{12} deficiency)
		Organic brain syndromes
		  Alcoholic dementia
		  Korsakoff's syndrome
		  Wernicke's encephalopathy

Respiratory	Respiratory depression/hypoxia Aspiration pneumonia	Pulmonary edema (from CHF) Bronchitis/COPD(from smoking)
Cardiovascular	Peripheral vasodilation → syncope	Cardiomyopathy Congestive heart failure Gastroesophageal varices

Gastrointestinal	Gastrointestinal hemorrhage
	  Mallory-Weiss tear
	  Ruptured gastric varices
	  Coagulopathy
	Acute pancreatitis
		Occult GI bleeding
		Chronic pancreatitis
		Peptic ulcer disease
		Oropharyngeal, esophageal, hepatic cancer

Hepatic	Acute hepatic failure with concurrent
	acetaminophen ingestion, hepatitis
	  Disulfiram reaction (Antabuse)
	  Metronidazole, cefotetan, INH, griseofulvin
		Chronic liver failure, ascites
		Hepatic encephalopathy
		Hyperbilirubinemia, coagulopathy
		Hypoalbuminemia, hypoproteinemia,
		Hypercholesterolemia, hypertriglyceridemia

Renal	—	Hepatorenal syndrome
Metabolic	Alcoholic ketoacidosis Hypoglycemia, hypokalemia, hypomagnesemia	Malnutrition Vitamin B_{12}/folate deficiency Thiamine (vitamin B_1) deficiency Vitamin K deficiency (coagulopathy)
Endocrine Genitourinary	—	Gynecomastia, impotence, testicular atrophy, infertility, menstrual irregularities
Hematologic	Anemia from acute hemorrhage	Pancytopenia
Dermatologic	Cigarette burns Traumatic bruising, lacerations	Ecchymoses (platelet dysfunction) Palmar erythema, spider angiomata, telangiectasia, jaundice
Musculoskeletal	Traumatic fractures, rhabdomyolysis	Osteopenia Peripheral atrophy, myopathy
Infectious	Aspiration pneumonia	*Klebsiella* or *Legionella* pneumonia Gram-negative sepsis
Psychiatric	Suicide or homicidal ideation Sexual assault Violence	Alcohol abuse/dependency Multidrug abuse/dependency Depression, anxiety disorder

Key Points

▶ Alcoholism is a common problem with significant effects on lifetime morbidity and mortality affecting every system in the body.

▶ The behavioral pathology of alcoholism stems from the development of alcohol tolerance and dependence due to metabolic, cellular, and behavioral adaptation; such dependence may subsequently result in social and occupational dysfunction with disease progression.

▶ Alcohol withdrawal results from the unmasking of the compensatory overactivity of the central nervous system to chronic alcohol intake; benzodiazepines suppress this overactivity.

Questions

1. TN is a 37-year-old man with a long history of alcoholism who is brought by ambulance to the emergency department severely agitated but oriented and cooperative. He is diaphoretic with vital signs stable at T 38.0°C; HR 98; BP 139/85; RR 24; Sao$_2$ 100%. He develops severe stuttering speech, a tongue wag, and generalized tremors, pronounced by intentional movement. He soon undergoes a generalized tonic-clonic seizure. Once he stops seizing, he is given longer-acting diazepam and is admitted to the hospital. He reports having had his last drink about 24 hours ago. What is his *most* likely diagnosis?

   A. Withdrawal tremors and seizure
   B. Delirium tremens
   C. Alcoholic hallucinosis
   D. Wernicke's encephalopathy
   E. Korsakoff's syndrome

2. NH is a 52-year-old woman with a long history of alcoholism who presents complaining of fatigue and palpitations. She notes having passed foul-smelling, black stool in the last 2 days. Her recent history is significant for three episodes of vomiting "coffee ground" emesis. Generally, she appears well, with a HR of 96 and BP of 125/87. Her exam is significant for general pallor, diffuse epigastric tenderness, and heme-positive stool. Laboratory findings are significant for Hct of 32%, Plt 150,000/μL, and MCV of 85 fL. What is the *most* likely cause of her anemia?

   A. Folate and vitamin B$_{12}$ deficiency causing a megaloblastic anemia
   B. Anemia of chronic disease from chronic alcoholism
   C. Iron deficiency anemia
   D. Occult bleeding from Mallory-Weiss esophageal tear
   E. Ruptured gastroesophageal varices

3. A 19-year-old boy is brought by ambulance after being found collapsed in his college dorm room by his roommate, "blue and not breathing on his own." On the field, he is found to have an O$_2$ saturation of 75% and is quickly intubated, which resolves his cyanosis, bringing his saturation to 100%. He has a heart rate of 55 and a blood pressure of 95/55, for which he is given fluids. He has a GCS of 3, glucose of 85. He smells of alcohol and shows no signs of trauma. His pupils are equal and reactive, and the rest of his exam is normal. What is his *most* likely diagnosis?

   A. Acute heroin overdose
   B. Acute alcohol toxicity
   C. Acute cocaine overdose
   D. Insulin overdose
   E. Acute benzodiazepine overdose

4. HM is a 72-year-old man with a long history of alcoholism who is brought in by ambulance after having collapsed in his chair at home. He is eventually diagnosed with a hemorrhagic stroke. What is the *most* likely cause of this stroke?

   A. Thiamine deficiency
   B. Hypoglycemia
   C. Korsakoff syndrome
   D. Hepatic encephalopathy
   E. Vitamin K deficiency

HPI: LW is a 37-year-old man who is brought by ambulance to the emergency room after having been found unconscious and unresponsive in his apartment by his sister. When emergency medical services arrived, he was found to have a heart rate of 60, breathing 8 breaths per minute, saturating at 89%, with other vitals signs normal. He had "pinpoint" pupils, unresponsive to light bilaterally. He was immediately intubated, given naloxone, thiamine, and vitamin B_{12}, to which he immediately responded with an oxygen saturation of 98% and Glasgow Coma Scale (GCS) of 12. The sister knew of no known ingestions he could have taken and had no suspicion of suicidality. His sister says LW has no significant medical history except for mild insomnia for which he takes a "sleeping pill." He is a registered nurse in the ward and has no known habits, including cigarettes, alcohol, or drugs.

PE: T 36.0°C   BP 112/75   HR 65   RR 22   Sao$_2$ 98% on oxygen
He is lying in bed, somnolent but arousable. His pupils were equally small and minimally reactive to light, and his head and neck exams were otherwise normal. He had a normal cardiac and abdominal exam. There was no evidence of track marks on his extremities or trunk.

Labs/Studies: Findings showed urine toxicology positive for opioids. Head CT showed no abnormalities.

Thought Questions

- What opioids are frequently used as drugs of abuse? How do they work?

- What are the definitions of *opioid abuse* and *dependence*? How does dependence develop?

- What are the clinical manifestations of opioid intoxication, overdose, and withdrawal?

- What are the complications associated with opioid addiction?

- How are opioid intoxication, withdrawal, and dependence managed acutely and chronically?

Basic Science Review and Discussion

Opioids are derived from the poppy plant *Papaver somniferum* and have been used for centuries as a sedative and analgesic. Today they are used for the same purposes medically, but also illicitly as drugs of abuse. A 1997 study reported a 1% lifetime prevalence of heroin use, about 800,000 opioid-dependent persons in the United States, with rates higher in males than in females. There are three main types of opioid abuses: (1) those who use illicitly obtained opioids (street drugs), (2) *health care professionals*

who have easy access, and (3) approximately 5% of patients with chronic pain syndromes. All opioids produce similar effects of euphoria, sedation, and analgesia, and can produce psychological and physical dependence over time (Table 35-1).

Mechanism of Action Opioids bind different opioid receptors, whose endogenous ligands include **endorphins** and **enkephalins**. These include μ-, δ-, and κ-receptors, which are inhibitory G protein–coupled receptors. The **μ-receptor** mediates analgesia, euphoria, reinforcement, constipation, hormone level modification, and respiration. This receptor is mostly responsible for the effects of reward, tolerance, dependence, and withdrawal. The κ-receptor mediates some of the preceding effects as well as mood. These drugs can be injected intravenously, which produces the most potent effect, as opioids are quickly metabolized by the liver and have a high first-pass metabolism if taken orally. With increasing purity of heroin, intranasal use is increasing. In addition, street heroin includes **adulterants,** nonopioid additives like powdered milk, sugar, caffeine, and even strychnine, which may produce unexpected effects to the injector.

The *Diagnostic and Statistical Manual of Mental Disorders,* 4th edition (DSM-IV), criteria for opioid abuse and dependence are the same as those for alcohol. Tolerance and

Table 35-1. Opioid Drugs and Their Effects on Opioid Receptors

Agonists		Mixed Agonist/Antagonists	Antagonists
Morphine	Propoxyphene	Buprenorphine	Naloxone
Codeine	Fentanyl (*most potent*)	Pentazocine	Naltrexone
Heroin	Methadone (*long-acting*)		
Oxycodone	Levomethadyl acetate		
Hydrocodone	(LAAM) (*longer-acting*)		
Meperidine			

dependence are thought to develop through similar neuro-chemical modifications of receptors and signaling pathways that opioids affect. Up-regulation of components of this pathway such as adenylyl cyclase and protein kinase A is thus implicated in the production of the withdrawal syndrome.

The primary effects of opioids are **sedation, analgesia,** and **euphoria.** Secondary effects include nausea, vomiting, and *decrease in gastrointestinal motility,* producing **constipation** and **anorexia.** It decreases secretion of luteinizing hormone (LH), causing **reductions in testosterone and sex drive** as well as **amenorrhea.** A particularly dangerous effect of opioids is **respiratory depression** with a reduction in brain-stem response to CO_2 tension. Opioids can also cause peripheral vascular dilation and orthostatic hypotension. However, the greater part of the morbidity and mortality of opioids is attributed to the risks of injection drug use, the criminal activity required to maintain the habit, and the generally poor social circumstances and functioning of some addicts. Injection drug use increases the risk of contracting hepatitis B or C, HIV, and bacterial endocarditis, each of which have their own short- and long-term complications.

Diagnosis   To recognize the stigmata of opioid depend-ence, signs and symptoms include constricted pupils that are poorly reactive to light **(pinpoint pupils)** and **needle marks** on the skin. In acute overdose, respiratory depression, bradycardia, and general unresponsiveness may subse-quently produce anoxic brain injury, cardiorespiratory arrest, and death. Withdrawal produces opposite symptoms, such as diarrhea, mydriasis as well as coughing, lacrimation, and rhinorrhea (*think secretions of* cranial nerve [CN] *VII*), sweating and piloerection ("goose bumps") (*think sympa-thetic effects on skin*), and increases in all vitals signs, especially temperature, blood pressure, and respiratory rate. Other diagnoses to consider of depressed level of con-sciousness include acute intoxication with benzodiazepines, alcohol, hypoglycemia, and other metabolic abnormalities, to name a few.

Treatment   Treatment of opiate overdose includes support for respiratory compromise and reversal of opioid effects with an **opioid antagonist** like **naloxone** or the longer-acting **naltrexone.** These antagonists may, however, precipitate withdrawal symptoms. Withdrawal symptoms, alternatively, are treated with an opioid such as **methadone.** Otherwise, **clonidine** may be useful for inhibiting autonomic hyper-activity with supplemental **benzodiazepines** to decrease agitation. In general, altered mental status can be empirically treated with glucose, naloxone, thiamine, and vitamin B_{12}. Other treatments may be considered, depending on their response to these empiric treatments and suspicion of other ingestions (e.g., flumazenil is an antidote for benzodiazepine intoxication).

Once stabilized, the patient requires either support of withdrawal symptoms for several days **(detoxification)** or long-term rehabilitation and pharmacologic support of opioid dependence with the long-acting opioid agonist **methadone** or the even longer-acting **levo-alpha-acetyl-methadol (LAAM),** administered through methadone maintenance programs. Counseling and psychotherapy can be provided in group settings or privately through residen-tial programs and clinics, which may include therapy for concurrent psychiatric illness. Alternatively, opiate-depend-ent persons may choose to achieve complete abstinence from opiates by undergoing treatment with opiate antago-nists (e.g., naloxone, naltrexone), although this has limited efficacy. Those with chronic pain syndromes are encour-aged to take nonopioid analgesics and limit their opiate intake with the advice that their pain can be minimized but not eliminated.

Case Conclusion   LW is monitored for the next 24 hours for overdose intoxication and withdrawal symptoms. After 3 hours, he demonstrated symptoms of opioid withdrawal and was started on methadone. During this time, he admits to having used intravenous opiate analgesics, oral morphine and fentanyl from the wards to relieve his stress and insomnia for several years and is now dependent on them for sleep. He agrees to undergo long-term rehabilitation with methadone treatment. Several months after this episode, he continues to attend group counseling and is on methadone maintenance.

Thumbnail: Behavioral Science—Opiate Drug Abuse and Dependence

Epidemiology	1% lifetime prevalence of heroin use; men > women
Molecular Biology	Agonists to μ-, δ-, κ-opioid receptors; μ-receptor acts to produce tolerance and dependence
Physical Exam	Track marks, constricted unresponsive pupils, tender liver edge (hepatitis)
Drug Intoxication	Sedation, analgesia, euphoria, constipation, ↓ LH leading to ↓ testosterone/sex drive, amenorrhea
Drug Overdose	Respiratory depression/arrest, orthostatic hypotension, hypoxic brain injury, death
Drug Withdrawal	Diarrhea, mydriasis, coughing, lacrimation, rhinorrhea, sweating, piloerection ("goose bumps"), yawning, and increases in all vitals signs (temperature, blood pressure, respiratory rate)
Drug Complications	Hepatitis B/C, HIV, bacterial endocarditis, cardiac valve disease, stroke, behavioral issues, skin cellulitis, abscesses, necrotizing fasciitis (skin infection with systemic spread and sepsis)
Treatment	*Overdose:* Intubation, oxygen, naloxone, naltrexone *Withdrawal:* Methadone, clonidine, benzodiazepines *Rehabilitation:* Methadone or LAAM (if refractory), counseling

Key Points

▶ Opioids primarily cause sedation, analgesia, and euphoria; secondary effects include constipation, nausea, and vomiting.

▶ Opioids exert their effects through opioid receptors and produce tolerance and dependence with continual use.

▶ Most of the morbidity and mortality of opioids come from the risks associated with injection drug use, criminal behavior, and generally poor social circumstances and functioning.

▶ Opiate addiction occurs not only in the stereotypical homeless heroin addict but in many individuals; therefore it is important to screen for opiate use in all patients.

Questions

1. BR is a 42-year-old homeless man who presents to the clinic complaining of 2 days of runny nose, cough, night sweats, and shortness of breath. He has also had 1 day of watery, nonbloody diarrhea. His vitals are T 38.4°C; BP 150/90; HR 104; RR 28; and Sao$_2$ 100%. On exam, he appears agitated and diaphoretic. He has a III/VI mid-systolic murmur at the right lower sternal border and a diffusely tender periumbilical abdomen without rebound or guarding. He has multiple track marks on his skin and has decreased skin turgor from apparent dehydration. What is the *likely* diagnosis?
   A. Acute gastroenteritis
   B. Bacterial endocarditis
   C. Upper respiratory tract infection
   D. Heroin withdrawal
   E. All of the above

2. TS is a 39-year-old woman who presents with severe lower back pain to the emergency room. She has a history of multiple back surgeries for chronic back pain without successful relief of the pain and is chronically taking meperidine for pain. She is currently screaming in agony, demanding pain medication. What is the best treatment strategy?
   A. Complete history of back pain, surgeries, pain management, and physicians from which she received pain medication.
   B. Review quickly her medical record and contact her primary physician.
   C. Administer intravenous morphine for her severe pain immediately and contact her primary physician.
   D. Give her intravenous ketorolac for her pain and contact her primary physician.
   E. Advise her to return to her primary physician for review of her pain symptoms and the appropriate pain regimen.

3. UN is a 57-year-old man. He presents with a painful skin infection on his right leg and states that he has been "feeling very, very sick" for the last 2 days. He has had this skin infection for 4 days, has recently felt "sick," and cannot elaborate except to say that this was unlike his normal withdrawal symptoms. He last injected heroin 6 hours ago. He has a temperature of 39.1°C, HR of 105, BP of 96/52, RR of 28, and Sao$_2$ of 99%. He appears ill and in mild distress. He has a 7-cm poorly circumscribed area of erythema and swelling on his right thigh that is extremely tender. It also has a questionable central area of fluctuance. His lungs are clear and his heart is regular, with no murmurs. What is the *most* important diagnosis to consider?
   A. Necrotizing fasciitis
   B. Cellulitis
   C. Abscess
   D. Opioid withdrawal
   E. Bacterial endocarditis

4. AL is a 40-year-old man who is brought by ambulance to the emergency room after being found collapsed on a park bench. He is breathing at a rate of 8 breaths per minute with an O$_2$ saturation of 85% on room air. He has no odor of alcohol on his breath and a Breathalyzer test shows an alcohol level of zero. He has multiple track marks and pinpoint pupils. He is given IV normal saline, naloxone, thiamine, vitamin B$_{12}$, and glucose with no response. He is given three more doses of naloxone with still no response. He is given flumazenil with improvement in his level of consciousness. What is the *most* likely etiology of his depressed level of consciousness?
   A. Hypoglycemia
   B. Heroin overdose
   C. Alcohol intoxication
   D. Hyponatremia
   E. Benzodiazepine overdose

HPI: MG is a 17-year-old girl who was brought by ambulance to the emergency room after her mother found her passed out and unresponsive on the bathroom floor after an evening out with her friends. Her mother was unsure of where she had gone but suspected that she had gone to a party or dance club. She did not smell of alcohol or vomit. She is otherwise healthy and has no significant medical or psychiatric history. Her mother does not know if she drinks, smokes, or takes drugs. She was found by emergency medical services to have a Glasgow Coma Scale (GCS) of 9, with equally dilated and responsive pupils bilaterally. She has a blood glucose of 75. She was given naloxone, thiamine, and vitamin B$_{12}$ and started on normal saline IV infusion with 5% dextrose, producing minimal improvement in her mental status.

PE: T 36°C   BP 98/65   HR 105   RR 32   Sao$_2$ 100% on room air
The patient is lying on the gurney and is tachypneic. She had no apparent head trauma, no meningismus. Her jugular venous pulsation (JVP) is flat and she is tachycardic, with occasional irregular beats. Her lungs are clear and her abdomen is benign. She now has a GCS of 10, localizing painful stimulus (5), responding to pain with a garbled "no" (3), and opens her eyes to painful stimulus (2). Her deep tendon reflexes are diminished but symmetric and with a negative Babinski's sign. She has diminished skin turgor diffusely and 2+ radial pulses.

Labs/Studies: CBC normal; Na 125; K 3.6; Cl 100; HCO$_3$ 20; BUN 40; Cr 0.7; glucose 100.; Ca^{2+}/Mg^{2+}/Phos normal. Serum osmolality low. LFT normal. PT/PTT/INR normal.
UA is negative; urine toxicology is negative; alcohol/acetaminophen/aspirin levels are zero.
ABG 7.37/36/100/20. EKG shows a sinus tachycardia with occasional premature atrial contractions. CSF findings are normal, cultures pending; head CT is normal.

Thought Questions

- What are the common drugs of abuse?

- What are the manifestations of intoxication and withdrawal for each drug?

- How does the body adapt to chronic drug exposure?

- What is the physiologic basis of reward, reinforcement, tolerance, and dependence?

Basic Science Review and Discussion

The common drugs of abuse can be divided into three main categories: (1) **stimulants**, (2) **sedatives**, and (3) **hallucinogens**. Any single drug will often have effects that fall into at least two categories; however, this helps one organize and narrow down the differential diagnosis in someone suspected of acute intoxication or withdrawal from a substance of abuse.

Stimulants   Stimulants include sympathomimetic drugs like **cocaine, amphetamines, phencyclidine (PCP)**, and **ketamine.** Roughly, these drugs stimulate excitatory neurochemical pathway components (e.g., NMDA receptor) in the central and peripheral nervous systems. For instance, cocaine acts by inhibiting the reuptake of the excitatory neurotransmitters **norepinephrine, dopamine**, and **serotonin.** Peripherally, this results in vasoconstriction, hypertension, tachycardia, dry mouth, and mydriasis due to its **sympathomimetic**

effects. Centrally, cocaine use produces subjective feelings of euphoria, alertness, increased confidence, and grandiosity. It may also produce anxiety and paranoid delusions. Other stimulant drugs will produce similar effects along with their own signature variations. PCP intoxication is distinguished by the associated hypersalivation and vertical nystagmus not present in intoxication due to other stimulants. These effects in overdose can produce severe vascular complications such as myocardial infarction and cerebral hemorrhage, or other neurologic complications such as seizure or coma. *Generally, symptoms of withdrawal from chronic use of any drug will produce effects opposite to those that the drug produces.* Therefore withdrawal from stimulants produces fatigue, hypersomnia, and depression.

Sedatives   On the other hand, sedatives produce central and peripheral autonomic depression. Common sedative drugs of abuse include **cannabis, benzodiazepines, barbiturates, ethanol, opiates** (e.g., heroin, narcotic analgesics) and a newer drug popular at clubs, **gamma-hydroxybutyrate (GHB).** Such drugs enhance the inhibitory gamma aminobutyric acid, type A (**GABA$_A$**) receptor and inhibit the excitatory N-methyl-D-aspartate (NMDA) receptor, or target other receptors that mediate sedative effects (e.g., cannabinoid and opioid receptors). Centrally, these drugs produce subjective feelings of sedation, cognitive depression, and dyscoordination (e.g., ataxia, dysarthria). Autonomic manifestations include the **parasympathomimetic effects** of pupillary miosis and relative bradycardia and hypotension. In severe overdose, central nervous system (CNS) depression produces *respiratory depression* due to decreased central responsiveness to the CO_2 content in the blood. Clinically, these intoxications can be distinguished by their differing pharmacokinetics and dynamics (i.e., duration of action, severity of effect) and even the order in which neurologic functions are depressed. For instance, GHB can produce severe coma with a GCS of 3 (the lowest possible) without producing respiratory depression. The withdrawal symptoms of sedatives include restlessness, anxiety, insomnia, and autonomic instability, including tachycardia and hypertension. Severe withdrawal can produce seizures and **delirium tremens,** a life-threatening withdrawal syndrome consisting of tremors, delirium, and severe autonomic instability. Often these symptoms require reintoxication with the offending drug (often as self-medication by the user) or with an analog (e.g., benzodiazepines).

Hallucinogens Lastly, hallucinogens, such as **lysergic acid diethylamide (LSD)** and 3,4-methylenedioxymethamphetamine **(MDMA, ecstasy),** are marked by their ability to produce vivid and bizarre visual, auditory, and tactile hallucinations. They can also produce unusual sensory perceptions, or **synesthesias,** such as colors producing the perception of different sounds. They have mild autonomic effects and tend to be sympathomimetic. With LSD, the main adverse effects result from the patient's inability to handle the state of altered perception. Impaired decision making can cause a person to engage in risky and at times life-threatening behavior. For instance, ecstasy, a popular club drug, produces a relatively benign syndrome of euphoria, enhanced mood, and perception of increased energy, often leading to continuous dancing and exertion for several hours. However, this can subsequently produce the more dangerous conditions of dehydration, hyponatremia (due to replacement of fluid loss with pure water), hyperthermia, rhabdomyolysis (from muscle breakdown), and renal failure.

Lastly, included in the list of drugs of abuse are legal drugs, which can produce the same phenomena of tolerance and of psychological and physical dependence. These include caffeine, alcohol, and tobacco. In addition to physical dependence, the latter two produce significant long-term medical complications. In fact, some of the most prevalent causes of morbidity and mortality in the United States are associated with chronic alcohol ingestion or tobacco use.

The unifying characteristic of all these drugs is that they produce some form of **euphoria,** a very rewarding stimulus. It is hypothesized that the experience of **reward** is mediated by the release of **dopamine** from the presynaptic terminals of the **ventral tegmental area** via the **median forebrain bundle** to the **nucleus accumbens, amygdala,** and **medial frontal cortex** of the **mesocorticolimbic dopamine system,** otherwise known as the reward center of the brain. The rewarding stimulus produces a compulsion or **craving** to repeat the drug use, that which is called **psychological dependence.** With repetitive use, neurons adapt by altering receptor and ion channel function and expression, signal transduction, gene expression, and synaptic connectivity. For instance, chronic ethanol exposure down-regulates the expression of NMDA receptors. These changes are thought to mediate the development of **tolerance,** wherein a user requires progressively higher doses of a drug to produce the same level of intoxication. These adaptive changes are also responsible for the development of **physical dependence,** wherein real pathophysiologic responses occur if the drug is withdrawn. All drugs of abuse, by definition, produce psychological dependence, but only a subset produce real physical dependence. The latter require not only behavioral modification therapy but also medical management to lessen the severity of the withdrawal syndrome, which at times can be life-threatening.

Cessation and rehabilitation are difficult tasks to accomplish. The barriers that a user must overcome are manifold and include intense craving, withdrawal, environmental stimuli that promote use, social pressures, life stresses, and lack of resources to help in quitting. It becomes the responsibility of every physician to screen for drug use and offer support and advice for quitting, even among those who openly express their unwillingness to quit (e.g., patients in the **precontemplation** phase). Once a person is thinking about quitting (i.e., **contemplation** phase), it becomes crucial to follow up with immediate referral to counseling and perhaps medical support for withdrawal symptoms. Pharmacologic agents are increasingly being used as adjunctive therapy in the treatment of addictions. For nicotine addiction, nicotine replacement and treatment with bupropion (an antidepressant) or clonidine have been used with good efficacy. Pharmacologic therapies for other drugs are listed later.

Case Conclusion The patient probably took the popular club drug ecstasy, which is not usually available in the urine toxicology screening. She probably developed a hyponatremia from prolonged exertion, followed by fluid loss and simultaneous free-water intake. During her fluid resuscitation with normal saline, her vital signs are monitored and stabilized. Her fluids and electrolytes are corrected. She is referred to drug counseling and is sent home, having suffered no long-term sequelae.

Thumbnail: Behavioral Science—Substances of Abuse and Common Symptoms

Narcotic	Routes/Mechanism	Effects	Withdrawal Signs
		Sedatives	
Benzodiazepines *Clonazepam* *Diazepam*	Oral, physical dependence* **GABA modulators** Rx: **Flumazenil**	Cognitive difficulty, ataxia, pinpoint pupils, *lateral gaze nystagmus,* respiratory depression	Insomnia, restlessness, nightmares, *less severe than symptoms for barbiturates*
Barbiturates	Oral, physical dependence **GABA agonist**	Similar to alcohol and benzodiazepines with *worse outcomes*	Insomnia, seizures, *delirium tremens,* hallucinations
Cannabis (THC) *Marijuana, hashish*	Smoked, oral **Cannabinoid agonist (CB$_1$, CB$_2$)**	Altered perception, "*amotivational syndrome,*" conjunctival injection, increased appetite, dry mouth	No significant withdrawal syndromes; some insomnia and restlessness in heavy users
Gamma hydroxybutyrate (GHB)	Oral, liquid form Physical dependence Unknown MOA	Similar to alcohol, seizures, **coma** *followed by respiratory depression,* death	Insomnia, tremor, ↑HR/BP, diaphoresis, *mild delirium tremens*
		Stimulants (Sympathomimetics)	
Cocaine *Free-base cocaine, crack*	Intranasal, IV, oral, smoked **Blocks reuptake of NE, DA, and 5-HT** Short duration of effect	*Hypervigilance,* paranoid delusions, chest pain, ↑T/HR/BP, arrhythmias, mydriasis, dry mouth, death	Fatigue, nightmares, insomnia/ hypersomnia, increased appetite, psychomotor retardation, agitation
Amphetamines and methamphetamine *Speed, meth, ice, crystal, crack*	Oral, IV, intranasal, smoked **Increased NE, DA, 5-HT release** Long duration of effect	*Enhanced concentration and physical performance,* grandiosity, anorexia, paranoid psychosis, ↑T/HR/BP, hemorrhagic stroke, seizure, death	Intense fatigue, agitation, anergia, hypersomnia, prolonged mental depression, suicidal ideation
Phencyclidine (PCP) *Angel dust*	Oral, IV, inhalation **NMDA receptor modulator, ↓ reuptake, and ↑↓ production DA, NE**	Hypervigilance, ataxia, ↑HR/BP, myoclonus, analgesia, psychosis, *hypersalivation, vertical nystagmus,* coma, death	No significant stereotyped withdrawal syndrome
Ketamine *Special K*	Oral, intranasal, smoked Physical dependence **PCP derivative, similar mechanisms**	"*Dissociative anesthesia,*" immobility, *nightmares,* mood elevation, sedation, amnesia, ↑HR/BP	Flashbacks with visual disturbances weeks after exposure; associated with risky sexual behavior
		Hallucinogens	
Lysergic acid diethylamide (LSD) *Acid*	Sublingual, smoked, intranasal, injected **Acts on 5-HT, DA receptors**	*Bizarre hallucinations,* altered perception and mood, anxiety, nausea, vomiting, diarrhea ↑HR/BP, mydriasis	No significant withdrawal symptoms; rare, persistent psychosis; *flashbacks*
MDMA *Ecstasy, XTC, E, X (popular at raves)*	Oral (intranasal) Increases 5-HT release and decrease 5-HT reuptake	Increased confidence, *empathy,* ↑HR/BP, *hyperthermia, dehydration, rhabdomyolysis, renal failure*	No significant withdrawal symptoms; associated with risky sexual behavior

*All addictive drugs, by definition, produce psychological dependence and tolerance with repetitive use. Only some drugs produce physical dependence, which are marked by adverse physiologic effects if withdrawn. Those drugs that produce physical dependence are noted as such; otherwise, they only produce tolerance and psychological dependence.

†Alcohol and opiates are not included in this table but should fall under the category of sedatives.

DA, dopamine; 5-HT, serotonin; GABA, gamma aminobutyric acid; MDMA, 3,4-methylenedioxymethamphetamine (ecstasy); MOA, mechanism of action; NE, norepinephrine; NMDA, *N*-methyl-*D*-aspartate; THC, Δ-9-tetrahydrocannabinol (marijuana).

Key Points

▶ Substances of abuse fall under three main categories: sedatives, stimulants, and hallucinogens; this simplification can aid with the diagnosis of a patient presenting with acute intoxication.

▶ The effects of drugs are varied and may even be benign in isolation. However, intoxication may pose secondary dangers to the user due to impaired judgment, altered perception, and perhaps the unsafe social contexts within which the drug is used.

▶ Reward and reinforcement of repetitive use are mediated by dopamine release in the mesocorticolimbic dopamine system; this produces psychological dependence.

▶ Tolerance, physical dependence, and withdrawal syndromes are produced by the neurochemical adaptations that develop from chronic exposure to a drug.

Questions

1. AT is a 16-year-old young man who is brought in by ambulance after being found by his mother "acting like he is on drugs." According to his mother, he was fighting with his 13-year-old brother and threatening to hit him for no apparent reason. He subsequently punched in the dry wall. When asked why he wanted to hit his brother, he said that his brother "wanted to steal his car and run off with his girlfriend." In the emergency department his vital signs were the following: T 37.5°C; HR 105; BP 148/89; RR 22; Sao$_2$ 98% RA. He is found pacing the exam room and answering appropriately but is at times tangential in his response. His pupils are equally dilated and minimally responsive to light; his extraocular movements are intact with a vertical nystagmus; his mucosal membranes are moist. He has diffusely exaggerated deep tendon reflexes. Which drug did he *most likely* take?

   A. Phencyclidine (PCP)
   B. Cocaine
   C. MDMA (XTC)
   D. Amphetamines
   E. Methamphetamine

2. MA is a 35-year-old man who arrives in the emergency department agitated and tremulous. He is unable to give a history due to his altered mental status. His vital signs are as follows: T 37.5°C; BP 150/100; HR 105; RR 24. He has no stigmata for alcoholism and his physical exam is otherwise normal. During evaluation, he develops a generalized tonic-clonic seizure. He is later given 4 mg of lorazepam, a benzodiazepine, to which he responds quickly with decreased agitation, tremulousness, and normalizing vital signs. Which of the following could be the *likely* cause of his presentation?

   A. Alcohol withdrawal
   B. Benzodiazepine withdrawal
   C. Barbiturate withdrawal
   D. Methamphetamine overdose
   E. All of the above

3. SJ is a 28-year-old woman who is brought in by ambulance after collapsing in the middle of a dance club. According to the bartender, she was noted to have three drinks that evening over the 3 hours she was in the club. A man who may have already left the bar bought one of those drinks for her. On the field she was unresponsive, with a GCS of 3, with the following vital signs: T 38.0°C; BP 135/85; HR 95; RR 20; Sao$_2$ 98% on RA. The rest of physical exam and laboratory studies are normal. What is her *most* likely diagnosis?

   A. Benzodiazepine overdose
   B. Alcohol intoxication
   C. Barbiturate overdose
   D. Gamma-hydrobutyrate overdose
   E. Ketamine overdose

4. IL is a 21-year-old woman complaining of a recent episode of acute-onset 8/10 nonradiating, dull, substernal chest pain while at rest lasting for 30 minutes. She had one previous episode of such pain last night before going to bed. She denies having shortness of breath, nausea, vomiting, or diaphoresis. She was previously healthy and only taking an oral contraceptive (a low-dose estrogen-progesterone combination). Her vital signs are T 37.7°C; BP 147/82; HR 105; RR 24; Sao$_2$ 100% on RA. She is in mild distress and her exam is otherwise normal. She currently has a normal EKG. What is the *most* important thing to ask her to help uncover the etiology of her chest pain?

   A. Prior history of asthma
   B. History of cocaine use
   C. History of hypertension
   D. Dosage of her oral contraceptive
   E. Family history of early myocardial infarction

HPI: CD is a 37-year-old man who presents complaining of 2 weeks of **nonproductive cough.** He denies having had a fever, chills, malaise, or runny nose. He denies having asthma, allergies, or any other chronic diseases. When asked about cigarette smoking, he reports having restarted smoking 1 month ago after a year of abstinence due to recent job stress and currently smokes one pack a day.

PE: T 36.5°C   BP 135/78   HR 79   RR 24 Sao_2 96%
He smells of cigarette smoke and otherwise appears healthy. His physical exam is normal.

Labs: WBC count 6500/μL with a normal differential. Hct 45%.

Thought Questions

- What is the mechanism of action of nicotine and how does it produce addiction?

- What are the medical complications associated with chronic tobacco use?

- What are the strategies employed to help a patient quit smoking?

Basic Science Review and Discussion

Nicotine addiction is obviously widely prevalent. The average person with nicotine addiction has neither presenting stigmata nor social dysfunction enough to draw attention to this insidiously dangerous disease. Although those with histories of long-term tobacco use are easy to detect, a significant number of patients who require intervention have not yet developed any pathology. In the United States, 40% of all smokers die prematurely unless they quit. Annually, 400,000 people die prematurely because of cigarette use, representing *one out of every five deaths.* Cigarette smoking is associated with the highest-ranking causes of death in the United States, including myocardial infarction, cerebrovascular accidents, chronic obstructive pulmonary disease, and lung cancer.

It is important to distinguish between different forms of tobacco use, as each form leads to different pathology. Cigarette smoking is the most prevalent, but the smoking of cigars, cloves, and pipe tobacco are also widely popular. Pipe and cigar tobacco have a more alkaline pH, which facilitates nicotine absorption through the oral mucosa; therefore pipe and cigar smokers tend to keep the smoke within the oral cavity. Similarly, chewing tobacco and moist snuff allows for absorption of nicotine through the oral mucosa. Therefore the diseases associated with these forms of tobacco use include oral, pharyngeal, and laryngeal squamous cell carcinoma. In some parts of Asia, "reverse smoking" (i.e., smoking with the lit side of the cigarette inside the mouth) has become widely popular, causing increased incidences of oropharyngeal and laryngeal carci-

noma as well. Cigarette tobacco, on the other hand, has a more acidic pH, requiring inhalation deep into the pulmonary tree to allow sufficient absorption across a greater surface area. This form of tobacco use has subsequently led to an epidemic of heart and lung disease in the United States.

The addictive component of tobacco is nicotine. Nicotine acts on the **nicotinic acetylcholine receptor (nAchR),** which classically resides in the *preganglionic postsynaptic membrane.* Thus it produces a mix of sympathetic and parasympathetic effects, which include vasoconstriction and heart rate reduction. Centrally, nicotine activates nicotinic acetylcholine receptors of dopaminergic **ventral tegmental area** neurons subsequently stimulating dopamine release from the **nucleus accumbens.** This is thought to mediate the reinforcing properties of nicotine, as biochemical blocking of this pathway attenuates addictive behavior in animal models. Although nicotine itself is largely benign, it leads one to repetitively expose oneself to the other components of tobacco, collectively called "tar." Tar includes greater than 40 carcinogens, carbon monoxide, respiratory irritants, and ciliotoxins. Over time, exposure to these components leads to the characteristic parenchymal changes, tissue damage, secondary hypoxia, and malignancy associated with cigarette smoking.

The long-term medical complications of tobacco use include several major organ systems producing ischemic, infectious, reproductive, neoplastic, and otherwise degenerative complications. Chronic obstructive pulmonary disease (COPD) results from the inflammatory changes and parenchymal damage induced by chronic smoke exposure; such changes develop as soon as 1 year after the start of routine smoking. The risks of cardiovascular and cerebrovascular accidents are associated with the pro-coagulopathic and vaso-occlusive effects of cigarette smoking. This also explains the higher rates of graft occlusion and coronary artery restenosis after vascular bypass surgery and angioplasty, respectively, in those who continue to smoke. The mechanisms that mediate the reproductive sequelae are thought to be mediated by poor placental functioning due to the microvascular compromise associated with cigarette smoking. Finally, the development of malignancy arises from the chronic exposure of the oral, upper, and lower respiratory tracts to the carcinogens in tobacco. The ability of inhaled carcinogens to spread systemically is evidenced by the association of cigarette smoking to neoplasms of remote organs like the kidney, bladder, and pancreas. Table 37-1 lists complications associated with tobacco use.

Approximately one-third of current smokers attempt to quit each year. Greater than 90% of unassisted attempts at smoking cessation fail. This figure emphasizes that there is currently an interest among smokers to quit and that a significant number of attempts can be made successful with enough support. Treatment of nicotine addiction and chronic tobacco use requires a multidisciplinary approach. Two of the most important and effective interventions are physician screening and counseling. Physician advice to quit, especially around the time of acute illness, can trigger a serious attempt at cessation. Physicians can review with the patient the particular triggers that cause them to go back to smoking. In a recent survey of smokers, 73% of smokers attempting to quit cited life stress as the biggest challenge. It is thus important for the physician and patient to come up with alternatives to smoking for those times when the patient is particularly tempted to smoke. Other environmental stimuli that encourage smoking cessation include advertising campaigns, higher costs of cigarettes, and work/public policy to prohibit smoking in the workplace, restaurants, and bars. Particular attention needs to be paid to adolescent patients, as most long-term smokers begin smoking in their teenage years, a time when they are particularly vulnerable to social pressures to smoke as a result of poor self-image and desire to be accepted. Some smokers may try to switch to "lower tar" cigarettes to reduce the risk of developing smoking-related diseases, but studies have shown no clinically significant benefits from such a strategy. It may simply delay attempts at full abstinence and thus should be discouraged as a strategy for cessation.

The benefits of quitting include reducing the risks of first myocardial infarction and sudden cardiac death within the first few years after cessation. It reduces the risk of a secondary coronary event within 6 to 12 months following cessation. After 15 years, a previous smoker's risk of new myocardial infarction and death are similar to those who have never smoked. Smoking cessation reduces the risk of developing cancer, although a low level of increased risk persists. Smoking cessation is the most effective intervention in chronic obstructive pulmonary disease, which slows the decline of pulmonary function.

Once patients resolve to quit, they should set a quit date by which date they will have stopped smoking completely. This quit date should be met with telephone follow-up counseling by a practitioner with special expertise in smoking cessation. Pharmacologic support for smoking cessation has also been shown to be efficacious and to include **nicotine replacement, clonidine,** and **bupropion.** Nicotine replacement comes in many doses and in many forms (e.g., transdermal patches, chewing gum, nasal or oral inhaler) and is available over the counter. It is used to reduce cravings by supplementing patients with the substance to which they are actually addicted. Bupropion is an antidepressant with the added side effect of reducing the subjective pleasure of cigarette smoking. Combination treatment with behavioral therapy and drug therapy may yield the highest rates of success.

Table 37-1. Medical Complications of Chronic Tobacco Use by System

Respiratory	• Chronic obstructive pulmonary disease
	  • Chronic bronchitis
	  • Emphysema
		• In children: respiratory infections, chronic otitis media, asthma, or exacerbation

Cardiovascular	• Coronary artery disease • Peripheral vascular disease • Myocardial infarction	• Aortic aneurysm • Carotid artery disease • Sudden cardiac death
Cerebrovascular	• Cerebrovascular atherosclerosis	• Ischemic stroke
Neoplastic *(roughly from highest to lowest relative risk)*	1. Lip, oral cavity, pharynx (with chewing) 2. Lung (squamous cell and small cell) 3. Larynx 4. Esophagus	5. Kidney 6. Bladder 7. Pancreas
Reproductive	• Women: low birth weight, premature rupture of membranes, abruptio placentae, placenta previa, preterm delivery, higher perinatal mortality, small for gestational age, sudden infant death syndrome, developmental lag • Men: impotence	
Miscellaneous	• Delayed wound healing • Osteoporosis • Senile cataracts • Pulmonary embolism	• Macular degeneration • Skin wrinkling • Gallstones and cholecystitis

Case Conclusion Given the lack of evidence of infection, you conclude that this cough is probably smoking related. You subsequently advise him to think about quitting. He expresses regret over his smoking but states that it is difficult to overcome such triggers as life stress, and often feels tempted to smoke at social occasions. You offer alternatives to smoking at those times, which include simple things such as exercise, partaking in other activities he enjoys, and, if necessary, removing himself from any situation that tempts him to smoke. He is started on nicotine replacement and bupropion. The patient sets his quit date for 1 week after his clinic visit. This is followed up with a telephone call from the smoking cessation counselor on his quit date.

Thumbnail: Behavioral Science—Tobacco Use

Contents of tobacco	Nicotine, carcinogens, carbon monoxide, respiratory irritants, ciliotoxins
Routes of use	Inhalation of cigarette to lungs Transmucosal absorption from chewing tobacco, cigar, and pipe tobacco
Mechanism of action	Nicotinic acetylcholine receptor agonist Acts centrally to enhance dopamine release from the nucleus accumbens Acts peripherally on the preganglionic nAchRs of the autonomic nervous system
Short-term effects	Alertness, anxiety, relaxation for chronic users
Long-term effects	Dependence, COPD, CAD, MI, CVA, pulmonary embolism, lung/oral/bladder cancer
Withdrawal symptoms	Irritability, headache, craving, weight gain
Signs of chronic tobacco use	Cigarette odor, burn marks on hands, digital clubbing; signs of COPD: pursed-lips breathing, barrel chest, supraclavicular/intercostal retractions, generalized cyanosis/flushing, suspicious oral lesions, hyperaeration on chest x-ray
Treatment	**Behavioral:** physician counseling, telephone follow-up counseling, group counseling **Pharmacologic:** nicotine replacement, clonidine, bupropion

Key Points

▶ Chronic tobacco use is an insidiously dangerous health problem and requires aggressive screening and intervention by health practitioners.

▶ Nicotine is a highly addictive component of tobacco, and the chronic exposure to the tar in tobacco produces a wide variety of disease, depending on the mode of tobacco use and the sites exposed to the components of tobacco.

▶ Successful smoking cessation programs include, first and foremost, motivation from the patient, followed by physician advice, follow-up clinic counseling, support from social networks, and pharmacologic intervention.

Questions

1. LC is a 15-year-old young man who presents for a general physical exam needed to participate in sports. What is an effective strategy for discouraging teenagers to smoke?
   A. Nicotine patches
   B. Lower tar cigarettes
   C. High cigarette taxes
   D. Clonidine
   E. Bupropion

2. DL is a 53-year-old man with known COPD who presents with shortness of breath diagnosed as acute exacerbation of COPD. After stabilization of his acute illness, what is the single most effective long-term therapy in preserving this man's lung function and reducing his mortality?
   A. Oxygen supplementation
   B. β_2-agonist
   C. Atropine
   D. Smoking cessation
   E. Ipratropium

3. BA is a 32-year-old woman who presents to the emergency room with acute-onset shortness of breath and pleuritic chest pain. She also noted recently having developed right leg pain and swelling. She was previously healthy and has no significant medical history. She is taking oral contraceptive pills. She had recently returned from a cross-country road trip. She also admitted to smoking one pack/day for the past 10 years. She is afebrile, breathing at a rate of 32 breaths per minute with a room air O_2 saturation of 93%. Her lungs are clear with no rales or wheezes, and cardiac auscultation reveals a loud S2. Her exam is otherwise unremarkable. Her chest x-ray is normal. What is the *most* likely cause of her shortness of breath?
   A. Chronic bronchitis
   B. Emphysema
   C. Community-acquired pneumonia
   D. Pulmonary embolism
   E. Asthma

4. ST is a 47-year-old man who presents for evaluation of his depression. He has been struggling with depression since the death of his late wife 2 years ago. He also notes decreases in appetite, inability to enjoy his usual hobbies, chronic insomnia, and poor energy. He has a medical history significant for hypertension, hypercholesterolemia, and type II diabetes mellitus; he had a myocardial infarction at the age of 43. He is taking several medications for his various conditions, although he admits to not taking them every day. He also notes that he had started smoking again after this event and has not been able to quit despite his cardiologist's advice. What is the *most* appropriate pharmacologic therapy for this man's depression?
   A. Fluoxetine
   B. Citalopram
   C. Bupropion
   D. Venlaxafine
   E. Olanzapine

HPI: MR is a 7-year-old boy who has been brought to the clinic by his parents, who are concerned that he might be "a little slow or something."

His parents say that their son is a happy little boy who started school 2 years previously. His teacher reported that he has severe difficulties with reading, attention, and even memory. These difficulties are accompanied by episodes where he became very frustrated at his inability to understand the written word.

His parents tell you that he is the youngest of five children and that he had a normal birth. He achieved his developmental milestones, though some may have been a "little behind the others," and was slow to master language. He did not attend preschool, as his mother preferred to have him at home, but he had a year of kindergarten. They said that he never appeared to have problems with hearing or vision. He had the usual childhood illnesses of chicken pox and the mumps. His parents describe him as a happy kid who enjoyed playing with his toys. He still occasionally wets the bed. His father recollects that his brother may have had difficulties learning to read as a child.

There is no other significant family history. His father is 50 years of age, his mother is 49; both appear to be in good health. Their oldest is 19 and attends junior college. None of their other children had any difficulties.

PE: Within normal limits except for low-set ears; there were no abnormalities on neurologic exam.

Thought Questions

- How does mental retardation differ from learning disorders?

- What do you think is wrong with this child?

Basic Science Review and Discussion

Mental retardation is defined as significantly below-average intellectual functioning that begins before the age of 18 years and is associated with impairments in adaptive functioning. It is coded on Axis II. The IQ is approximately 70 or below (approximately two standard deviations) and is divided into four categories in the *Diagnostic and Statistical Manual of Mental Disorders,* 4th edition (*DSM-IV*):

1. Mild mental retardation: IQ between 50–55 and 70

2. Moderate mental retardation: IQ between 35–40 and 50–55

3. Severe mental retardation: IQ 20–25 and 35–40

4. Profound mental retardation: IQ below 20 or 25

These individuals also have deficits in more than two of the following skill areas: communications, self-care, home living, social/interpersonal skills, use of community resources, self-direction, academic skills, leisure, work, health, and safety. The IQ can be measured using standardized tests such as the Stanford-Binet or the Wechsler Intelligence Scales for Children.

Epidemiology Mental retardation is found in approximately 1% of the population. This translates to 2.5 million people living in the United States. It is reported to be more common in boys than in girls; this may be due to higher rates of congenital abnormalities, X-linked conditions, and complications of prematurity among boys.

Mild mental retardation accounts for approximately 85% of those with the disorder. These children may not be diagnosed until 5 to 10 years of age and with special education techniques can achieve academic levels of approximately a sixth-grade level.

With suitable supports these individuals can live in the community. Some can manage more independent living situations, but others need supervised settings.

Moderate mental retardation accounts for approximately 10% of those with the disorder. These individuals have communication skills and with vocational training and supervision can attend to some self-care. Educationally, they may reach a second-grade level. They may be able work in sheltered workshops and live in supervised settings in the community.

Approximately 3% to 4% of those with mental retardation fall into the **severe** category. They can talk but cannot read adequately. They can manage to live in group homes or with their families unless they need specialized care. **Profound mental retardation** is found in approximately 1% to 2% of individuals with this disorder. Most of these individuals have an underlying neurologic disorder. They need constant supervision and help. Some may be able to perform simple tasks if training is successful.

Etiology of Mental Retardation Of those who are severely impaired approximately 32% have Down's syndrome; genetic causes or associated malformations, perinatal injury, infections, and inborn errors of metabolism account for smaller percentages (see Thumbnail). Those individuals who reside in long-stay facilities have higher rates of behavioral disturbances.

A specific cause of mental retardation can be identified in approximately two-thirds of cases. The more severe the impairment is, the more likely it is that a cause will be identified. Individuals with mild mental retardation have an identifiable cause in approximately 30%. More than 500 genetic disorders are associated with mental retardation (see Thumbnail), and chromosomal disorders are responsible for 10% of all cases of mental retardation. Chromosomal abnormalities occur in 1 in 200 births and in 50% of first-trimester miscarriages.

Fetal Alcohol Syndrome   **Fetal alcohol syndrome** is the most common recognizable cause of mental retardation and is thought to occur in between 1 in 300 and 1 in 1000 newborns. The children have shallow philtrums without vertical ridges and short palpebral fissures. They also have growth retardation, particularly head circumference. The average IQ is approximately 65. These individuals often have problems with impulsivity, attention, psychiatric problems, and substance abuse. This may occur with exposure to more than two units of alcohol a day during pregnancy. Milder variants of the disorder may be referred to as fetal alcohol effects.

Other nongenetic causes of mental retardation include the following:

1. **Toxic/nutrition:** Placental insufficiencies, malnutrition (includes neglect), lead encephalopathy, infantile hypoglycemia, teratogens, such as medications (anticonvulsants), drugs (cocaine), fetal alcohol syndrome, and exposure to radiation.

2. **Infection:** Toxoplasmosis, *Listeria,* rubella, cytomegalovirus, syphilis, and herpes simplex in the mother; meningitis and encephalitis in the child.

3. **Trauma:** Perinatal trauma, accidental and nonaccidental injury, including asphyxia.

Prenatal factors account for the majority of individuals with severe mental retardation but less than half of those with mild retardation. Perinatal factors likely cause less than 10% of all cases of mental retardation, being more associated with cerebral palsy. Postnatal insults lead to approximately 5% to 10% of the cases of mental retardation.

Neurologic disorders are often associated with mental retardation. Seizure disorders are found in 15% to 30% of individuals with mental retardation; sensory impairments, in 10% to 20%; and motor abnormalities, in 20% to 30% of individuals. Mental retardation is found in approximately 50% of those with cerebral palsy.

Chromosomal abnormalities may be diagnosed by prenatal testing, such as amniocentesis, chorionic villus sampling, maternal serum alpha-fetoprotein, or ultrasound. Genetic counseling is offered to high-risk populations. Individuals with mental retardation should live as independently as possible, avoiding institutionalization and pursuing education and vocational training.

Learning Disorders   Difficulties in attaining intellectual skills at the same rate as others are known as **learning disorders** and were previously referred to as academic skills disorders. Learning disorders are diagnosed when the discrepancies between standardized tests in math, reading, or writing are more than two standard deviations behind those expected for age, schooling, and IQ. Learning disorders may also be referred to as learning disabled. Other disorders that affect academic performance include language and motor skills disorders. Difficulties can arise from inputting information (visual and auditory perception), integration of this input (sequencing and organizing), remembering of this information (short-term and long-term memory), and output (language). There are three types of learning disorders: **disorders of written expression, reading, and mathematics.**

Prevalence   It has been estimated that between 5% and 10% of the population have learning disorders, 4% of schoolchildren have a reading disorder, and 1% have a mathematics disorder. Studies have reported that boys have a higher prevalence than girls, but more boys may be referred for treatment as they are acting out. Approximately 40% of children with learning disorders drop out of school.

Comorbid psychiatric disorders include conduct disorder, oppositional defiant disorder, major depression, dysthymia, attention-deficit/hyperactivity disorder (ADHD), and borderline personality disorder. These disorders may also lead to social problems, as they cause difficulties in peer group activities. These young people may also have problems with social skills. Between 20% and 25% of individuals with learning disorders have ADHD, and between 70% and 80% of those with ADHD have a learning disorder. Approximately 60% of those with Tourette syndrome have a learning disorder. Learning disorders may be caused by a variety of prenatal, perinatal, or postnatal insults. Studies have revealed a family pattern in between 40% and 50% of children, and monozygotic twins are more likely than dizygotic twins to have academic problems.

The differential diagnosis must include poor performance due to a lack of opportunity, poor teaching or cultural factors, impaired vision or hearing, mental retardation, and developmental disorder. These conditions may also coexist with a learning disorder.

Treatment of these disorders may include psychological, educational, and social skills training. These disorders are not cured but the individuals with these disorders and their families can be helped. Remedial methods are used to help those with reading disorders, which may have difficulties in decoding, comprehension, or a combination of both.

Case Conclusion You arrange for MR to have IQ testing. It reveals a nonverbal IQ in the normal range and a verbal IQ in the low normal range, with some problems with vocabulary and language. Other testing found no difficulties with math but significant problems with reading skills in both recognition and comprehension. You persuade the parents to enroll him in extra individual reading classes three times a week; a year later he is doing well.

Thumbnail: Behavioral Science—Genetics Causes of Low IQ and Mental Retardation

Prenatal Causes	Examples
	Genetic disorders: 32% of cases
(1) Trisomies	Trisomy 21–22 (Down syndrome) Trisomy 17–18 (Edward's syndrome) Trisomy 13–15 (Patau's syndrome)
(2) Microdeletions	Cri du chat Wolf's syndrome Prader-Willi syndrome Angelman's syndrome Williams syndrome
(3) Multifactorial	Fragile X syndrome Familial mental retardation Tuberous sclerosis Metabolic disorders (PKU, Hunter's, Lesch-Nyhan syndrome, galactosemia, Tay-Sachs, Niemann-Pick, etc.) Congenital hypothyroidism
	Malformations of unknown cause: 8% of cases
(1) CNS malformations	De Lange's syndrome Sotos' syndrome Neural tube defects Holoprosencephaly
(2) Multiple malformations	
	Prenatal external causes: 12% of cases
(1) Maternal infections	Toxoplasmosis, rubella, cytomegalovirus, *Listeria*, syphilis, and HIV
(2) Toxins	Fetal alcohol syndrome
(3) Placental insufficiency and toxemia	Prematurity Intrauterine growth retardation
(4) Miscellaneous	Radiation Traumatic injury
	Perinatal causes: 11% of cases
(1) Infection	Herpes simplex II Meningitis
(2) Obstetric complications	Hypoxia Trauma
(3) Miscellaneous	Hyperbilirubinemia
	Postnatal causes: 8% of cases
(1) Infection	Encephalitis Meningitis
(2) Toxic	Lead poisoning
(3) CNS disease and disorders	Trauma Tumors Cerebrovascular accidents
(4) Psychosocial problems	Poor nutrition, lack of stimulation, and abuse

Key Points

- Academic skills disorder may appear similar to mild mental retardation, visual or hearing impairments, or neurologic deficits.
- Five percent to 10% of the population in the United States has learning disorders.
- Four percent of schoolchildren have reading disorder, and 1% have a mathematics disorder. Studies have reported that boys have a higher prevalence than girls.

- Approximately 40% of children with learning disorders drop out of school.
- Mental retardation affects approximately 1% of the population.
- Approximately 85% have mild mental retardation, 10% have moderate retardation, and 3% to 4% have severe retardation.

Questions

1. Which of the following statements concerning learning disorders is accurate?
   A. Between 30% and 40% of those diagnosed with reading disorder are males.
   B. Approximately 0.5% of schoolchildren have reading disorder.
   C. Approximately 5% of schoolchildren have mathematics disorder.
   D. It is rare to have a disorder of written expression without another learning disorder.
   E. They are not often found in association with general medical conditions.

2. A 32-year-old primigravida has just delivered a full-term baby girl. The midwife asks you to examine her more closely because she is concerned that the baby may have Down syndrome. Which of the following features would you expect to find in an infant with Down syndrome?
   A. Brushfield's spots; high, arched palate; and floppy ears
   B. Brushfield's spots; high, arched palate; and hypertonic muscles
   C. Prognathism, epicanthic folds and protruding tongue
   D. Prognathism, single palmar crease, and blue eyes
   E. Epicanthic folds, protruding tongue, and single palmar crease

3. The parents of an 8-year-old boy with mild mental retardation bring him for his annual physical. They are concerned about planning for his future. Which of the following could you tell them?
   A. The mortality rates are four times that of the general population for all those with mild mental retardation under 20 years of age.
   B. The life expectancy is directly related to their IQ.
   C. Most individuals with mental retardation develop seizures.
   D. There is no increased risk of developing psychiatric disorders.
   E. They should plan for institutional care.

4. Which of the following features are associated with Rett's disorder?
   A. Microcephaly, gait abnormalities, increased purposeful hand movements
   B. Macrocephaly, gait abnormalities, decreased purposeful hand movements
   C. Microcephaly, loss of previously acquired skills, and stereotyped movements
   D. Microcephaly, loss of previously acquired skills, equal sex distribution
   E. Microcephaly, loss of previously acquired skills, increased male distribution

HPI: FP is a 27-year-old male who comes to your clinic with his wife for assessment. His wife reports that he "is just not himself." He has become very apathetic and depressed over the previous month.

PE: Unremarkable except for increased reflexes and the presence of a grasp reflex.

MSE: He is casually dressed with fair hygiene. Eye contact and rapport are also fair. He describes his mood as "down" and his affect is somewhat flattened. Thought processes are logical and goal directed but slowed. He denies hallucinations, SI, or HI. There was no evidence of delusions. On a brief assessment of cognitive function he had deficits in attention and concentration and short-term recall. Abstract reasoning was also impaired. Insight and judgment were impaired.

Labs/Studies: Within normal limits. CT scan revealed a 2-cm ring-shaped lesion in his right frontal lobe.

Thought Questions

- What do you think is going on with this young man?

- What psychiatric symptoms may be seen in this condition?

- What are the individual lobar syndromes associated with such pathology?

Basic Science Review and Discussion

Brain tumors may present initially with either focal or nonfocal symptoms and signs, but these are not mutually exclusive and a combination may occur together. Symptoms may appear gradually or more suddenly with a seizure. Nonfocal symptoms are caused by raised intracranial pressure. The headaches associated with a brain tumor have classically been described as occurring in the morning and are associated with nausea, but more important, they are associated with behavioral changes (personality, mood, and cognition), seizures, and focal signs. Focal signs include seizures (presenting symptom in between 20% and 40% of patients), cranial nerve palsies, motor or sensory dysfunction (see Thumbnail). Tumors in neurologically "silent" areas such as the frontal or parietal association cortices may reach large sizes before symptoms or signs are present.

The differential diagnosis would include conditions such as a cerebral abscess, granuloma, aneurysm, vascular malformations, multiple sclerosis, degenerative neurologic disease, hydrocephalus, pseudotumor cerebri, or subdural hematoma. It is rare for the clinical presentation to occur so rapidly as to suggest a stroke.

The work-up for a brain tumor should include careful medical and neurologic examinations, assessments of mood, behavior, and cognitive function. Neuroimaging may include CT or MRI scans (with contrast material), but biopsy may be necessary for a definitive diagnosis. MRI is more useful to view posterior fossa structures and generally provides better-quality images.

Brain tumors may be primary or metastatic in nature. Primary brain tumors are outlined in Table 39-1.

Metastatic brain tumors are 10 times more common than primary brain tumors and spread mostly from lung, breast, skin (melanomas), kidney, colon, and rectal tumors. Approximately 20% of all patients with cancer will have metastases to the skull, meninges, or brain during their illness.

It has been reported that up to 50% of patients with brain tumors develop **psychiatric symptoms** at some stage of their illness. These symptoms are determined by the location and characteristics of the tumors. Psychiatric symptoms that may be seen include changes in personality, cognition (confusion or decline in intellect), mood, psychosis (delusions and hallucinations), and dissociative phenomena (derealization or depersonalization). Changes in **behavior** may include inertia, lack of spontaneity, apathy, forgetfulness, poor insight, anxiety, or irritability. These symptoms are most likely to be caused by tumors in the frontal lobe, temporal lobe, and corpus callosum. The personality changes seen in frontal lobe tumors are described in the Thumbnail. Disinhibited, euphoric behaviors are related to lesions in the orbitofrontal region, whereas depression and apathy are related to lesions in the dorsolateral region of

Table 39-1. Primary Brain Tumors

Intra-axial types	Astrocytomas
	Oligodendrogliomas
	Ependymomas
	Pineocytomas/pineoblastomas
	Glioblastomas
	Medulloblastomas
	Lymphomas
	Gangliocytomas/gangliogliomas
	Neuroblastomas
Extra-axial types	Meningiomas
	Pituitary adenomas
	Acoustic neuromas

the frontal lobe. Tumors involving the hypothalamus may cause reactions of violent rage. Bilateral tumors affecting the limbic structure may cause a placid demeanor.

Mood changes include depression and mania. Depression is most commonly associated with tumors affecting the left frontotemporal area. Mania may occur with right-sided tumors in the region of the hypothalamus or the inferomedial frontal lobes.

Psychosis may present with hallucinations or delusions. Visual hallucinations may occur more commonly with temporal lobe or brainstem tumors, and more rarely with frontal lobe tumors. Olfactory hallucinations may occur with tumors affecting the olfactory pathways. Auditory hallucinations may occur with tumors of the temporal lobes. Temporal lobe tumors may cause persecutory delusions.

Delirium and dementia may also be associated with brain tumors. However, these are usually associated with signs of raised intracranial pressure or focal neurologic signs or symptoms. A paraneoplastic syndrome may present with cognitive deterioration and cerebellar signs without actual metastatic spread. Tumors reported to be associated with this syndrome include tumors of the breast, tumors of the lung (oat cell), and Hodgkin's disease.

Most tumors causing psychiatric symptoms are located in the frontal lobe. Patients may present with changes in motor function (including bladder and bowel incontinence), cognition (attention and memory), personality, or language. Other physical signs may include papilledema, gait abnormalities, increased tendon reflexes, frontal reflexes such as grasp and sucking/snout reflexes. Treatment of brain tumors includes dexamethasone or, more rarely, mannitol to decrease intracranial pressure and edema. Patients with posterior fossa or acoustic neuromas do not usually require treatment with anticonvulsants, unlike patients with other tumors. Anticonvulsants include valproic acid, carbamazepine, and phenytoin. Surgical success depends on the tumor's location, preoperative level of neurologic functioning, and surgical skill. Stereotactic procedures allow for surgery in areas that were previously avoided, such as the brainstem, basal ganglia, language areas, and corpus callosum. The aim is to remove the maximum amount of tumor while preserving function. Other treatment modalities include radiation and chemotherapy.

Radiation is administered in smaller daily doses, which build up over time into the total dose.

Treatment of the psychiatric and behavioral symptoms with psychotropic medications requires extra care, as these patients may be more sensitive to side effects such as sedation or decreased seizure threshold. Supportive psychotherapy can help maintain the patient's self-esteem and sense of control. Patients may need help to grieve.

Case Conclusion   A stereotactic brain biopsy was performed that confirmed a glioblastoma multiforme, which unfortunately is the most malignant variant of all primary brain neoplasms. FP was treated by surgical resection followed by postoperative external beam radiotherapy. However, his tumor continued to progress despite all treatments and he succumbed a year later.

Thumbnail: Behavioral Science—Brain Region Lesions: Possible Symptoms and Signs

Frontal lobe	**Personality changes** may present with either (1) disinhibition, facetious humor, euphoria or (2) depression, apathy, loss of initiative, slowing of thought, and motor activity. Cognitive dysfunction may present with inattention, distractibility, and perseveration of actions; difficulty in problem solving; programming/planning sequences of behavior; urinary incontinence. Judgment, memory, abstract reasoning, concentration, and attention may also be affected. **Motor and premotor cortex:** Contralateral paraparesis, truncal ataxia, reduced fine motor control; grasp reflex; reduced verbal fluency; impaired spelling. Generalized or focal motor seizures. Common cause of pseudobulbar symptoms. Lesions of the falx can cause weakness of both lower limbs and urinary retention. Broca's area (dominant premotor cortex)—expressive dysphasia.
Parietal lobe	Contralateral sensory loss, with or without mild contralateral (CL) hemiparesis. Lower quadrant contralateral homonymous hemianopia. Astereognosis (inability to recognize objects by touch). Sensory Jacksonian fits, crude visual hallucinations. **Disorders of body schema:** **Dominant lobe:** Alexia, agraphia, constructional disorders, Gerstmann's syndrome (right-left disorientation, finger agnosia, dyscalculia, dysgraphia), astereognosis, pain asymbolia, ideomotor apraxia, and receptive/fluent aphasia. **Nondominant lobe:** Hemisomatognosia (failure to recognize a body part as one's own), anosognosia (denial of the disorder), dressing apraxia, proposagnosia, topographic agnosia, constructional apraxia.
Temporal lobe	**Personality/psychosis:** Formed visual hallucinations, complex partial seizures, memory disturbances (e.g., déjà vu). **Motor/sensory:** Contralateral hemiparesis with deep lesions with or without corticospinal tract with a weak face, and 3rd nerve palsy. **Auditory functions:** Impaired auditory sensation—verbal (dominant), musical (nondominant), auditory agnosia. Sensory dysphasia (Wernicke's area— dominant) with or without writing difficulties. **Visual functions:** Contralateral upper quadrant, homonymous hemianopia. **Dominant:** Impaired verbal memory, visual object agnosia, color agnosia, ataxia or simultanagnosia (inability to comprehend more than one element of a visual scene at a time or to integrate the parts into a whole). May cause a schizophreniform illness or decreased IQ functioning. Emotional lability, aggressive behavior changes similar to frontal lobe lesions may also occur. **Nondominant:** Impaired nonverbal spatial memory, agnosia for sounds, dysprosody, and amusia. **Kluver-Bucy syndrome**—extensive **bilateral** lesions: Loss of fear and aggression, visual agnosia, blunt affect, hypersexual, hyperorality, amnesia, and hypermetamorphosis.
Occipital lobe	Cortical blindness (bilateral), contralateral homonymous hemianopia (unilateral), scotoma (focal), loss of visual perception, visual object agnosia, alexia. **Dominant lobe:** Color agnosia. **Nondominant:** Prosopagnosia, metamorphosis, visual/spatial agnosia, and complex visual hallucinations.
Hypothalamus	Appetite disturbance, elevation of temperature, obesity, amenorrhea or impotence (altered sexual development in children), polydipsia, and polyuria.
Thalamus	**Sensory:** Contralateral sensory loss **Dominant:** Poor verbal memory, anomia, and apathy **Nondominant:** Poor nonverbal memory and mania
Corpus callosum	Mental symptoms often present first with apathy, drowsiness, decreased memory, depression, or anxiety. Lesions may cause a severe and rapid deterioration of IQ with local neurologic signs.

Key Points

- Brain tumors may present with focal or nonfocal symptoms, signs, or a combination of both.
- Nonfocal symptoms are caused by raised intracranial pressure.
- Focal signs include seizures, cranial nerve palsies, motor or sensory dysfunction.
- Metastatic brain tumors are 10 times more common than primary brain tumors.
- Up to 50% of patients with brain tumors develop psychiatric symptoms.

- Symptoms include changes in behavior, personality, cognition, mood, psychosis, or dissociative phenomena.
- Most tumors causing psychiatric symptoms are located in the frontal lobe.
- Frontal lobe signs include changes in motor function (including incontinence), cognition, personality, or language. Physical signs include papilledema, gait abnormalities, increased tendon reflexes, frontal reflexes such as grasp, and sucking/snout reflexes.

Questions

1. When evaluating the possibility of a brain tumor in FP, which of the following other nonfocal symptoms would you consider?
   A. Nausea, vomiting, and diarrhea
   B. Nausea, vomiting, and florid manic symptoms
   C. Nausea, vomiting, headaches, confusion, and lethargy
   D. Hemianopia
   E. Cranial nerve palsies

2. Six months after completion of his treatment FP returns for follow-up with his wife and she reports that he seems to be having more difficulties with memory. You advise them that which of the following may be an irreversible cause of cognitive dysfunction?
   A. Steroids
   B. Effects of radiation
   C. Anticonvulsants
   D. Depression
   E. Metabolic disturbances

3. Which of the following disorders is associated with parietal lobe dysfunction?
   A. Depression
   B. Schizophrenia
   C. Obsessive-compulsive disorders
   D. Delirium
   E. Conduction aphasia

4. BQ is a 24-year-old male brought to the emergency room after a motorbike accident. He has an open head injury. Which of the following complications of traumatic brain injury must you consider?
   A. Cognitive outcome is related to the Glasgow Coma Scale score.
   B. Recovery from diffuse injury is related to hypoxia.
   C. Seizure disorder may develop in approximately 5% of those with an open head injury.
   D. The majority of neuropsychiatric complications are mood disorders.
   E. The likelihood of a neuropsychiatric disorder is not influenced by premorbid conditions.

Answer Key—Part II: Neuroscience, Psychiatry, Psychopharmacology, and Psychopathology

Case 20
1. B
2. D
3. C
4. E

Case 21
1. C
2. D
3. E
4. C

Case 22
1. A
2. C
3. E
4. D

Case 23
1. A
2. B
3. D
4. D

Case 24
1. D
2. C
3. B
4. B

Case 25
1. D
2. A
3. E
4. B

Case 26
1. D
2. A
3. C
4. C

Case 27
1. C
2. B
3. E
4. B

Case 28
1. C
2. C
3. E
4. A

Case 29
1. C
2. B
3. E
4. B

Case 30
1. D
2. E
3. D
4. D

Case 31
1. A
2. B
3. C
4. D

Case 32
1. C
2. B
3. A
4. C

Case 33
1. B
2. C
3. C
4. E

Case 34
1. A
2. D
3. B
4. E

Case 35
1. E
2. D
3. A
4. E

Case 36
1. A
2. E
3. D
4. B

Case 37
1. C
2. D
3. D
4. C

Case 38
1. D
2. E
3. B
4. C

Case 39
1. C
2. B
3. E
4. A

Part III

Epidemiology, Biostatistics, and Health Policy

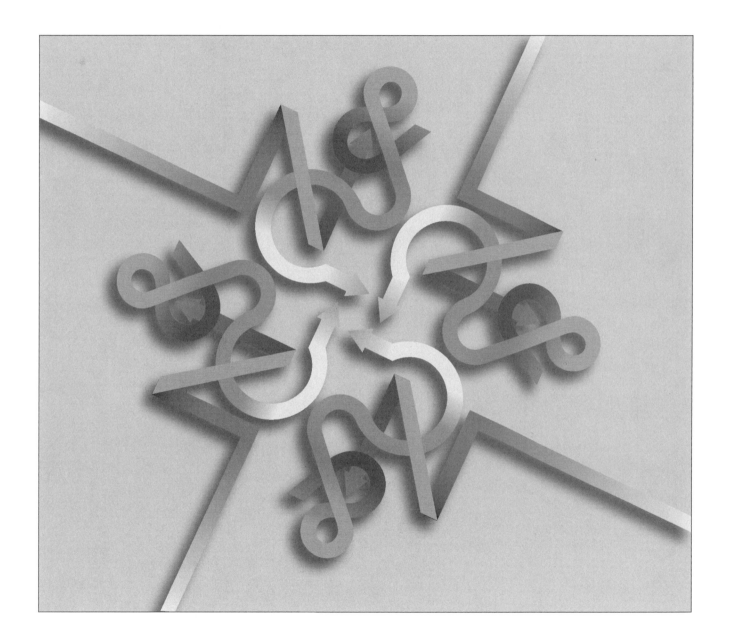

> **HPI:** MM is a 56-year-old white male who presents for management of hypercholesterolemia to you, his primary physician. You offer to start him on your favorite statin of choice and tell him that the mean reduction in total cholesterol is 15 points. MM then asks, "Does that mean that half the people who use the medication experience an even greater reduction in their cholesterol level?"

Thought Questions

- What is the answer to MM's question?

- What are the three different measures of the center of a distribution?

- What are two ways that the dispersion of a distribution is measured?

Basic Science Review and Discussion

The measurement of most outcomes in a population of subjects will vary. Whether you are measuring height, weight, blood pressure, or the change in any of these, there is usually variation between subjects. The collection of data on one of these variables is known as a distribution. We are often interested in some central tendency of a distribution, or what subjects experienced, "on average." The three standard measures of the center of a distribution are the mean, median, and mode. The mean (also known as the arithmetic mean or average) is the weighted sum of all measurements in a distribution. For example, if there are N subjects, the mean is the sum of all of the measurements divided by N. Denoted by

$$\bar{X} = \frac{\Sigma x_i}{N}$$

where $\bar{X}$ is the symbol for the sample mean, Σ is the symbol for a sum, and x_i represents each of the measurements as i varies from 1 to N. The median of a sample is that value that falls directly in the middle of all of the measurements; that is, 50% of them are above the median and 50% are below. If there are an even number of measurements, then the median is the average of the middle two values. The mode is that value that occurs most commonly in a distribution.

Variation of Distributions Although the mean and median give a feeling of the middle of a distribution, one also needs a measurement to describe the dispersion of the data. That is, while the data sets {49, 50, 51} and {1, 50, 99}

have the same mean, they are very different data. The variance, σ^2, or its square root the standard deviation, σ, are used to describe the dispersion of a distribution around its mean. If these values are higher, then the data are dispersed further away from the mean. In the most commonly assumed shape of a distribution, the normal distribution, the interval ranging from one standard deviation below the mean to one standard deviation above the mean, contains 68% of the data. If expanded to 1.96 standard deviations above and below the mean, 95% of the data is contained by the interval. A classic way to present data is the mean plus or minus 1.96 standard deviations, giving a 95% confidence interval (CI). If the analysis is part of a comparison of a study result to a null hypothesis, commonly 1 or 0, if the null hypothesis is not contained in the 95% CI, then it can be rejected.

Since the median measures the point at which 50% of the data are above it and 50% below, the dispersion measures used echo this technique; the most commonly used are the 25th and 75th centile points. This is where 25% of the data are below and above these points. Any centile mark can be used; 5th, 10th, 90th, and 95th are the most common after the 25th and 75th.

Types of Distributions In a symmetric distribution (i.e., the distribution is a mirror image of itself when folded over on the mean), the mean and median are the same value. Symmetric distributions include the normal distribution, or bell-shaped curve, and uniform distributions where any value in the possible range has the same probability of occurring. Other distributions may not be symmetric and can be described as skewed to the right or to the left (Figure 40-1), meaning that there are values that are farther away from the mean or median to the right or to the left, respectively. Another type of distribution seen commonly in medicine is the bimodal distribution (Figure 40-2), where two disparate results are seen much more commonly than the others. Other common distributions include the Poisson, Bernoulli, and binomial, which are further described in the Thumbnail.

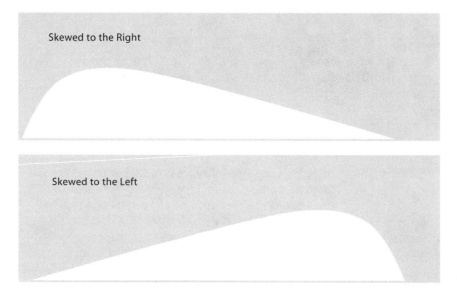

Figure 40-1: Asymmetric distributions

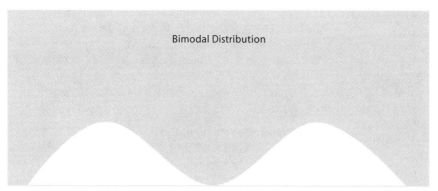

Figure 40-2: Biomodal distribution

Case Conclusion Given the preceding information, you discuss with MM that the mean decrement of 15 points means that the average person will lose 15 points off of their total cholesterol measurement. However, because the distribution is skewed to the left, toward 0, that more than 50% will actually experience a less than 15-point drop, but a few people will experience a very large drop.

Thumbnail: Biostatistics—Common Distributions and Their Mean and Variance

Distribution	Parameter(s)	Formula	Mean $[E(X)] = \bar{X}$	Variance
Uniform: defined over an interval (a,b), where probability of outcomes is equal	a,b	$P(X < c) = (c - a)/(b - a)$, where c is between a and b	$(a + b)/2$	$(b - a)^2/12$
Bernoulli: trial with binary outcomes 0 or 1	p	$P(X = 1) = p$ $P(X = 0) = 1 - p$	p	$p*(1 - p)$
Binomial: number of occurrences x in a series of n Bernoulli trials	n,p	$P(X = x) = (nCy) * p^y$ $(1 - p)^{n - y}$	np	$np(1 - p)$
Poisson: number of occurrences x in a given time period t	$\lambda = x/t$	$P(X=x/\lambda) = e^{-\lambda} \lambda^x/x!$	λ	λ

Note: $P(X = \#)$ is the probability that $x = \#$
p = probability of an event occurring (e.g., probability of outcome 1 in a Bernoulli trial)
x! = x factorial = x(x − 1)(x − 2) . . . (1)

Key Points

▶ The most common summary statistics utilized are the mean, or arithmetic average, and the median, which marks where 50% of the values are above and below.

▶ The variance 6^2 (and its square root, the standard deviation 6) give information about the spread of a distribution around its mean.

▶ When looking at a distribution around a median, more commonly, percentiles such as the 75th or 95th are used to communicate about the distribution.

▶ The most common distribution assumed and used in biostatistics is the normal distribution (or bell-shaped curve).

Questions

1. Given the following collection of data {1,2,4,6,7,8,9}, which is correct?
   A. The mean is 5.0.
   B. The median is 5.0.
   C. The median is 5.5.
   D. The median is 6.0.
   E. The mean is 6.0.

2. Given the following collection of data {1,1,1,1,2,3,5,5,6,6,7,7,9,9}, which of the following is correct?
   A. The mode is 1.
   B. The mean is 4.5.
   C. The median is 6.
   D. a and b are correct.
   E. a and c are correct.

3. Which of the following statements is true about a 95% confidence interval?
   A. There is a 95% chance that the true value is in the interval.
   B. Ninety-five percent of the time, the true value will fall in the interval.
   C. If you repeated the study 20 times, the true value would be in the interval at least once.
   D. If the interval does not contain the null hypothesis, you can be 95% certain that your result is the true value.
   E. If you repeat the study an infinite number of times, the results would fall in the interval 95% of the time.

4. You are told that your patient has a cholesterol result that is the mean of that in the population. Which of the following distributions would also mean that his result is necessarily greater than half of the population?
   A. Skewed to the left
   B. Skewed to the right
   C. Uniform
   D. Normal
   E. Bimodal

HPI: ST is a medical student who is working with you in an outpatient clinic. She comes to you with a research paper regarding an issue on a patient you saw together the previous day. The patient had high cholesterol and was asking to be treated with a drug that he saw in an advertisement. You had told the patient that there is no evidence to suggest that the drug is any better than the current medication he is on. The paper that ST brings to you found that in two groups of patients the mean value of total cholesterol points lowered was 12 for the new drug and 10 for the old drug in a study with a total of 40 patients. ST asks, "Doesn't this study show that the new drug is better than the old drug?"

Thought Questions

- What is the answer to ST's question?

- What test is used to compare two means?

- What test is used to compare two proportions?

- What test can be used to compare more than two groups?

- When these tests are used, how do you know what kind of errors in the findings might be made?

Basic Science Review and Discussion

One of the fundamental purposes of biostatistics is to be able to compare the summary statistics of two or more groups and determine the likelihood that the two groups are different. In the preceding case, we are interested in whether the mean values of 10 and 12 are statistically different. A number of factors go into this. The most important is how different the numbers actually are. In this case, 12 and 10 are relatively close together in that the total difference is 2 and, proportionately, 12 is only 20% more than 10. Nearly as important is the size of the study. In a study with thousands of patients in each group, these findings are likely to be statistically different. In this study with 40 patients, they are less likely to be statistically different, but this needs to be examined.

It is equally important to ask, when considering a finding such as the preceding, not only whether the results are statistically significant, but whether the findings are clinically significant. Essentially, one must ask whether the difference suggested by the results is enough to make a difference in clinical outcome. In the preceding case, it is unclear whether two more points lowered by a cholesterol-lowering agent are likely to make a clinical difference.

Finally, when considering studies, it is important to think of the results not as absolute, but as possibly making one of two types of errors. Results can essentially fall into one of four categories, true positive, true negative, false positive, and false negative (see Thumbnail). The first two mean that the results indicated by the study are correct. A false-positive result is known as type I error. This is what researchers attempt to avoid by having the null hypothesis be rejected only if it falls outside of a 95% confidence interval, or a $p < .05$ standard used in statistical tests. A false-negative result is known as type II error. Unfortunately, the standards used to examine type II error are poorer. Many studies with negative results do not report the probability of a type II error. The probability of not making a type II error is known as power. As compared with the less than 5% chance of making a type I error, commonly the standard for making a type II error is 20%, or only 80% power. One of the reasons for this is that many times to ensure a negative finding it is not worth the cost of increasing the sample size to ensure greater power. For the purposes of clinicians, it is important to understand these issues and the statistical tests used to compare outcomes.

Comparison of Two Groups   The two common summary statistics that will be compared between two groups are the mean of some measurement and the proportion of the group that is positive for some characteristic. When comparing means, the test used is called the Student's t test. The t test takes the difference between two means, divides it by a pooled estimate of the variance, and compares the result against a table of values dependent on the degrees of freedom. When comparing two proportions, the z test is commonly used. This test statistic is normally distributed, so it resembles the t test with an infinite number of degrees of freedom.

The t *Test*   An example of a situation in which the t test would be used is to compare the mean effect of an agent to lower cholesterol. Let us assume there are two agents, A and B, and we are comparing their effects in a small trial of 40 patients with the following results:

	A ($n = 18$)		B ($n = 22$)	
	Mean	SD	Mean	SD
Cholesterol difference	12	3	10	2

(where SD is standard deviation)
The formula for the t test is

$$t = \frac{(X_A - X_B)}{\sqrt{(s^2/n_A + s^2/n_B)}} \quad (s^2 = \text{pooled variance})$$

Where the pooled variance,

$$s^2 = \frac{(n_A - 1)(SD_A{}^2) + (n_B - 1)(SD_B{}^2)}{(n_A + n_B - 2)}.$$

So

$$s^2 = \frac{(18 - 1)(3^2) + (22 - 1)(2^2)}{(18 + 22 - 2)}$$

$$= \frac{(17 \times 9) + (21 \times 4)}{38}$$

$$= \frac{237}{38} = 6.24$$

and the t test is

$$t = \frac{12 - 10}{\sqrt{(6.24/18 + 6.24/22)}}$$

$$t = \frac{2}{\sqrt{(0.3467 + 0.2836)}}$$

$$t = \frac{2}{\sqrt{0.6303}} = \frac{2}{0.79} = 2.53$$

We then examine the t test table for 38 degrees of freedom (dof) and find the following:

t test probability	0.5	0.2	0.1	0.05	0.02	0.01	0.005	0.001
38 dof t value	0.681	1.304	1.686	2.024	2.429	2.712	2.98	3.57

So our value of 2.53 leads to a p-value just under 0.02, or more than 98% certainty that the two means are different.

Interestingly, even with this relatively small sample size, these findings were statistically significantly different. Another way to examine these findings would be to see what proportion of patients experienced a certain outcome.

The z Test   Now let us assume that instead of comparing the mean values in the two groups we care about the proportion of patients whose cholesterol was decreased by 10 points or more. Examining the same group studied earlier, we find

	A($n = 18$)	B ($n = 22$)
Number > 10 points	14	10
Proportion (p)	0.78	0.45

Now, when comparing sample proportions we need the proportions, sample size, and standard errors. Since these types of proportions are simply Bernoulli trials, that is each subject either does or does not meet the criteria proposed, an estimate for the standard error can be used from the Bernoulli distribution. That is,

$$\text{Std error, } s = \sqrt{[p(1 - p)/n]}$$

So the estimated standard errors for the preceding would be

$$s_A = \sqrt{(0.78 * 0.22/18)} = \sqrt{(0.00953)} = 0.098$$

$$s_B = \sqrt{(0.45 * 0.55/22)} = \sqrt{(0.01125)} = 0.106$$

And the z test is: $z = \dfrac{p_A - p_B}{\sqrt{s_A{}^2 + s_B{}^2}}$

$$z = \frac{(0.78 - 0.45)}{\sqrt{(0.00953 + 0.01125)}} = \frac{0.33}{0.144} = 2.29$$

Since this is a z test, it is comparable to a t test with an infinite number of degrees of freedom and is based on the normal distribution.

z test

Probability	0.5	0.2	0.1	0.05	0.02	0.01	0.005	0.001
z value	0.675	1.282	1.645	1.96	2.326	2.576	2.807	3.291

So the results of the test are that it is almost 98% certain that the proportion of subjects in group A that had a 10-point or greater drop in diastolic blood pressure is greater than that in group B. This comparison is done using a two-tailed test, since there is no initial assumption regarding which group is assumed to have a higher proportion. Of note, instead of a z test, commonly the chi-squared test is used to compare proportions. Interestingly, the z-distribution and chi-square distribution are related, in that as the sample size becomes large, the z-distribution squared is the chi-square distribution. One major advantage of the chi-square distribution is that it can be used not only to compare two proportions, but to analyze a study with multiple proportional results.

Case Conclusion   Going through the study with ST, you find that indeed there was a statistically significant difference in the two cholesterol-lowering agents. However, from a much larger clinical study you know that the difference of two points actually does not seem to make a long-term difference in rates of myocardial infarction (MI) or stroke. Thus you opt to wait for more evidence about the possibility that the drug will lower cholesterol more than this initial study or that this small difference will make a clinically significant difference in outcomes.

Thumbnail: Biostatistics—Types of Error Made in Research

Study Results	True Results	
	Positive	**Negative**
Positive	True positive	False positive Type I error
Negative	False negative Type II error	True negative

Key Points

▶ When comparing two means, commonly the Student's *t* test is used.

▶ When comparing two proportions, either the *z* test or chi-square test may be used.

▶ The chi-square test can also be used to compare more than two proportions.

▶ It is important to consider whether findings are both statistically significant and clinically significant.

Questions

1. You read a paper where the null hypothesis was not rejected with *p* = 0.18. A power analysis was done revealing 96% power. What is the probability that a type II error was made?

   A. 0
   B. 0.04
   C. 0.18
   D. 0.82
   E. 1

2. You are designing a study to investigate whether ethnicity is associated with type 2 diabetes. You have a cohort of 1000 patients of Asian, African American, Caucasian, and Latino ethnicity. Which of the following tests would be the best to compare the results of the study?

   A. Student's *t* test
   B. Power analysis
   C. *z* test
   D. Chi-square test
   E. Bonferroni correction

3. Which of the following best describes type I error?

   A. There is a positive result on a screening test, but the patient does not have the disease.
   B. There is a positive result on a screening test, and the patient does have the disease.
   C. There is a negative result on a screening test, and the patient does not have the disease.
   D. There is a negative result on a screening test, but the patient does have the disease.
   E. None of the above.

4. The following results from a screening study are available (Table 41-1). What are the rates of type I and type II errors, respectively?

   A. 0.15, 0.05
   B. 0.85, 0.05
   C. 0.95, 0.15
   D. 0.05, 0.85
   E. 0.05, 0.15

Table 41-1

Study Results	True Results	
	Positive	**Negative**
Positive	True Positive 85	False Positive 50
Negative	False Negative 15	True Negative 950

HPI: AM is a 35-year-old G1P0 woman at 14 weeks of gestation. She comes for a routine prenatal visit. At the end of her visit she tells you that she saw a genetic counselor and despite his recommendation to obtain an amniocentesis she would prefer to avoid the risk of this procedure if possible. You validate her decision and ask if she would like to obtain a triple-marker screening test for Down syndrome, which has an 80% sensitivity in women 35 or older. She is interested in this test because it involves only drawing blood and she will be quite happy to avoid the amniocentesis if the test is negative.

Her screening test returns the following week and is negative using a 1:190 cutoff. You tell her the happy news, and she asks, "Does this mean my baby does not have Down syndrome?"

Thought Questions

- What is the answer to AM's question?

- What are the sensitivity and specificity of a screening test?

- What are positive and negative predictive values?

- What are likelihood ratios?

Basic Science Review and Discussion

Often in medicine there are two possible pathways to a diagnosis. One method, illustrated earlier by amniocentesis, involves a risky, often more expensive diagnostic test. The second often involves utilizing a much less risky, often cheaper screening test to identify the high-risk patients within a population in order to determine who should undergo the more invasive test. Which pathway to use is dependent on the importance of the diagnosis, the baseline risk of the patient, the risk of the diagnostic procedure, and the test characteristics of the screening test. The two classic test characteristics reported are usually the sensitivity and specificity, and these, in addition to the other attributes of the situation, are used to determine whether a patient will benefit from being screened.

Test Characteristics **Sensitivity** is defined as the percentage of cases identified by a screening test. If among 100 cases, a screening test identifies 93 of them, then it has a 93% sensitivity. In a 2 × 2 table it is the number of true positives

divided by the total number with disease (Table 42-1). **Specificity** is the percentage of people without disease that are correctly identified as not having disease. For example, if in the same population above, there were 100 people who were not cases, and 96 of them were identified as not being cases, then the test has 96% specificity. In a 2 × 2 table this would be the number of true negatives divided by the total number of individuals without disease (Table 42-1). Of importance is the relationship between sensitivity and specificity. Most screening tests return a value that is either above or below a threshold. Where the threshold is set determines the sensitivity and specificity. If the threshold of the test is set quite low, then the sensitivity will be high but the specificity low. Conversely, if the threshold is set quite high, then the sensitivity will be low but the specificity high. When the sensitivity versus 1 minus specificity are plotted for a series of possible threshold values for a test, it is called a receiver-operator curve (ROC). The ROC can be examined to look for an optimal point where the trade-off between sensitivity increase and specificity decrease is equalized (Figure 42-1).

Predictive Value of Screening Tests Although the trade-off between sensitivity and specificity is an important consideration, another is how useful the test is to differentiate

Table 42-1. Sensitivity and Specificity in a 2 × 2 Table

Test Result	Disease	
	Present	**Absent**
Positive	a = TP true positive	b = FP false positive
Negative	c = FN false negative	d = TN true negative

Sensitivity = a/(a+c)
Specificity = d/(b+d)

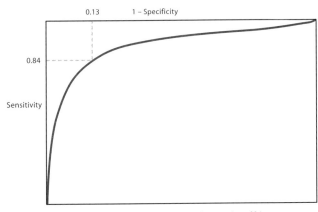

Figure 42-1: The ROC diagram illustrates the trade-off between sensitivity and specificity. In the ROC above, the point chosen illustrates where the sensitivity is 84% and the specificity is 87%.

Table 42-2. Calculating Predictive Value

	Disease	
Test Result	**Present**	**Absent**
Positive	a = TP true positive	b = FP false positive
Negative	c = FN false negative	d = TN true negative

PPV = a/(a+b)
NPV = d/(c+d)

individuals with a diagnosis from those without. One way to use the results of a screening test is to use its predictive value. The **positive predictive value** (PPV) is the proportion of screen-positive patients who actually have the diagnosis. These are the true positive patients divided by all those who test positive or $a/(a + b)$ in a 2 × 2 table (Table 42-2). The **negative predictive** value (NPV) is the proportion of screen-negative patients who do not have the diagnosis. These are the true negatives divided by all who test negative, or $d/(c + d)$ in a 2 × 2 table (Table 42-2). In the example of the triple marker screen, because the test is positive for all women with a risk greater than or equal to 1:190, the positive predictive value is poor, only about 1%. The negative predictive value, on the other hand, is quite good at 1:700 or better. This is because the baseline risk in the population is low.

Likelihood Ratios   The PPV and NPV of tests can also be calculated by using likelihood ratios (LR). A likelihood ratio is the probability of a particular test finding in a patient with disease divided by the probability of the same test finding in a patient without the disease. Thus a likelihood ratio can

be calculated for both positive and negative tests. A positive likelihood ratio, LR(+), is equal to the sensitivity divided by 1 − specificity, whereas the negative likelihood ratio test is equal to 1 − sensitivity divided by the specificity. This is shown here:

$$LR(+) = \frac{Prob(pos\ test\ given\ disease)}{Prob(pos\ test\ given\ no\ disease)} = \frac{a/(a + c)}{b/(b + d)}$$

$$= \frac{sensitivity}{1 - specificity}$$

$$LR(-) = \frac{Prob(neg\ test\ given\ disease)}{Prob(neg\ test\ given\ no\ disease)} = \frac{c/(a + c)}{d/(b + d)}$$

$$= \frac{1 - sensitivity}{specificity}$$

Now that we know how to calculate likelihood ratios, we need one more concept in order to use them to calculate posttest probabilities. What we need is odds as opposed to probability. Odds is a ratio of probabilities, defined as the probability of an event occurring divided by the probability of the event not occurring.

$$Odds = \frac{p}{1 - p} \text{ and } p = \frac{Odds}{Odds + 1}$$

The likelihood ratio is actually multiplied by the pretest odds to calculate the posttest odds. So the pretest probability can be converted to odds using the first of the preceding equations, then multiplied by the likelihood ratio, and converted back to probability using the second equation. Of note, when the pretest probability is small, less than 1%, odds and probability are almost equal.

Case Conclusion   You explain to AM that, despite a negative test, there is a small chance that her baby has Down syndrome, though using an LR(−) of 0.5, the probability is only half of what it was before having the test. Because she had not wanted an amniocentesis to begin with and now knows that her probability is lower, she decides to do without the diagnostic test. Her healthy 46XX baby girl is born 5 ½ months later.

Thumbnail: Biostatistics—Example of How to Use a 2 x 2 Table

Let's assume we are given the following 2 × 2 table for Down syndrome screening:

Test Result	Disease	
	Present	**Absent**
Positive	$a = 10$	$b = 980$ false positive
Negative	$c = 10$	$d = 9000$ true negative

Sensitivity = $a/(a + c) = 10/(20) = 0.5$
Specificity = $d/(b + d) = 9000/(9980) = 0.90$
PPV = $a/(a + b) = 10/(990) = 0.01$
NPV = $d/(c + d) = 9000/(9010) = 0.999$
LR(+) = sens/(1 − spec) = 0.5/0.1 = 5
LR(−) = (1 − sens)/spec = 0.5/0.9 = 0.56

Example of Using LR(+)
In this case, the pretest probability is 20/10,000 = 0.002
Odds = 0.002/(1 − 0.002) = 0.002
Posttest odds = 0.002 x (5) = 0.01
Posttest prob = 0.01/(1.01) = 0.01 = PPV

Key Points

▶ Any screening test has a trade-off between sensitivity and specificity.

▶ Because most screening tests are noninvasive, usually the goal is to get a maximum sensitivity.

▶ The predictive value of a test tells you what the probability of disease is in someone with that test result.

▶ The likelihood ratio can be used in a setting where you do not have a 2 × 2 table to calculate the predictive value of the test.

Questions

1. You are interested in developing a screening program to identify patients at high risk for a hematologic disease. The diagnostic test (bone marrow biopsy) for this disease is expensive, is painful, and has associated risks. There is no treatment at this time for the disease, but you feel it would be of some benefit to know whether you do have the disease earlier rather than later. If you are to be screening the general population, what test characteristics would you consider to be the best?
   A. 99% sensitivity and 10% specificity
   B. 98% sensitivity and 20% specificity
   C. 96% sensitivity and 40% specificity
   D. 90% sensitivity and 75% specificity
   E. 86% sensitivity and 99% specificity

2. A screening test is performed and there are 10 positive results. Of these, six are false-positives. Of note, there are exactly 10 people with disease in the population screened. Which of the following is true?
   A. This test has a 40% sensitivity.
   B. This test has a 60% sensitivity.
   C. This test has a 100% sensitivity.
   D. This test has a 60% specificity.
   E. This test has a 40% specificity.

3. A screening test for diabetes is being evaluated. You know that 900 nondiabetics and 100 diabetics are being screened. There are 100 positive tests, and of these, 90 have diabetes. Which of the following is true in this population?
   A. The negative predictive value of the test is 0.9.
   B. The negative predictive value of the test is 0.5.
   C. The negative predictive value of the test is 0.1.
   D. The positive predictive value of the test is 0.1.
   E. The positive predictive value of the test is 0.9.

4. In the screening test in question 3, what is the LR(+)?
   A. 1
   B. 8
   C. 81
   D. 99
   E. 990

HPI: One of the residents, RC, who works with you in the department of internal medicine meets with you to discuss a research project. RC says that she and many of her colleagues have been treating patients with pyelonephritis as outpatients throughout the past 6 months. She wants to study whether this treatment is as good as the inpatient treatment used earlier. Because they had made a conscious decision to change management, she wonders if this can be considered a prospective study.

Thought Questions

- Is RC's study prospective?

- What sort of studies could RC perform to examine this question?

- What are the differences between a case control and cohort study?

- When are retrospective studies preferable to prospective ones?

Basic Science Review and Discussion

Epidemiologic studies are undertaken to ascertain disease frequency, distributions, and determinants within populations of subjects; to identify risk factors for disease; and to examine whether different treatments are effective. Many types of studies can be performed, each having different strengths and weaknesses.

Descriptive Studies   These studies describe the general characteristics of the distribution of a disease in relation to personal demographic factors as well as other factors, such as diet or medication use. They are used to provide clues (hence generate hypotheses) about the possible determinants of a disease. They are also used to provide useful information for those planning health care services. **Descriptive studies** may be divided into individual-based studies and those that are population based.

Individual-based studies include (1) case reports of single patients, (2) case series where the characteristics of several patients with the same disease are reported, and (3) cross-sectional surveys in which individuals are studied with respect to both an exposure and a disease at a particular point in time. However, such studies cannot tell if the exposure preceded the disease or if the disease itself affected the patient's level of exposure. They are useful for questioning an association but not for testing an actual hypothesis. Further, although cross-sectional studies can give an idea about disease prevalence at a particular time, they do not provide information about the incidence of new cases of disease. For example, a disease with a high incidence but also a high mortality rate may have a low prevalence.

Population-based descriptive studies are used to examine different groups within an entire population and to compare the frequency of a disease at the same time, or the same population can be studied at different points in time. These are also called **correlational** studies.

Observational Studies   While a descriptive study is useful to determine baseline disease frequency, often we are interested in examining risk factors for disease as well as treatment. Analytic studies are explicit in nature as the investigator examines groups of individuals to ascertain if the risk of disease is different among those exposed to a factor from that among those not exposed. Hence hypotheses may be tested. They may be divided into observational and interventional studies. Observational studies can be retrospective or prospective and include case–control and cohort studies.

Case–control studies begin with collecting a group with the disease (cases) and a group without the disease (controls). Other data can then be collected about these patients, particularly concerning exposure to a particular factor of interest, and compared. These designs are useful when studying relatively rare diseases. Case–control studies are more commonly retrospective in nature, as the outcome of interest has already occurred and can be identified.

In **cohort studies** subjects are initially classified concerning the presence of an exposure and then followed for a length of time to ascertain the development of a particular disease. This design is best to investigate relatively common diseases or the risks associated with rare exposures, as enough data may be gathered in a relatively short time. These types of studies may be retrospective or prospective in nature. In retrospective studies, the study may be started after both the exposure and the disease have occurred, whereas in prospective studies exposed and nonexposed subjects are identified and then followed over time to ascertain disease development. Prospective studies are by their nature more complex, time-consuming, and expensive to perform but are very useful in identifying possible risk factors.

Interventional Studies   Whereas in the studies described thus far, patients are primarily observed to determine how they have fared in a nonexperimental clinical setting, in interventional studies, the investigator purposely intervenes. The study may entail the allocation of a particular exposure, but more commonly examines the efficacy of a particular treatment. Patients are then followed prospectively and their outcomes are measured, noted, and analyzed.

An interventional study may just involve the treatment of all patients with a particular disease to determine how they respond; however, these studies are often randomized so that some patients are treated and others are not. This allows the results of the study to show that the efficacy of the treatment is related to the treatment itself rather than to confounding factors.

The "gold standard" of these types of studies is the prospective, double-blinded, randomized, placebo-controlled trial. In this study design, the subjects are randomized into either an exposed (treatment) group or a nonexposed group (placebo), which allows these types of studies to provide reliable evidence regarding causation or prevention. A placebo should be identical to the treatment medication or procedure in shape, size, and color as well as how the treatment is performed. Randomization allows for control of other factors that may affect investigation except for the specific exposure under investigation. These factors are controlled for whether the investigator can identify them or not. The differences in survival rates between the two treatment groups are then compared. The double-blinded description refers to the concept that neither the patient nor the physicians running the study know who received the treatment. This can be difficult to do when there are obvious side effects from medications or particularly involved surgeries. The blinding of a study is important since it has been shown that simply being told you will be receiving a treatment can have an effect on outcomes. Additionally, by blinding the care-providers they will treat patients the same other than the intervention.

Since prospective, randomized, controlled trials (RCTs) are clearly much more reliable than case–control and cohort studies, why are they not the only types of clinical studies performed by medical researchers? There are a number of problems with RCTs beyond study design. The first is that they are quite expensive to administer and run, often costing millions of dollars. Second, it may not be ethical to offer a placebo control for many interventions where there is already an established treatment. In these cases, safety studies are often performed, and then a head-to-head study comparing one treatment to another is performed. Finally, prospective studies can take much longer to get an answer, whereas if retrospective data are available, it may be more reasonable to get an answer by collecting the data from charts and analyzing.

Case Conclusion   You discuss these possibilities with RC. After understanding the study designs a bit better, she would like to design a prospective RCT. However, given her time frame, she decides to begin with a retrospective case–control. She is going to identify all the patients treated as outpatients over the past 6 months and then find an equal number of inpatient controls in the time period prior. This will give her some safety data to support the idea of a prospective study in the future.

Thumbnail: Epidemiology—Study Design

Study Design	Aim of the Study	Outcome Measures	Strengths/Weaknesses
Cross-sectional studies	Information is gathered on possible risk factors and health status at a specific point in time	Prevalence rates	No information on incidence, nonanalytic
Case–control (often retrospective)	Prior exposure to risk factors is investigated	Odds ratios are used to quantify relative risk	Useful when disease is rare, inexpensive
Cohort (prospective or retrospective)	Follow those exposed to a risk factor and those not exposed to see who develops disease	Relative risk May be used to calculate attributable risk	Usually more powerful than case-control to identify risk factors, less expensive than interventional studies
Interventional studies (often RCTs)	To determine efficacy of intervention as compared to placebo or other intervention	Odds ratios, relative risk, cure rates	Controls for both identified and unidentified confounders.

Key Points

▸ A variety of study designs examine research questions in medicine. The one chosen depends on funding, timing, safety, and ethics of the treatment.

▸ When examining risk factors for a particular outcome, it is important to control for other possible confounding factors.

▸ Because case–control studies do not represent the true diseased versus control population ratio, an odds ratio rather than a relative risk is calculated.

Questions

1. Interventional trials can be too expensive and unwieldy to perform, whereas cross-sectional studies are much easier. Which of the following would be a problem in the design of a cross-sectional study?
   A. Selection bias
   B. Placebo selection
   C. Sampling bias
   D. Blinding
   E. Poor randomization

2. Which of the following is correct?
   A. Prevalence ratio is the number of persons who have a specific disease over a specific time period.
   B. Incidence rate is the number of persons who develop a disease in a specific time period divided by the total number at risk of developing the disease during the same time period.
   C. Prevalence equals the incidence divided by the average duration of the disease process.
   D. Prevalence is less than the incidence if the disease is long-lasting.
   E. If a disease is rapidly fatal or resolves quickly, the incidence is less than the prevalence.

3. You wish to study how diet and exercise are associated with the development of heart disease. Given that you have as much time as you need, the best study to perform would be
   A. A retrospective case–control study
   B. A retrospective cohort study
   C. A prospective case–control study
   D. A prospective cohort study
   E. A cross-sectional survey

4. There is a rare disease that occurs in 1 in 10,000 patients each year. You are interested in studying associations between the disease and patient demographics. You want to present the results of the study within the next year at a conference. The best study for this is:
   A. A retrospective case–control study
   B. A prospective, randomized control trial
   C. A retrospective cohort study
   D. A case series
   E. A prospective cohort study

HPI: CP is a 24-year-old woman who presents to the hospital for the management of her first labor and delivery. During her labor, her fetus begins to show nonreassuring signs on the fetal heart tracing known as late decelerations, but the fetal heart rate variability is still excellent. Suddenly, the fetal heart rate drops down to the 80s (normal is between 120 and 160). The staff moves the patient to the operating room for an emergent cesarean delivery. This is accomplished with delivery of the fetus 14 minutes from the time the fetal heart rate decreased. Upon delivery, there was noted to be a complete placental abruption with extreme maternal blood loss and the development of a consumptive coagulopathy. CP is given blood products and is stabilized without need for hysterectomy. However, her baby has seizures on the first day of life several hours after delivery.

Thought Questions

- Was this a case of malpractice?

- What factors might affect the probability of whether this will lead to a lawsuit?

- How can physicians decrease the chance that they will be sued?

Medical-Legal Review and Discussion

To determine whether the actions of a health care practitioner are consistent with malpractice, they need to be compared to existing national and local standards of practice. Medicine is not practiced in a vacuum, and what is considered standard practice can vary throughout the country (and certainly around the world). For instance, the procedure that is most commonly performed for an acute myocardial infarction, angioplasty, stent placement, or coronary artery bypass graft may vary between institutions and have regional trends. However, national standards also may be put forth by an accredited body such as the American College of Surgeons, or research literature may be used to substantiate a particular clinical pathway.

In the preceding case, it is difficult to know from the description how long the fetal heart rate tracing showed the nonreassuring late decelerations. Even in light of these, fetal heart rate variability is more predictive of current fetal status, and that description did not necessarily merit action on the part of the obstetrician. Once the acute sign of fetal distress, the fetal bradycardia, occurred, the obstetrician and labor and delivery team acted quickly and were able to deliver the fetus in 14 minutes. The American College of Obstetricians and Gynecologists has used the standard of 30 minutes, and research suggests that the most serious fetal morbidity occurs once bradycardia is 15 minutes or longer. Given these two aspects of support for the care given, as well as the excellent care for CP intraoperatively and postoperatively for her coagulopathy, there is no evidence of malpractice in this case. However, whether a lawsuit will result in this setting is a different story.

Risk Factors for a Lawsuit Of course, the principal risk factor for a lawsuit in medical practice is a bad patient outcome. Even if a physician makes errors in the care of a patient but they do not result in a bad patient outcome, the patient is unlikely to sue. Moreover, if the patient wants to sue, it is unlikely that such a suit would yield much, since there are little or no damages. Given this, what patients may define as a bad outcome can be quite varied, and often more pain and suffering or mental anguish than might have been experienced in another health care setting can be considered a bad outcome for litigious patients. While having a bad outcome is an almost necessary risk factor for a lawsuit, it is not sufficient. Bad outcomes occur constantly in the health care setting. In fact, it is estimated that even among patients who do have bad outcomes and experienced some degree of substandard care, 5% or fewer of these patients proceed to a lawsuit. Given these low numbers, what other factors may be predictive of lawsuits?

One clear factor that is predictive of whether a patient will sue is the type of relationship that the patient and the care provider enjoy. Thus patients are more likely to sue physicians who they have only interacted with for a short time than they are to sue those with whom they have longstanding relationships. Another factor is the nature of their relationship. If the physician has provided what the patient perceives as excellent care for a long time, then the patient is less likely to sue than if he or she perceives that the physician has made other mistakes or provided care different from what he or she would have liked in the past.

Another factor related to the relationship is that of the communication between the physician and the patient. Often physicians who are overworked and dealing with several ill patients simultaneously may be rushed in their communication with a patient and the patient's family. Furthermore, it is common that once a bad event or outcome occurs that the physician may avoid that patient either for feelings of guilt or simply because talking to patients about bad outcomes is difficult. It has been shown that physicians who simply spend more time with patients communicating about their disease, the plan of treatment, and the possible outcomes are sued less often. Similarly, physicians are also less likely to be sued if they seek to communicate to the patient and the family frequently after a bad outcome and explain what happened and what the plan of care is now.

It seems that certainly these two risk factors are the most important to a physician or a physician-in-training, as they are what can most easily be affected by physician behavior. However, other risk factors exist as well, such as patient demographics and socioeconomic status (wealthy > poor), region of the country (northeast > midwest), and the field of medicine (obstetrics > internal medicine) being practiced. However, a physician cannot affect these factors other than by moving or changing the field of medicine being practiced.

Evidence-Based Practice Opposed to Defensive Medicine
Because of concerns for lawsuits, many physicians practice defensive medicine. An example of this would be ordering a CT for every patient with a headache, or at least those who ask for one. It results in the waste of medical resources, causes unnecessary tests, and rarely results in better outcomes. In fact, because tests all have false-positive rates, it can lead to further risky diagnostic tests that may lead to complications.

A better way to practice that is also likely to avoid lawsuits, or at least avoid malpractice, is to practice evidence-based medicine. This seems obvious; however, with the number of medical journals and advances in medicine in the pharmaceutical, diagnostic technology, and procedural fronts, it can be difficult to keep abreast of all of the changes in medical practice once a physician completes training. Continuing Medical Education (CME) credits are required to maintain licensure, but one or two courses per year rarely update the clinical knowledge necessary to stay at the forefront of medical practice. Another way to maintain excellence is to attend weekly grand rounds and morbidity and mortality rounds at a university teaching hospital. Practicing in a group of physicians rather than in solo practice is another way to stay on top of changes in the practice of medicine, as is reading the current journals as much as possible. Usually, summaries of important journal articles and updates on clinical practice are published by medical societies. These are excellent substitutes for failing to read three or four journals per month and provide an idea of national standards.

Case Conclusion   After CP's cesarean section, her physician meets with her family to describe what happened to her and her baby, and answers their numerous questions. In the following 5 days, CP's physician sees her every morning and evening while she recovers from her cesarean delivery and coagulopathy. He also checks in with the neonatologists frequently to determine how her baby is doing and communicates this information to CP. An MRI of CP's baby's brain shows no evidence of anoxic brain injury. CP is discharged home on postoperative day 5 and her baby is able to go home on day of life 10. A week later, she sees her obstetrician in the clinic and they discuss the events that led to her emergent cesarean delivery again. A year later, she presents to her obstetrician's office with a positive pregnancy test for care again. She reports that her baby is slightly delayed, but making progress on all of his developmental milestones.

Thumbnail: Medical-Legal Issues—Decreasing Risk of Lawsuit

Risk Factor	Description
Relationship	Forming longstanding relationships with patients does decrease the risk of a lawsuit; however, this is impossible in an acute setting. A strong immediate relationship can be formed by acknowledging patient concerns, discussing tests and treatments before they are ordered, and breaking down some of the professional barriers that stand between a physician and patient in terms of power, paternalism, and information asymmetry.
Communication	It is important to communicate with patients regarding their diagnosis, tests, treatment, and prognosis in an unhurried fashion, allowing patients and their families to ask questions. It is also important to follow up with patients after bad events to make sure that they do not feel abandoned and to ensure that they are able to understand why a particular outcome has occurred.
Knowledge	More than in any other profession, updating medical knowledge by a practitioner is paramount in medicine. The available data change rapidly, and keeping up with national standards is difficult, but this above all else is the foundation for competent medical care.

Key Points

▶ Malpractice is providing health care in a way that does not meet local or national standards.

▶ Many cases of malpractice go unnoticed because they do not necessarily lead to bad outcomes.

▶ Even in cases of malpractice with bad outcomes, 5% or less actually lead to lawsuits.

▶ Lawsuits occur less often when physicians have a good relationship with a patient; communicate thoroughly, allowing all questions to be answered; and do not avoid patients after bad events occur.

Questions

1. You are a surgeon taking care of three patients in the emergency department. One has chronic back pain, one has abdominal pain suspicious for appendicitis, and one has a laceration of her hand requiring sutures. You are seeing your third patient who wants to discuss the possibility of scarring and is quite concerned; however, you are paged by the radiologist regarding the CT results on your abdominal pain patient. Which of the following is the likely the best provision of care?

A. Because you are currently with your third patient, continue your discussion with her and answer all of her questions.
B. Tell your third patient, "I will be right back," and go see your first patient, who has been waiting the longest.
C. Tell your third patient, "Let me go arrange a consultation with plastic surgery after I answer this page" and go to answer the page from radiology.
D. Tell your third patient, "Don't worry; no one will notice this scar," and go to answer your page.
E. Tell your third patient, "Don't worry; no one will notice this scar" and suture her hand.

2. You are an obstetrician providing care for a patient in labor. A nurse informs you that the fetal heart rate is experiencing a bradycardia, and on examination there is an umbilical cord prolapse. The patient is being moved to the operating room for an emergency cesarean section. Which of the following describes optimal documentation of this event?

A. Immediately write down your impression of the situation and your plan of action.
B. Go to the patient's bedside and facilitate the move to the operating room; after the cesarean, write a note documenting what occurred and when.
C. Tell the nurse your plan of action, then postoperatively, time your note for when you told the nurse of the plan.
D. Write a quick note, and then postoperatively, make changes to the note that reflect what actually occurred.
E. There is no need to document what occurred, because nursing will do the documentation.

3. A patient you are seeing for the first time has chronic back pain. He wishes to have an immediate MRI and a referral to a neurosurgeon. He tells you this is what his last doctor was going to do. Your best course of action is to

A. Order the MRI and make the referral.
B. Tell the patient that because this is the first visit, you need to start the work-up of his back pain from the start.
C. Give the patient ibuprofen and order an x-ray of the back.
D. Ask the patient for the name and number of his prior physician and ask him to obtain his prior medical records and reschedule him in 1 or 2 weeks.
E. Order a CT and refer him to an orthopedic surgeon.

4. A physician is caring for a patient with atrial fibrillation and is prescribing medication to anticoagulate her blood. Which of the following actions is most likely to increase the risk of lawsuit?

A. Physician prescribes twice the necessary dosage of medication, but there are no complications and a month later, the dosage is decreased.
B. Physician prescribes the appropriate medication, but the patient experiences a stroke despite the treatment. Physician sees the patient daily in the hospital.
C. Physician prescribes the appropriate medication, but the patient experiences a stroke despite the treatment. Physician explains how medication does not always work.
D. Physician prescribes the appropriate medication, but the patient experiences a stroke despite the treatment. The physician allows the hospital team to provide excellent care for the patient and plans to see the patient back in the office after discharge.
E. Physician prescribes the appropriate medication, but the patient experiences a stroke despite the treatment. Physician updates the patient's family with daily changes in her status.

MH is a 32-year-old woman who presents for an annual exam to you, her primary physician. When she comes into your office she appears a bit angry. You ask her what is wrong and she replies, "My health insurance plan has added copays to the visits, so now I have to pay $15 for this appointment. It annoys me that I am paying more out of pocket for the same health insurance." You say, "Do you have dental insurance?" She answers affirmatively. "Don't you pay a portion of the bill at that office?" "Twenty percent" she replies, "but I don't have to pay it until later, whereas here, I have to pay it up front, and your office doesn't take credit cards. Also, I don't have to pay anything for the annual cleaning, just when I have a cavity filled. For my health care, I pay to come to the annual exam, but wouldn't have to pay if I was admitted to the hospital." You agree with her that this seems a bit odd but remind her that it is a small amount of money and that in the long run, it is likely cheaper than paying a portion of a hospitalization.

Thought Questions

- What is the purpose of health insurance in the United States?

- Why have many health plans started charging copays for office visits?

- What are moral hazard and adverse selection?

- What is the difference between copays and coinsurance?

Basic Science Review and Discussion:

Health insurance that would pay for hospital costs and/or physician fees has been around since the turn of the twentieth century in the United States. With the advent of unions representing workers to large industrial firms, health insurance coverage was one of the benefits that was demanded for workers. For retired workers, **Medicare** was created in the late 1960s to provide health insurance. Similarly, **Medicaid** was created for those who were near the poverty level. Increasingly, having health insurance is equated with having access to health care. This is worrisome, since the number of the uninsured or underinsured continues to increase in the United States and is currently thought to be approximately 40 million.

While Americans rely primarily on health insurance to pay for health care services, most westernized nations have national health care systems that permit their citizens to receive treatment without fees. Of note, most of these countries also have private physicians who the wealthy pay extra to see. Furthermore, many of the services we expect as part of health care are less available in these countries, and patients are generally managed in a less aggressive fashion.

Health Insurance and Adverse Selection   One of the important aspects of any form of insurance is the information asymmetry between the insurer and the insured. Generally, an individual knows his or her own health risks better than an insurance firm. This can lead to only the sicker, at-risk individuals purchasing health insurance. If only the sicker individuals who will use more health services purchase health insurance, this will lead to the cost of health insurance increasing. This cyclic process that results in only the most at-risk members of society purchasing health insurance is known as **adverse selection.** In the United States, because most members of society get their insurance through employment, there is minimal adverse selection because there is no decision involving the cost of insurance. Generally, health insurance for most is a benefit, received essentially free of charge (which leads to another problem, moral hazard). However, among those individuals who are purchasing their own health insurance, concerns for adverse selection may lead insurance companies to raise fees.

Health Insurance and Moral Hazard   When the consumption of an item, such as health care, is subsidized or paid for entirely, we are more likely to consume more than we would want if we were bearing the costs. This complication of insurance is known as **moral hazard.** In the health insurance and health care sectors we see this occur at two levels. First, because health insurance is often a benefit of employment, we will have whatever insurance plan that is offered by the company, despite what we would want if we had to pay for it. Since health insurance also covers spouses, many two-income families have double the insurance, clearly much more than anyone would need.

Second, once insured, the individual bears no or minimal financial cost of the health care services consumed. For example, if there are two drugs for a treatment, one that costs $1000 that is just taken one time and another that costs $20 but requires three doses per day for a week, most individuals would chose to purchase the cheaper treatment despite the inconvenience of the longer dosing. However, if the price is the same to the patient (say, a $10 copay for either), then the patient is likely to chose the more convenient dosing. Thus, without bearing any of the cost of consumption, patients will overutilize health care, driving costs up for the entire society.

Copays and Coinsurance   One way to have patients bear some of the costs of the consumption of health care is for them to pay for part of the costs. Two ways this is done are **copays** (a set amount per service or product) and **coinsurance** (a fixed percentage of costs up to a certain amount). Since the 1990s, copays have been increasing in the usage of clinical services and pharmaceuticals and usually range from $5 to $25 per visit. The copay for an emergency room visit is usually higher, at $50 or so, to discourage use in a nonemergent condition. However, there are usually no copays for hospitalizations and diagnostic tests, which is where the largest costs are incurred. Thus it is unclear whether copays actually decrease costs in any appreciable way.

Coinsurance is most commonly seen with dental insurance, where the individual might pay approximately 20% of all services obtained, possibly up to a certain **deductible**. This provides a disincentive to overutilize services. In the preceding example, one interesting point made by MH is that as a society we might want to encourage the use of preventive care, such as annual exams. This is commonly done with dental and vision packages, where the annual exams are covered, but more services have a deductible or coinsurance attached. However, in most health plans, patients pay the copay to obtain preventive care, but do not do so for hospitalizations.

Because of the concern for overinsurance and rising health care costs ($1.4 trillion in 2002) forms of insurance with larger coinsurance, higher copays, and greater deductibles are being suggested to decrease the moral hazard within the health care system.

Case Conclusion   MH undergoes her annual exam and you notice a 2-cm breast lump. She undergoes a mammogram, ultrasound, and breast biopsy (approximately $3000 cost). You see her after the work-up and point out that her health insurance only cost her the two office copays ($30), whereas she would have paid $600 if it was similar to her dental insurance. This cheers her up considerably, along with the news that the mass was just a benign cyst.

Thumbnail: Health Policy—Methods to Decrease Moral Hazard

Method	Description
Copay	A small fee paid in conjunction with services or product obtained, although much less than the actual cost of health care, has been shown to decrease utilization.
Coinsurance	A percentage of the amount billed or reimbursed— commonly, 10% to 20%. Currently seen most often with older indemnity insurance plans and with dental or vision insurance.
Deductible	A set limit of $100 to several thousand dollars or more paid by the insured, after which the charge is paid by the insurance company. This provides insurance against large costs, but still allows for cost-based decision making below these costs.

Key Points

- Most individuals obtain their health insurance through their or their spouse's employment.
- Medicare and Medicaid are national insurance plans designed to cover the elderly and poor, respectively.
- Despite these plans, approximately 40 million Americans are uninsured.
- Health care costs were $1.4 trillion in 2002.

Questions

1. Which of the following is moral hazard?
   A. Patient with diabetes pays for better drug coverage.
   B. Professional tennis player decides not to purchase health insurance.
   C. Insured patient with headache demands CT scan from physician.
   D. Patient without insurance buys only half the medication prescribed.
   E. Patient with chest pain goes to emergency room.

2. Which of the following is a component of adverse selection?
   A. Patient with diabetes pays for better drug coverage.
   B. Professional tennis player decides not to purchase health insurance.
   C. Insured patient with headache demands CT scan from physician.
   D. Patient without insurance buys only half the medication prescribed.
   E. Patient with chest pain goes to emergency room.

3. Which of the following might be useful in decreasing moral hazard?
   A. $5 copay for office visits
   B. $500 deductible for pharmaceutical use
   C. 20% coinsurance for all health care bills
   D. A and B
   E. A, B, and C

4. Which of the following might help with adverse selection?
   A. $5 copay for office visits
   B. $500 deductible for pharmaceutical use
   C. 20% coinsurance for all health care bills
   D. Risk-adjusting health insurance premiums
   E. Providing health insurance at the same price to everyone

HP is a 64-year-old woman who you have served as her primary care physician for 12 years. She presents to your office for an annual exam. After the exam, you are going over her laboratory results, which were all within normal results. At the end of the visit, she thanks you for your care and informs you that she is not sure whether she will be able to continue to see you because her husband is retiring and their health plan is switching from one funded by his employment to Medicare. She has a list of plans that are available from Medicare that she and her husband can choose from and need to do so over the next month. She and her husband are worried about paying big deductibles and about pharmaceutical costs, so they have chosen a plan where they can see certain physicians without any copay or deductible, but if they see any other physician, they must pay 20% coinsurance.

Thought Questions

- What are the common health plan designs seen in the United States?

- What is managed care?

- What types of financial incentives do physicians in different plans have?

- What type of plan has HP switched into?

Basic Science Review and Discussion

The traditional way that health care was provided in the United States prior to the 1950s was on a fee-for-service basis. Patients would see a physician and pay for services rendered. However, as health care costs rose, particularly in the hospital sector, more individuals carried some form of health care insurance. This health care insurance by and large paid most or all of health care costs, but still on a fee-for-service basis. This insurance was of a standard indemnity type. Patients could choose their health care providers, and either the provider or the patient could submit the bill to the insurance company. As unions gained more strength in the workplace, one of the benefits they insisted upon was health insurance for the employees and their families. Thus, by the mid-1960s, most people had health insurance if they were employed by a large firm.

Managed Care Although standard indemnity insurance was fine when health care costs were reasonable, as they increased to larger sums, health insurance companies began to intervene in the actual services provided. This sort of insurance is known as managed indemnity. Thus, although the reimbursements are the same as fee-for-service, the insurance company may get involved with utilization review or preapproval of services. This became known as managed care, where nonclinicians were managing the provision of health care by clinicians. Needless to say, this has not been generally well received by physicians or patients.

Another route taken by a few firms was instead of paying for health insurance, they provided a company physician to care for their employees. In the case of one firm in particular, Kaiser, a physician was hired to care for employees working on a dam. Such physicians were paid on a salary or prospectively per capita (per employee in the firm). This sort of payment was entirely different from traditional fee-for-service, and some large firms felt that costs of this type were much more predictable. Kaiser expanded this form of the provision of health care that it offered to its own employees and began offering it to other firms' employees. This plan was known as a Health Maintenance Organization (HMO). It differed from traditional medicine in that the providers of health care were paid on a prospective, per capita basis and the focus was on preventive, cooperative, and large-group practice of medicine. The standard HMOs were either the group model, in which the HMO contracted exclusively with a collection of providers, or the staff model, in which the HMO hired physicians on a salaried basis to staff their clinics and hospitals. In the late 1980s and throughout the 1990s, these forms of medical practice were adopted on a widespread basis, incorporating several other components, utilization review and quality assurance, to control health care costs.

Health Plan Evolution In addition to the number of plans that became HMOs, a number of other types of health plan have been created and adopted over the past two decades. One of these is known as the preferred provider organization (PPO). A PPO endeavors to create a network of providers that a health insurance plan believes will help control costs better than other health care providers in the same area. In fact, the health plan may make a contract with providers that tells them what treatments can be used in certain situations, that they will undergo utilization review of some of their medical management, and that they may need preapproval for particularly expensive treatment plans. Then the patient in the PPO is able to receive care from network providers at no cost or a small copay. However, if they seek care outside the network, they must pay a much higher copay or a certain percentage of the bill.

Another plan resembles a PPO, in that it is based on having a network of providers; it is known as a point-of-service plan, or POS. A key innovation by the POS plans was to have primary care gatekeepers. Thus for a patient to see a specialist or have an emergency room visit covered, he or she would first need a referral from the primary care provider. This put a lot of the burden to control costs on the primary care provider, who was commonly paid via capitation, which created a financial incentive to minimize referrals.

Another health plan, which was created to compete with the large, vertically integrated HMOs in particular, is the independent practice association (IPA). Whereas some HMOs were just loosely associated networks of providers, not that dissimilar from a PPO, others were quite organized, having hospitals, physicians with exclusive relationships with these hospitals, and patients that received little or no reimbursement if they went outside the HMO. IPAs bound collections of individual and small groups of physicians together. Similar to other HMOs, these IPAs often paid the physicians on a prospective basis based on the number of patients who considered them their physician. Although IPAs increased in number in the 1990s, their numbers have decreased since 2000, possibly because they suffered from a lack of collegiality and collaboration that vertically integrated HMOs are able to facilitate.

One way in which PPOs and IPAs differ significantly from vertically integrated HMOs is the exclusivity of the relationship between the health plan and the physician. Thus, physicians can see patients who have a variety of different insurance plans. In a vertically integrated plan such as Kaiser Permanente Medical Group, physicians have an exclusive relationship with the plan.

Health Care Costs   Unfortunately, some of the initial reductions in health care costs accomplished by HMOs have not been maintained in the long term. Some of the cost reductions were not real, but were accomplished because the types of patients (employed, young) cared for by the HMOs were less expensive to care for than patients in other health plans. However, many of the cost reductions gained by shifting hospitalized patients to outpatient surgery, home health care, and short-term nursing facilities were one-time cost reductions now adopted by much of the health care system, but such measures do not continue to reduce costs. One method to reduce costs utilized by health plans in the 1990s was to give the physician reduced financial incentives to provide expensive care.

In the traditional fee-for-service practice of medicine, the more patients and procedures a physician sees and does, the more income is earned. However, in the most severe form of managed care, physicians' salaries and bonuses were tied to how much health care was utilized by their patients. Thus if a patient was hospitalized, needed several CTs, had an angiogram, and required expensive medical treatment, this was counted against a total amount of allowable expenses for the physician. This led to a backlash from both patients and physicians and to a number of bankrupt medical groups who attempted to bear the medical expenses of a panel of patients but failed. Increasingly today, physicians bear little of the financial risk of their patients' health care, but at the same time, they are reimbursed less for the sheer volume of health care provided. Thus neither the one-time cost reductions nor the financial incentives to physicians have been able to keep health care costs from rising without impacting quality of care. Meanwhile, costs continue to rise secondary to increasing technology and pharmaceuticals, reaching $1.4 trillion in 2002.

Case Conclusion   You discuss HP's new plan with her. It turns out to be a PPO of which you are a member. HP is relieved that she will be able to continue to see you, and actually schedules a visit with you for her husband who "hasn't seen a doctor in 10 years."

Thumbnail: Health Policy—Types of Health Plans

	Indemnity	Managed Indemnity	PPO	POS	IPA HMO	Group or Staff HMO
Premiums	High	High	Medium	Medium	Medium	Low
Deductible	High	High	Medium	0	0	0
Copays and coinsurance	High	High	Medium	Low	Low	Low
Gatekeeper	N	N	N	Y	Y	Y
Preapproval for care	N	Y	Y	+/−	+/−	+/−
Exclusive relationship with doctor	N	N	N	N	N	Y
Coverage out of network	Y	Y	Extra cost	Extra cost	N	N
Market share in United States	Minimal	Decreasing	Increasing	Minimal	Moderate, beginning to fall	Moderate, beginning to fall

Key Points

▶ Managed care was begun to help decrease health care costs.

▶ Forms of managed care included having primary care providers act as gatekeepers, requiring preapproval for some types of care, and only insuring care within a defined network of providers.

▶ Another form of health plan that evolved was the group or staff model HMO, which was an exclusive network of providers and often facilities just for their insured.

▶ Despite the variety of forms of health plans and financial disincentives placed on providers, health care costs continue to rise.

Questions

1. CC has had a cough for 3 days. She has no fever and no nausea or vomiting, but she does have some postnasal drip and sinus congestion. She visits a hospital emergency room that is nearest to her work without verifying if her insurance will cover the visit. Which form of health plan is most likely to charge her the most?
   A. Standard indemnity
   B. Managed indemnity
   C. PPO plan
   D. POS plan
   E. IPA model HMO

2. You are a primary care physician and see a patient in your office who has back pain, a fever of 102°F, chills, dysuria, and a urinalysis positive for white blood cells and bacteria. You decide to admit the patient to the hospital for intravenous antibiotics. Which health plan is most likely to allow the admission without preapproval.
   A. Managed indemnity
   B. PPO plan
   C. POS plan
   D. IPA model HMO
   E. Staff model HMO

3. A health plan is attempting to give a financial incentive to physicians to provide the least expensive care. Which of the following reimbursement schemes would best accomplish this?
   A. Fee-for-service payment (payment for every procedure performed)
   B. Prospective, capitated payment (payment to care for a patient the entire year)
   C. Flat salary (the same amount of money, regardless of care)
   D. Salary plus bonus for seeing more than 20 patients per session
   E. Fee-for-service plus bonus for seeing more than 20 patients per session

4. As discussed in the text, which of the following is in chronological order of the development of health plans?
   A. Indemnity, POS, PPO, IPA, HMO
   B. HMO, POS, indemnity, PPO, IPA
   C. Indemnity, HMO, PPO, IPA
   D. HMO, IPA, indemnity, PPO
   E. Indemnity, IPA, HMO, PPO

Case 40

1. D
2. D
3. E
4. B

Case 41

1. B
2. D
3. A
4. E

Case 42

1. E
2. A
3. E
4. C

Case 43

1. C
2. B
3. D
4. A

Case 44

1. C
2. B
3. D
4. D

Case 45

1. C
2. B
3. E
4. D

Case 46

1. E
2. E
3. B
4. C

Answers

Case 1

1. B Rapprochement was defined by Margaret Mahler as the process by which the child practices moving away from the parent or caregiver, coming back for reassurance and comfort. Separation anxiety typically occurs at 7 to 9 months, as does stranger anxiety. Exploration is not a stage, as it happens to everyone at all ages in differing forms. Attachment theorists, such as Mary Ainsworth, defined different types of attachment patterns in infants: secure, insecure, and unattached. The type of attachment defined how the infant interacted with the world, parents, and strangers.

2. C Children usually take their first steps around their first birthday. Usually by 18 months they can walk up steps.

3. C As this child is speaking in two-word sentences his age should be 2; thus he should be able to wash and dry his hands. Riding a tricycle is usually accomplished around age 3. Copying a +, hopping on one foot, and dressing without supervision are usually accomplished by age 4.

4. B This child has a social smile (1 to 2 months) and can grasp (4 months) but cannot sit unassisted (6 months). The stepping reflex (in which if the infant is held vertically with pressure on feet she will make stepping motions) disappears at 2 to 3 months. All the others except Babinsky are gone by 4 to 6 months. These include the moro reflex (movement causing extension, abduction, and then adduction of the extremities), grasp reflex (pressure on the palm causes infants to grasp), and rooting reflex (oral or perioral stimulation causing orientation toward the stimulus and sucking). Babinsky (scratching the lateral aspect of the sole [heel to toe] leads to dorsiflexion of the big toe and fanning of other toes) is consistently negative (flexor, downward) after 18 months.

Case 2

1. B Piaget—Preoperational. Piaget was the theorist who examined cognitive development, using the terms *sensorimotor, preoperational, concrete operations,* and *formal operations.* An "operation" is an action carried out through logical thinking. Thus children age 2 to 5 have not mastered logical reasoning. A classic example of this is failure of conservation (i.e., not understanding the concept that no matter what shape the flask, if you pour water from one to the other, the amount of water remains constant).

2. C Freud described the phallic phase or Oedipal phase from 3 to 6 years of age. It is characterized by the child's discovering that the genitals are a site for pleasure. This is a time of sexual curiosity. The Oedipus complex can be understood as a child's desire for the opposite-sex parent, and a conflictual wish for the same-sex parent (and any siblings) to be gone. The oedipal/phallic phase is followed by the latency phase (age 6 to 12), in which the child identifies with the same-sex parent and focuses on same-sex friendships. *Preoperational* and *sensorimotor* are cognitive stages from Piaget.

3. E From the developmental clues this child is about 4 years old. Erikson's basic stages are the following: (a) *Trust vs mistrust (birth to 12 months).* Meeting basic needs. (b) *Autonomy vs shame and doubt (12 months to 3 years).* The child is gaining confidence in his or her abilities (e.g., learning to walk, and mastering bowel and bladder control). Parents need to be supportive not disapproving. (c) *Initiative vs guilt (3 to 5 years).* The task is to be able to initiate and carry through on tasks, to achieve a sense of competence and mastery. (d) *Industry vs inferiority (age 6 to 11).* The child feels a sense of competence through mastery of skills in the context of school and culture. (e) *Identity vs role diffusion (11 years of age to the end of adolescence).* This involves a consistent sense of oneself in any situation and the ability to ask the questions and make the decisions that are necessary to become an adult.

4. B The stages that cover the first year of life are the following: (a) Oral (Freud—babies get their primary gratification through oral stimulation, sucking). (b) Trust vs mistrust (Erikson—infants depend on others for food, shelter, and affection, and therefore must be able to completely trust their parents or caregivers). (c) Sensorimotor (Piaget—the child's understanding of the world is based on sensory input and growing motor ability).

Case 3

1. A Testicular feminization syndrome is also called androgen insensitivity, as the body cells do not respond to this hormone. Inguinal masses may reveal testicles at puberty, and breasts develop normally. Development of the gonads depends on the Y chromosome. The testes secrete hormones, which cause the internal and external genitalia to develop as a male. If there are no secretions, then the internal and external genitalia develop as female. Prenatal exposure to these hormones leads to gender-specific differences in brain development. Congenital adrenal hyperplasia has a 46,XX genotype and a female phenotype though the genitals are masculinized. In this disorder the adrenal glands cannot produce enough cortisone, which leads to excessive adrenal androgen secretion. In Turner's syndrome the genotype is 45,X and the phenotype is a female with short stature, a web neck and cubitus valgus. These females are infertile, as their ovaries are nonfunctional.

2. C The use of serotonin reuptake inhibitors (SSRIs) is associated with increased rates of anorgasmia in females and impaired ejaculation. Levodopa causes an increase in libido and erectile performance. Neuroleptics have the opposite effect and may cause erectile failure. Yohimbine is an α_2-agonist and can be used to enhance sexual function in both males and females. Venlafaxine (Effexor) is thought to have few sexual side effects. Sildenafil (Viagra) inhibits phosphodiesterase, thus enhancing nitric oxide enhanced cGMP and causing vasodilatation. However, like trazodone, it may cause priapism (a persistent and painful erection that may require surgical intervention). Other medications that inhibit sexual performance include beta-blockers and chronic use of alcohol, marijuana, and heroin. Amphetamines and cocaine may increase libido. Alcohol and marijuana may increase libido by increasing disinhibition when initially used. Other prescription drugs that cause impaired sexual function include antihypertensives and other antidepressants such as tricyclics.

3. E Trazodone acts as both a serotonin and α_2-adrenergic antagonist and may be moderately helpful in about a third of patients with erectile dysfunction (ED), but it may cause unwanted sedation or priapism. Other treatments include sildenafil (Viagra), local injections of prostaglandin E1 intracavernosally, and intraurethral E1 suppositories. Sildenafil has become very popular, with success rates in up to 80% of men treated, but it is contraindicated in patients taking long-acting nitrate or nitroglycerin preparations, as it may cause cardiovascular collapse. ED is estimated to affect 2% to 3% of men in the United States, though this range may be low. The prevalence increases with age and while it can have a psychological component, it often has an organic cause. While hypertension and epilepsy do not themselves cause ED, the pharmacologic treatment of them may.

4. E Most female orgasm disorders are lifelong rather than acquired, because a female learns to have an orgasm and generally does not lose that capacity. As women age they increase their capacity for orgasm. Medical conditions such as a history of vaginal or vulval surgery, spinal cord injuries, multiple sclerosis, neuropathies, temporal lobe lesions, diabetes, hypothyroidism, hypofunctioning adrenal cortex, hyperprolactinemia, pituitary dysfunction, or vascular disease may cause impaired orgasmic function. Psychological/psychiatric causes include trauma, such as abuse or rape; relationship conflicts; poor sexual communication; and mood disorders. Occasional orgasmic dysfunction that does not cause marked distress is not considered to be a female orgasmic disorder. The normal pattern of the sexual response cycle involves Desire ⇒ Excitement ⇒ Orgasm ⇒ Resolution. Disorders of sexual response can occur at any of these phases. Estimates of sexual dysfunction rates of up to 50% have been reported in outpatient populations. Other causes of impaired sexual functioning in women include dyspareunia (pain on penetration) and vulvar vestibulitis (inflammation of unknown etiology causing redness and pain at the vaginal opening). Vaginismus is caused by painful involuntary muscle contractions of the perineum when penetration is attempted.

Case 4

1. C Predisposing risk factors for teenage pregnancy include depression, poor planning for the future, academic difficulties, and divorced parents. Teenage pregnancy is a serious social problem in the United States, with approximately 600,000 births and 400,000 abortions annually. Teenagers are not consistent in their use of contraception; only about a third use contraception regularly. The average age of first intercourse in the United States is 16 years. By 19 years, 80% of men and 70% of women have experienced intercourse. Teenagers are at high risk for obstetric complications because of their physical immaturity and lack of prenatal care. Almost 50% of unmarried mothers are teenagers.

2. B By the age of 30 years between 60% and 70% of those living in the United States are married and have children. Erik Erikson defined this period of psychosocial development as one of intimacy versus isolation. During this phase, there is pressure to develop intimate, stable relationships. If the individual lacks the capacity and ego strength to develop a mutually beneficial relationship, then emotional isolation may develop. During early adulthood (20 to 40 years) the individual's role in society is defined, independence is achieved, and physical development peaks. Daniel Levinson describes this transition phase as one in which a reappraisal of the individual's life occurs; this happens at approximately 30 years of age.

3. C Postpartum psychosis occurs in between 0.1% and 0.2% of women after delivery. This is the most severe of all the postpartum psychiatric syndromes and usually develops 2 to 4 weeks after delivery. The postpartum blues occurs in between 30% to 85% of women after childbirth. Crying, irritability, depressed mood, anxiety, and insomnia characterize the condition. It generally appears within the first week and is a self-limiting condition that usually responds to reassurance, support, and some education about the condition. However, it has been estimated that 20% of women with the baby blues go on to develop major depression. In postpartum depression, ambivalent or negative feelings toward the infant are often reported, as are doubts about the mother's ability to care for her infant. When severe, suicidal ideation is frequently reported, but suicide rates appear to be relatively low. Increased risk may be associated with stressful life events during pregnancy or near delivery. Marital dissatisfaction or inadequate social supports may increase the likelihood of developing a postpartum depressive illness. Rates of 26% among teenagers have been reported. Factors suggested that might place women at increased risk of depression at this time include the fall in serum estrogen, progesterone, thyroid hormone, cortisol, and psychosocial issues surrounding the adjustment to having an infant. Treatment involves antidepressant medications and psychotherapy.

4. D Approximately 50% of women have further episodes of psychosis. Postpartum psychosis occurs in 1.5 per 1000 deliveries. It is associated with primigravida females. Risk factors include a family history of psychiatric disorders, a history of bipolar or mood disorder in the mother. Psychological risk factors include the previous (or current) death of a child, poor social support, the quality of the relationships between the patient and her partner, his family, and her own mother. Most of these episodes are due to mood disorders. Very few are due to organic/medical causes. A prodromal period may begin 2 days after birth, with restlessness, insomnia, irritability, and changes in mood. This may be followed by confusion, overactivity, labile mood, and psychotic symptoms, including hallucinations and delusions (often focused on the baby). Approximately 5% of women with this disorder commit suicide and 4% commit infanticide. These women are at increased risk of developing further episodes of psychosis in the postpartum period or at any time.

Case 5

1. D Baseline examinations prior to starting lithium treatment should include the following: urea, electrolytes, creatinine, urine tests, thyroid function tests (TFTs), weight, EKG, and pregnancy test if of childbearing age. During treatment with lithium, levels should be drawn approximately every 8 weeks once the dose has been stabilized. Urea, electrolytes, creatinine, TFTs, and urine should be checked every 6 to 12 months. An EKG should be preformed annually. Lithium treatment can cause a benign leukocytosis with an increase in neutrophils.

2. D The side effects of valproic acid include nausea (25%), vomiting (5%), diarrhea, weight gain, hair loss (5% to 10%), sedation, ataxia, dysarthria, tremor (can be treated with beta-blockers if troublesome), elevated liver function tests (5% to 10%), thrombocytopenia, and platelet dysfunction, which can increase bleeding times and, more rarely, pancreatitis and fatal hepatotoxicity (0.85 per 100,000 patients). Use of valproic acid in the first trimester of pregnancy has been reported to cause neural tube defects in 1% to 2%. It is contraindicated in this situation (and breast-feeding) and in those with hepatic disease.

3. C Hypoparathyroidism does not influence the distribution of a drug. Edema can be caused by a variety of conditions, such as cardiac failure, cirrhosis, and nephrotic syndrome, all of which can both increase distribution and decrease clearance. Pregnancy causes an increase in blood volume, increasing distribution. Obesity increases the distribution of lipophilic agents and increases distribution and the half-life of such agents. Weight is of consideration when planning dosages of medications. Increasing age is associated with an altered volume of distribution, as lean body mass decreases and fat increases, which affects the volume of distribution.

4.C. Efficacy of a drug is a measure of the maximum effect a drug can produce. Potency is a measure of the amount of a drug required to produce a particular effect. Therapeutic indexes are used to measure the safety of drugs. (**The therapeutic index** is the ratio between a lethal dose and a clinically effective dose.) SSRIs usually have a high therapeutic index, and tricyclics have a lower one. A **therapeutic window** is the range in which a drug has a maximum clinical effect. Above and below this range decreased clinical effects may occur. The tricyclic nortryptiline has a therapeutic window.

Case 6

1. E Mental retardation is defined in the *Diagnostic and Statistical Manual of Mental Disorders,* 4th edition (*DSM-IV*), as significantly subaverage intellectual functioning with an IQ of 70 or below on individual IQ testing. There are deficits in at least two of the adaptive areas of functioning: communication, self-care, home living, social/interpersonal skills, the use of community resources, self-direction, academic skills, work, leisure, health, and safety. The correct classifications are as follows: mild—IQ 50–55 to approximately 70; moderate—IQ 35–40 to 50–55; severe—IQ 20–25 to 35–40; and profound—IQ below 20 or 25.

2. E Several sources of error may occur when using questionnaires or standardized interviews. These include response set, social acceptability, bias toward the center, and the halo and Hawthorne effects. The response set occurs when the subject always tends to agree or disagree with the questions. Social acceptability occurs when the subject chooses the acceptable answer rather than a true one. Bias toward the center occurs when the subject tends to

choose the middle response and avoid extreme answers. The halo effect occurs when answers are chosen to fit with previous answers. The Hawthorne effect is caused by researchers who by the nature of their presence alter the situation.

3. D Constructional apraxia is the inability to copy simple objects and is associated with lesions of the nondominant parietal lobe. Lesions of the dominant parietal lobe may cause finger agnosia (difficulties correctly naming fingers), dysgraphia (difficulties writing), dyscalculia (difficulties in calculation), and right-left disorientation. Lesions in the frontal lobe (Broca's area) cause expressive language problems, where the patient cannot speak language fluently. Lesions in the temporal lobe (Wernicke's area) cause receptive language problems, where the patient can speak but cannot understand language.

4. D The Halstead Reitan battery can be used to detect, localize, and assess the effects of localized brain lesions and would be useful in such a patient. The Minnesota Multiphasic Personality Inventory (MMPI) is a personality test, which is often used clinically to assess patients who may be malingering. The sentence completion test is used to assess personality, such as "I wish. . . ." Both the Stanford-Binet and the Wechsler Adult Intelligence Scale (WAIS) are used to assess intellectual functioning.

Case 7

1. B This is an example of classical conditioning. The nurse is the conditioned stimulus, which has become associated with an unconditioned stimulus, the injection and the ensuing discomfort provoking the conditioned response of crying. After a period of time when the conditioned stimulus has not been paired with the unconditioned stimulus, extinction of the conditioned response occurs.

2. B Biofeedback is a technique that is based on operant conditioning. Patients are trained to control peripheral skin temperature using galvanic measure and have been reported to decrease migraine attacks. Biofeedback techniques are also used to help control hypertension, tension headaches, asthma, and generalized anxiety. Each uses a physiologic parameter, which can be measured, and continuous information is provided to the patient who learns to alter these parameters using relaxation techniques. Patients must have a high level of motivation, as these techniques take a lot of practice to master.

3. E Positive reinforcement of the undesired behavior is occurring. Most likely this is due to the increased attention from the mother that this behavior evokes. You recommend that she try ignoring this behavior if possible to cause extinction and also to reinforce the desired behavior.

4. B Modeling is used in social skills training and assertiveness training, where a live model demonstrates appropriate behaviors during role-playing exercises. Observational learning is enhanced by models that have high status, social power, competence, and some common characteristics with the observer. Aversive therapy uses classical conditioning to link a discomfort (e.g., electric shock) with an undesired behavior. Aversive therapy may be temporarily effective. Token economies are examples of operant conditioning and are used to modify behaviors in ward settings, particularly with psychiatric patients. Flooding is used to treat phobias by keeping patients in the feared (but harmless) situation until their anxiety and fear decrease. Systematic desensitization is used to treat phobias and other irrational anxieties. It begins with imagining a graded hierarchy of anxiety-provoking stimuli while practicing relaxation techniques. An example would be the patient who is fearful of flying but who imagines buying an airline ticket, packing his or her bag, going to the airport, and so on.

Case 8

1. E. Suppression along with sublimation, altruism, anticipation (planning for future internal discomfort or adverse outcomes), asceticism (removing basic pleasurable aspects of experiences), and humor are the mature defense mechanisms. The others are immature defense mechanisms.

2. D In phobias unacceptable internal affects are displaced onto external objects. In hysteria, there is denial, projection, and identification. Obsessional conditions display isolation, reaction formation, and magical undoing. Paranoid conditions are associated with splitting and projection, whereas depression is associated with turning against the self.

3. C A woman who was physically abused as a child and then starts abusing her children is an example of identification. An example of splitting would be a patient who believes his or her doctor to be wonderful until the doctor is late for an appointment and then decides the doctor is awful. The woman who was sexually abused and then develops multiple personalities provides an example of dissociation. The man who is attracted to his sister-in-law and starts believing that his wife is having an affair is an example of projection. An example of reaction formation would be a man who unconsciously resents his wife and buys her expensive gifts. The man with bowel cancer who decides to worry about it for only 20 minutes a day is an example of suppression. However, denial is an important defense mechanism used by those with serious illness.

4. C Primary process thinking is associated with the unconscious mind; it involves primitive drives or impulses without logic or a sense of time and is common in young children. Secondary process thinking is logical and is involved with reality; it is associated with the preconscious mind. Transference is the shifting of unconscious emotional attitudes from the patient's past experience of people or objects onto the therapist. These reactions are examined and interpreted in psychoanalysis. Countertransference refers to the therapist's emotional attitude toward the patient and may not be interpreted in the patient's analysis, but it should be closely examined by the therapist. Freud referred to dream work as the process whereby the hidden or latent (unconscious) content of dreams is converted into the reported manifest (actual) content of the dream. He believed that dreams represented wish fulfillment and the gratification of unconscious impulses.

Case 9

1. C Narcolepsy appears to affect both sexes equally. This disorder causes an irresistible desire to fall asleep. There may be up to six "attacks" a day, and each may last between 10 and 20 minutes. Although it usually appears during the second decade of life, it may not be diagnosed for many years. Animal studies have identified a gene that causes narcolepsy; it is called *hypocretin receptor 2* and codes for a protein that allows brain cells to receive messages from other cells. Abnormal versions of this gene cause these messages to be ignored, perhaps not taking into account wakefulness messages. This mutation has rarely been reported in humans with narcolepsy, but studies have reported that there is a large reduction in neurons containing hypocretins in the brains of those with this disorder, compared with controls. However, the exact cause of this deficiency is unknown. Hypocretin-based medications and sodium oxybate are under investigation. Two-thirds of those suffering from narcolepsy have reported falling asleep while driving, and up to 80% have reported falling asleep at work.

2. E Hypnotics and anxiolytics are not used to treat this disorder; in fact, stimulants such as methylphenidate (Ritalin), pemoline (Cylert), dextroamphetamine (Dexedrine), and modafinil (Provigil) are used. The first three agents may cause headaches, nervousness, irritability, mood changes, insomnia, irregular heartbeats, and tolerance to their effects. Drug holidays may decrease the development of tolerance. Scheduled daytime naps are also helpful. Antidepressants such as tricyclics or selective serotonin reuptake inhibitors (SSRIs) are used to treat cataplexy by suppressing rapid eye movement (REM) sleep. Monoamine oxidase A inhibitors (MAOIs) are not generally used in this condition.

3. D Sleep apnea is the cessation of breathing for 10 or more seconds while sleeping and is associated with cardiac arrhythmias and hypoxia. It can be caused by obstruction of airways, a central lack of respiratory effort, or mixed pattern of central lack of respiratory effort followed by an obstructive apnea. Risk factors for obstructive sleep apnea include male gender, middle age, obesity, jaw and nasopharyngeal abnormalities, as well as an endocrine cause, such as hypothyroidism and acromegaly. Treatment includes weight loss, continuous positive airway pressure (CPAP) administered by nasal mask, and surgical treatment of airway obstructions and malformations. Parasomnias are disorders characterized by abnormal physiology or behaviors of sleep and include nightmares, sleep terrors, or somnambulism (sleep walking). Dyssomnias include narcolepsy, insomnia, hypersomnia, sleep apnea, and circadian rhythm sleep disorders (sleeping at inappropriate times). These disorders are characterized by abnormalities in the timing, amount, or quality of sleep.

4. C Noradrenaline decreases the amount of REM sleep and the total amount of time spent asleep. Acetylcholine activity in the reticular formation increases both REM sleep and the total sleep time. Dopamine antagonists actually improve sleep. Serotonin increases both the amounts of slow-wave and total time of sleep. Histamine increases active wakefulness, and antihistamines cause sleepiness or sedation.

Case 10

1. D Approximately 30% of people who attempt suicide will have anther attempt, and 10% will succeed. The greatest risk is in the 3 months following an attempt.

2. A Whites are at higher risk than blacks for suicide. Otherwise age, being male, chronic medical illness, recent loss of a spouse, and access to a weapon all increase the risk for completed suicide. Women have more attempts (4:1), but men have a higher percentage of completed suicides.

3. A Fluoxetine is an SSRI and is rarely lethal in overdose. Acetaminophen is associated with hepatic failure; aspirin, with bleeding and metabolic acidosis; imipramine, a tricyclic antidepressant, with QT prolongation and potential heart block or arrhythmia; ibuprofen, with nausea, vomiting, gastrointestinal (GI) bleeding, renal insufficiency, and so on.

4. B At least 10% of schizophrenics die by suicide, and 25% to 50% attempt suicide. Risk factors include male gender, youth, substance abuse, high aspirations/lost expectations, multiple relapses, depressed mood, and living alone.

Case 11

1. B Anniversary reactions may be provoked by the actual anniversary of the death or another reminder, such as a birthday or when the bereaved reached the same age as the deceased when they died. These reactions tend to diminish over time. Grief may begin before the actual death and may be referred to as anticipatory grief. This is usually seen when the death is slow, and although anticipatory grief may soften the blow of the loss, it does not decrease the risk of later grief. Most grief does not resolve completely and may re-emerge with certain triggers, such as hearing the deceased's name or seeing his or her picture. Sudden unexpected deaths may lead to the development of traumatic stress reactions. Chronic grief is abnormal, and here the deceased may be idealized and the bereaved may become angry or bitter. Very close, ambivalent, or dependent relationships with the deceased are associated with its development, along with poor psychosocial supports. Loneliness may be the most lasting symptom of grief and may continue for years after the death of a spouse or partner. Feelings of guilt or worry about not having done enough for the deceased may occur when grieving.

2. E Characteristics in the bereaved personality associated with complicated grief include the following: low self-esteem, dependence, insecurity, and difficulties coping with stress. Other risk factors in the bereaved include a history of substance abuse, depression, poor health, and multiple stressors at the time of loss. Other risk factors for developing complicated grief include sudden, unexpected, traumatic deaths; deaths associated with a stigma such as due to AIDS; ambivalent and dependent relationships with the deceased; and the loss of a child. Age and gender remain controversial as risk factors.

3. C Complicated grief may be delayed in onset and there may have been no evidence of grief during the expected phase of mourning. It is associated with denial, anger, and guilt, which may be prolonged in nature. Hypertrophic grief is extremely intense in nature, is often provoked by an unexpected sudden death, and may take a long time to improve. Chronic grief is the most common form of complicated grief. Bereavement may be associated with increased medical and psychiatric illness in the bereaved. Particularly seen in men under the age of 65 years, this increased risk of mortality may continue until the man remarries. The increase in mortality in men is due to the increased risk of death by suicide, cardiovascular disease, accidents, and even some infections. Psychiatric illness may include depression, anxiety, substance abuse, posttraumatic stress disorder, and suicide.

4. B Loss of appetite is common in bereavement, and there is no significant weight loss. Feeling hopeless, feeling worthless, and experiencing significant sleep disturbance, weight loss, and suicidal ideation are characteristic of depression. See Table 11-1.

Case 12

1 D In fact, continued occupational and physical activities are associated with increased longevity, as are marriage, a family history of longevity, higher education, and sleeping 6 to 9 hours a night. Marriage is one type of social support, as are family and friends, that are associated with increased longevity. Retirement is a critical phase in the life cycle and changes in income can lead to increased anxiety about coping with future medical costs. Other factors associated with longevity include suburban living (as opposed to urban) and a calm personality.

2 C Deaths from diabetes, chronic lung disease, and AIDS are increasing, whereas those from cardiovascular disease, stroke, homicide, and accidents have decreased. Deaths from heart disease (34%) and cancer (23%) still account for most deaths. Lung cancer causes most cancer deaths in both sexes, followed by prostate cancer in men and breast cancer in women. The third most common cause of cancer deaths in both sexes is colorectal cancer. Life expectancy at birth has decreased since 1980 from 75.8 years to 75.5 years. This is thought to result from increased deaths from influenza, pneumonia, infection, and unintentional injuries. AIDS is the ninth leading cause of death in the United States and is the leading cause of death among men 25 to 44 years of age. It is the third leading cause of death among African American women and the sixth among white women in the same age group. In the United States 80% of people reach 60 years of age. It has been estimated that by 2020 more than 20% of the population will be more than 65 years of age, with the greatest increase expected in those more than 80 years of age. The age adjusted death rate in 2000 was 873.1 per 100,000 population.

3. C The most common medical conditions in the elderly are arthritis, hypertension, and heart disease. More than 75% of those beyond 65 years of age suffer from at least one chronic medical condition. About 5% of those more than 65 years of age require nursing home care. The elderly currently account for approximately 30% of all health care costs, but as the population of the elderly continues to increase in the United States, this is expected to increase to 50% by the year 2050. Although cognitive abilities such as recall and new learning may be impaired with age, cognitive decline is not inevitable. Approximately 5% of those 65 years of age have dementia. This increases approximately 5% every 5 years thereafter until a plateau is reached at 95 years, where approximately 50% are demented.

4. C Tubular function is decreased along with renal blood flow and actual kidney mass in older persons and may decrease a drug's elimination. Distribution is decreased due to decreases in body mass, water, and albumin levels. Increases in body fat may affect the storage of lipophilic drugs. Noncompliance is not associated with aging. In fact, studies have shown that the average person aged 80 years and older may be on six or more medications. Therefore the possibility of interactions affecting absorption, distribution, metabolism, or elimination should be considered. Older persons should be asked carefully about their use of over-the-counter preparations. Gastric secretions are also decreased and thus may affect absorption of medications.

Case 13

1. D Denial is the most likely reason for his not looking for medical care. Denial is a common defense mechanism that may delay access to care. Although major depression causing apathy or hopelessness and/or suicidality could cause a person to not seek medical care, there is no indication in this case. Despite his busy schedule, this patient made time to come in now and could have done so in the past.

2. D In this scenario there are a number of ways to address the patient's behavior, which can range from addressing psychosocial factors that may be influencing the behavior, gently explaining that it would not be appropriate for you to meet socially, to having someone else present during the exam and trying to diffuse the situation by ignoring it. Neither dating the patient, lying to the patient, nor abruptly confronting him or her is appropriate or will allow the physician-patient relationship to continue. Not doing a physical exam would be negligent.

3. B Since he seems so anxious about this, it is important to understand why and what he is afraid of. It could be something as simple as not knowing what might cause the rash or as complicated as his having unacknowledged HIV risk factors and being petrified that this is a sign of AIDS. Being straightforward, explaining the etiology and treatment in simple language, is the best course to reassure him. Laughing may well alienate him; speaking in medicalese, being overly simplistic, not explaining the cause or treatment, or being overly dramatic may make him more anxious.

4. C A number of factors increase compliance: a good physician-patient relationship; an experienced, knowledgeable, and enthusiastic clinician; a patient with an acute illness or who feels ill; written instructions; and working with the patient to define goals within the context of his or her life. In this case, since there are many things that the patient will need to address to improve her overall medical condition, it is important to let the patient help in setting realistic goals and priorities. Setting unrealistic

goals or having too many goals concurrently often makes the patients feel hopeless or inadequate and decreases the likelihood of achieving anything. Scaring or threatening the patient and giving instructions without seeing how they will fit into the patient's life are not likely to be useful, especially at this time. In the context of discussing the diagnosis it is important to review the prognosis and why the interventions are being recommended, but not in a threatening manner. Of note, things that decrease compliance are poor physician-patient relationships, complex schedules, or multiple behavioral changes, verbal instructions, and chronic illness.

Case 14

1. E In fact, those who abuse the elderly are often the closest family member, such as a spouse (almost 60%) or child (almost 25%) of the victim. They often have a history of mental or emotional problems, abuse alcohol or illicit substances, are socially isolated, and are in financial difficulty. Characteristics of the victim include physical dependence on others and cognitive impairment, and they tend to deny the abuse for fear of the consequences. It has been reported that up to a third of demented elderly are abused.

2. D In fact, more premature, low-birth-weight infants are abused (approximately 25%) than full-term infants (8%). These children may require more attention from their parents. These children may have mild physical disabilities and may be hyperactive or described as "slow." Most children who are physically abused are under 5 years of age. Often these children do not report their injuries to others outside the family unit. Persons who abuse family members are likely to have a personal history of abuse or neglect as a child themselves. Figures reported are as high as 80%, but most abused children do not grow up to be abusive parents themselves. Some of these abused parents may abuse their children if under stress.

3. C The average number of children being born to women in the United States has decreased from 3.6 in 1960 to 2.0 in the early 1990s and these decreases are seen in both single and married women. About 25% of families are led by a single parent (55% in African American families), and 90% of these single parents are women. Approximately 60% of children in the United States under 18 years of age have both parents who work outside the home. Approximately 25% of couples are childless, due equally to choice and fertility impairments. The actual percentage of children in the population has decreased from 35% in 1960 to 25% more recently. Approximately 40% of new marriages will divorce, half of these within 5 years.

4. B Studies have reported that up to 40% of women seen in general practice have been victims of domestic violence. The risk is increased for women who are pregnant. Dangers to the unborn child include poor prenatal care (women may avoid going to the doctor to avoid detection of abuse), miscarriage, ante partum hemorrhage, prematurity, low birth weight, and even stillbirth. Studies have shown that physicians fail to identify these women. The violence tends to follow a three-phase cycle, which starts with increasing levels of tension and criticism, possibly with shoving.

The second phase includes increasing anger and violence. This phase is followed by a third phase of apologies and promises to change. Usually the violence continues and may become more severe. It is important that the physician express concern and compassion but not be too controlling or directive. More than a third of female murder victims are killed by their partners. It is important not to pressure patients into filing police reports, as they are able to judge their own safety in this regard. These women should be encouraged to develop a safety plan, which may involve having a bag packed with clothing and important papers (ID, passport, etc.). Domestic violence advocates and social workers can help the patient plan for the future. Legal aid and domestic violence programs are available. It is probably better if both partners attend different group therapies.

Case 15

1. B Serotonin neurons may play a role in behavioral inhibition. Impulsive or aggressive behaviors have been reported to be related to low levels of cerebrospinal fluid (CSF) 5-hydroxy indoleacetic acid (5-HIAA). Studies with fenfluramine have shown that low levels of serotonergic responsiveness correlate with scores of impulsive aggression. Postmortem studies of suicides reported reduced brainstem levels of serotonin and reduced imipramine binding, which is thought to be associated with reduced presynaptic serotonergic binding sites. This was accompanied by an increase in postsynaptic 5-HT$_2$ receptors (N.B. the prefrontal cortex). Patients with lesions bilaterally in the prefrontal cortex may have a chronic pattern of impulsive aggressive behavior. Pet studies have reported selective reductions in glucose metabolism in the prefrontal and frontal cortex of patients with impulsive aggression.

2. D Risk factors for divorce include premarital pregnancy, short courtships, young age of marriage, significant parental disapproval of the marriage, poor social supports, and fairly broad differences in background. However, the history of a previous divorce does not increase the risk of a second divorce. Approximately 40% of new marriages will end in divorce, and half of these will end within 5 years.

3. D This boy has conduct disorder with symptoms of aggression toward animals, destruction of property, and breaking rules. Oppositional defiant disorder (ODD) does have some shared features, such as disobedience and opposition to authority, but excludes the more serious types of behavioral problems. Attention deficit hyperactivity disorder (ADHD) patients may have hyperactive and disruptive behaviors, but these do not violate societal norms. Both ODD and ADHD can be diagnosed together. Adjustment disorders can occur with either disturbances of conduct or mixed disturbances of emotions and behaviors. These disorders are associated with psychosocial stressors. Individuals with a manic episode may have irritability or behavioral disturbances, but these follow an episodic course.

4. C Higher rates of antisocial disorder among first-degree relatives have been reported particularly for females with antisocial disorder. Increased rates of somatization disorder, depression, and substance abuse are also reported. Studies have reported bilateral slow theta waves on the EEG in individuals with antisocial personality disorder as well as soft neurologic signs. Patients with antisocial personality disorder have increased risk of developing major depression, substance abuse/dependence, anxiety disorders, and impulse control disorders (e.g., gambling) but not obsessive-compulsive disorder (OCD). Those with narcissistic personality disorders have a need for excessive admiration.

Case 16

1. A Competence is a legal determination. Thus a physician cannot declare her incompetent. The decision about competence is often made using information from a capacity assessment that is done by a physician. Psychiatrists are most often called upon, but any physician can perform a capacity assessment. Patients require capacity to make any medical decision, whether they are "going along with the doctor" or not. Health care proxies can be used to intervene only when the patient lacks capacity or cannot speak for him- or herself. In this case the patient is severely demented, cannot manage her activities of daily living, and has significant aphasia. She lacks capacity to make treatment decisions, and her health care proxy can override her "refusal." Finally, unless her cousin's husband has been designated her proxy, he has no legal right to intervene in her health care decisions, especially when the patient's wishes have been clearly documented.

2. C There are four D's of malpractice: Demonstrating negligence or **dereliction,** demonstrating that the physician did have a relationship and therefore a **duty** to the patient, demonstrating that **damages** occurred (that the patient was injured in some way) and that the damages were caused **directly** by the negligence. Malpractice is a tort, or civil wrong, not a criminal matter. It is unnecessary to prove malicious intent or to show that the physician was paid or that the hospital was vigilant in its hiring practices.

3. C A Christian Scientist, who does not believe in medical or surgical intervention, may refuse medication or surgery for him- or herself. Although parents are allowed to make medical decisions for their minor children (under age 18), they cannot refuse life-saving treatment (e.g., an emergency appendectomy). Adult Jehovah's Witnesses who are cognitively intact may refuse blood transfusion even if it means death. Patients with early-stage Alzheimer's disease often retain capacity, especially for less complex decisions. They may not be able to manipulate large quantities of complex information, but may well be able to consent to a biopsy, to appoint a health care proxy, and even to make a living will. Having a motor deficit (hemiplegia) does not imply anything about capacity.

4. B A 35-year-old patient with widely metastatic ovarian cancer who declines further treatment probably has capacity. The 5-year survival for stage IV ovarian cancer is less than 5%, and with no response to chemotherapy the decision to halt treatment would not be inappropriate. The other patients all have psychiatric symptoms that are interfering with their ability to make these decisions. The anorexic is denying the severity of her illness and cannot control her weight, the person with depression inappropriately feels that life is hopeless and there is no reason to remove a skin cancer, the schizophrenic has incorporated the treatment into his delusions, the man with moderate dementia needs significant homecare but believes that he can manage his postoperative course on his own. In addition, he may be unable to fully understand other risks of that procedure.

Case 17

1. B According to the *DSM-IV,* the correct way to categorize his diagnoses is Axis I: major depression, Axis II: mental retardation, Axis III: hypertension. To review:

Axis I: Clinical disorders or conditions requiring clinical attention

Axis II: Personality disorders and mental retardation

Axis III: General medical conditions

Axis IV: Psychosocial and environmental problems and stressors

Axis V: lobal assessment of the patient's functioning (100-point scale)

2. C Psychomotor retardation is a common finding in severe major depressions. Pressured speech is most commonly associated with mania, as is flight of ideas. Circumstantiality may be seen in a variety of disorders, including mania or schizophrenia. Suspiciousness could be associated with a psychotic disorder such as delusional disorder, paranoid type, or schizophrenia.

3: D Mania is most often associated with flight of ideas (thought process) and grandiosity (thought content), which may take on delusional proportions, pressured speech, and psychomotor agitation. Manic individuals may be well groomed, disheveled, or inappropriately groomed. The affect of persons who are manic is often expansive, not flat. Flat affect may be seen in severe depression or sometimes in schizophrenia. Loosening of associations, which may also be seen in schizophrenia, is an example of thought process.

4. E Fixed false beliefs are delusions and are commonly seen in schizophrenia. Hypnagogic and hypnopompic hallucinations are seen upon going to sleep or waking, respectively, and may be associated with certain sleep disorders such as narcolepsy. Illusions refer to misunderstanding real stimuli, such as seeing a shadow and thinking it is a person or a small animal. One place that illusions are seen is in the visually impaired. Intrusive ego dystonic thoughts refer to obsessions, which are seen in obsessive-compulsive disorder. Schizophrenics may well have intrusive obsessive thoughts, but they are usually not ego dystonic. Delusions are a much more prominent and common symptom in schizophrenia.

Case 18

1. B Long-term effects of anorexia include cardiac and renal impairments, renal calculi, osteoporosis, impaired fertility, increase rates of perinatal mortality, and dental problems. More than 10%

of those with anorexia will die. Some will recover completely, but others will follow a more chronic course of relapse and remission.

2. B The associated physical features of bulimia may be divided into two types.

(a) Signs and symptoms: Vomiting leads to callused hands (also called Russell's sign), dental erosions, and enlarged parotid glands. Menstrual abnormalities, even amenorrhea, may occur. More severe complications include cardiac/skeletal myopathy from the regular use of ipecac, torn esophagus, and gastric rupture from vomiting. Cardiac arrhythmias may also occur. Those with the non-purging type have fewer medical complications. Weights may be near normal in most with the disorder.

(b) Investigations/labs: Purging may lead to hyponatremia, hypochloremia, and hypokalemia. Vomiters may develop a metabolic alkalosis, and those who abuse laxatives may develop a metabolic acidosis.

Lanugo hair is associated with anorexia and starvation. Alopecia is not characteristic of bulimia.

3. C In the intergenerational-experiential school of family therapy the dysfunctional behavioral problems are viewed as arising from a family developmental fixation. The view of the behavioral-psychoeducational school is that current environmental events shape, maintain, and control interpersonal behaviors. The structural-strategic approach is based on general systems theory as outlined in the text. Some therapists focus on correcting the structure of the family; others focus on the organization and processing of the family.

4. C Yalom described several curative factors found in groups, including instillation of hope, universality, catharsis, insight, group cohesiveness, altruism, modeling of behavior, development of socializing techniques, and corrective formation of a family group.

Group think happens when there are cohesive group members within a group with a strong leader. This can lead to decisions being made without consideration of other intragroup wishes or external opinion. Triangulation is a communication style of a leader-led group. Scapegoating is described in the discussion. None of these are curative factors in a group. Humor is a mature defense mechanism.

Case 19

1. B Bariatric surgery is not an available option to patients with body-mass indexes (BMIs) of less than 40. However, with a BMI of 29 and concurrent obesity-related medical conditions, she is eligible for pharmacologic therapy if she desires. Of course all patients can benefit from a low-fat, high-fiber diet regimen with moderate exercise. Rigorous exercise can lead to higher rates of injury.

2. C It is important to assess the degree to which obesity affects the family in order to properly address a child's obesity. Childhood obesity is most commonly affected by eating and exercise habits of the family. No treatment that isolates the child as the sole target of therapy will ever be effective in reducing his weight. Therefore family counseling is often employed and has been shown to be an effective means of treating childhood obesity. Although a child's family may have a strong propensity for obesity, investigating inherited leptin deficiency may not be appropriate, as this is a very rare cause of obesity, and serum leptin tests are very expensive and only available through special labs. In addition, such investigations rarely lead to changes in management. Lastly, medication and surgery have not been approved for use in children.

3. D There are many possible causes of dyspnea in an obese person. These include upper airway obstruction, decreased lung volumes from chest wall compression and increased intra-abdominal pressure, and congestive heart failure. Given LC's history and physical, he is probably experiencing congestive heart failure, a condition associated with obesity. Although this is the most likely cause, other possible causes must be investigated, such as sleep apnea, restrictive lung disease, and coronary artery disease. These can be evaluated with the use of a sleep study, a pulmonary function test, and a stress test (probably pharmacologic testing instead of treadmill testing, given his chronic knee pain). He is probably not having an acute myocardial infarction, given his EKG and negative troponin tests.

4. C Sympathomimetic drugs are contraindicated in those who have hypertension or cardiac disease, as they may worsen both conditions. However, diet and exercise are always appropriate therapies for obesity. He is also eligible for treatment with orlistat, given his BMI. Finally, with proper medical clearance, he may also be eligible for surgical treatment.

Case 20

1. B SSRIs are reported to have fewer side effects and to be safer than either tricyclics or MAOI agents. They do not act as α-adrenergic receptors and hence do not cause orthostatic hypotension. They also do not act as sodium channel inhibitors and therefore do not cause cardiac toxicity. As a group, the SSRIs may cause nervousness, agitation, insomnia, nausea, and headaches. Sexual dysfunction is a common adverse effect of all SSRIs and may cause delayed orgasm or anorgasmia in females and delayed ejaculation in males. Strategies suggested to help with this sexual dysfunction include drug holidays, decreasing the dosage, using agents with shorter half-lives, and the addition of agents such as buspirone, bupropion, yohimbine, or cyproheptadine. Nausea can be minimized by taking the agent with food; insomnia, by taking it in the morning. Sertraline, paroxetine, and fluoxetine are highly protein bound. Therefore care should be taken in patients who take either digitoxin or warfarin and their levels should be closely monitored. SSRIs should not be combined with MAOI agents to avoid serotonergic syndrome. SSRIs also inhibit the cytochrome P450 isoenzyme system.

2. D Although antidepressants are generally used to treat depression, they have a variety of other uses, including the treatment of anxiety (imipramine and SSRIs), bulimia (fluoxetine), enuresis

(imipramine), obsessive-compulsive disorder (clomipramine, fluoxetine, and fluvoxamine), narcolepsy (MAOIs and imipramine), and panic disorder (imipramine and SSRIs), and pain management (amitryptiline). Serotonergic noradrenergic reuptake inhibitors (SNRIs) have not been shown to be useful in the treatment of bulimia. Antidepressants may also be used in the treatment of encopresis and attention deficit disorder in children. Trichotillomania is compulsive hair pulling and has been reported to respond to clomipramine.

3. C Tricyclics have several common side effects related to their mechanism of action. Anticholinergic effects may cause dry mouth, blurred vision, urinary retention, and constipation. These agents should be avoided in those with acute angle glaucoma and prostatic hypertrophy. Antihistaminergic effects may cause sedation, and effects at adrenergic receptors may lead to orthostatic hypotension. Tricyclics are concentrated in conduction tissue and may be fatal in overdose. Priapism is a persistent painful erection that is a surgical emergency. It may be caused rarely by trazodone, which can also cause agranulocytosis. Recent reports have been made of acute liver failure with the newer agent Serzone.

4. E MAOIs may interact with other central nervous system (CNS) active agents such as other sedatives. Opiates, anesthetics, stimulants, and tricyclic antidepressants (TCAs) can cause serotonergic syndrome with SSRIs. MAOIs also bind irreversibly to the MAO enzyme. It may take 2 weeks for new enzymes to be formed. MAOIs also cause a reduction on platelet MAO activity, and this can be used to monitor therapeutic efficacy. Tyramine is contained in a variety of foods, such as aged cheeses, beer, wines, meat, yeast extracts, chicken liver, pickled herring, and broad bean pods. MAOIs may block the degradation of tyramine and cause a release of catecholamines, leading to a hypertensive crisis. (Symptoms may include head and neck pain, palpitations, and hyperprexia, and may lead to convulsions, coma, and death.) Other side effects of MAOIs include anticholinergic side effects, postural hypotension, paresthesia in the limbs, ankle edema, tremor, myoclonus, nausea, and insomnia or precipitation of mania. Atypical features of depression or dysthymia include mood reactivity; significant weight gain or increase in appetite; increased sleeping; heavy, leaden feelings in the limbs; and a long-standing sensitivity to personal rejection.

Case 21

1. C The risk factors reported in bipolar disorder include age (average age of onset is 30 years), marital status (higher prevalence of bipolar disorder among separated or divorced than among singles), a positive family history of mood disorders, stressful life events, and poor social support. Gender distribution is equal in this disorder, and although there is a strong association between bipolar disorder and substance abuse, it has not been shown to be a risk factor.

2. D Family members of patients with bipolar disorder have a higher incidence of other psychiatric disorders than members of the general population. Particularly of note are the increases in both schizoaffective disorder and depression, which has led some researchers to believe that these conditions are in the same spectrum of disorders. None of the other conditions have been shown to be significantly associated with bipolar disorder.

3. E There have been preliminary reports linking chromosome 18 and bipolar disorder with positive lod scores in an analysis of 22 pedigrees, but this remains controversial. Monozygotic twins have identical genetic genomes, but dizygotic twins share only 50% of their genomes. If monozygotic twins have a higher concordance rate for a disorder than dizygotic twins, then genetic factors are implicated in the development of the disorder. If monozygotic and dizygotic twins have similar concordance rates for a disorder, then environmental factors may play an important role in the development of the disorder. Some psychiatric conditions, such as Alzheimer's disease, appear to have a small number of cases explained by autosomal dominant transmission. Otherwise, most psychiatric disorders are thought to have polygenic modes of transmission. The diseases shown to be associated with trinucleotide repeat expansions include Huntington's disease, fragile X syndrome, myotonic dystrophy, spinal and bulbar muscle atrophy, and dentatorubral-pallidoluysian atrophy, but family pedigrees in both bipolar disorder and schizophrenia are being investigated for a trinucleotide repeat expansion. In these families there was evidence of anticipation, with increased severity of disease phenotype and earlier onsets of illness in subsequent generations. Early linkage studies in bipolar disorder have not been well replicated (e.g., linkage to 11p15 in an Old Amish pedigree).

4. C Several medical conditions can cause manic symptoms, but if the mood disturbance is thought to have been directly caused by a medical illness, then it should be diagnosed as a mood disorder due to a general medical condition. The following illnesses may present with manic symptoms: Cushing's syndrome, hyperthyroidism, multiple sclerosis, and brain tumors. This may also be referred to as secondary mania and may be induced by a variety of other conditions [hemodialysis, surgery, infection (e.g., HIV), neoplasms, and epilepsy) and agents (steroids, isoniazid, levodopa). Patients with this condition tend to be older and do not usually have a family history of bipolar disorder.

Case 22

1. A You would advise her to consider other methods of contraception, as some mood stabilizers induce the hepatic induction of estrogens. Patients taking mood stabilizers may use progestin-only oral contraceptives or alternative methods of contraception. You would warn all females taking mood stabilizers about the possible teratogenic effects, particularly with lithium, valproic acid, and benzodiazepines. Mood stabilizers do not generally cause photosensitivity. Cimetidine, not ranitidine, interferes with the metabolism of valproic acid and may cause toxicity. Valproic acid also may cause alopecia; zinc and selenium supplements may help stimulate hair growth.

2. C Early side effects of lithium include nausea, vomiting, diarrhea, dry mouth, thirst, tremor (on voluntary movements), drowsiness, fatigue, metallic taste, and stuffy nose. Later effects include diabetes insipidus, nephropathy, edema, hypothyroidism, goiter, acne, alopecia, T-wave flattening on the EEG, short-term

memory deficits, and other neurologic symptoms, such as tardive dyskinesia and ataxia. Signs of lithium toxicity include tremor, lack of coordination, slurred speech, confusion, ataxia, disorientation, seizures, coma, and death.

3. E Topiramate decreases glutamate, as does carbamazepine and lamotrigine. Valproate increases gamma aminobutyric acid (GABA), as does gabapentin. Lithium, carbamazepine, and valproate all decrease second messengers and G proteins. Nimodipine decreases calcium. High-potency benzodiazepines increase chloride ion influx. Typical neuroleptics block D2 receptors, whereas atypical agents block D1, D2, D4 receptors and 5-HT2 receptors.

4. D Patients with rapid cycling may respond to thyroid hormone (Cytomel) augmentation. Lithium has a success rate of approximately 50% in the prophylaxis of bipolar disorder and is the standard maintenance treatment. An alternative is valproic acid. Carbamazepine is the third alternative. Lithium levels should be maintained between 0.5 to 1.2 mEq/L. Patients with bipolar disorder should be advised to avoid periods of insomnia, as these may provoke a manic episode. Lamorrigine (Lamichal) has recently received FDA approval for the long-term maintenance treatment of Bipolar I disorder.

Case 23

1. A Given her pervasive fear of humiliating herself in social situations, her likely diagnosis is social phobia. The probable course of social phobia is chronic and long-standing. People often suffer for years before seeking help.

2. B The treatment of generalized social phobia is usually an antidepressant, usually an SSRI, and cognitive behavioral therapy. Propranolol is only useful in the limited form of social phobia (e.g., in those with performance anxiety). Long-standing use of high-dose benzodiazepines is not the treatment of choice for any disorder, although clinically one may encounter patients on those regimens. Buspirone may be effective in generalized anxiety disorder.

3. D Lorazepam is a benzodiazepine. Benzodiazepines bind to the GABA-A receptor, allosterically modifying it so that with GABA binding there is an increase in Cl⁻ ions. Benzodiazepines cannot open the chloride channel without the presence of GABA. Lorazepam is only glucuronidated and does not have active metabolites.

4. D Withdrawal seizures. Benzodiazepines are associated with ataxia, drowsiness, tolerance, physical dependence, risk of withdrawal seizures, dizziness, and amnesia. Headaches, constipation, and weight fluctuations are not prominent side effects of these medications.

Case 24

1. D This man meets criteria for posttraumatic stress disorder (PTSD). He was traumatized and has nightmares, hyperarousal, and avoidance. The death of his wife was probably a trigger that brought many of the feelings of loss to the surface. Bereavement is a reaction to a death, which may include sadness and depressive symptoms. The duration of the symptoms varies, but if they remain severe more than 2 months after a loss, a diagnosis of major depression may be entertained. Certain symptoms are not usual for bereavement (such as inappropriate guilt, suicidal ideation, serious functional impairment, significant hallucinatory experiences), and if present should increase the index of suspicion for a major depression or other psychiatric disorder. Major depression requires depressed mood or anhedonia with a number of neurovegetative signs, such as decreased sleep, energy, and concentration, along with increased or decreased appetite. It may be accompanied by suicidality (see Case 20: Depression). Sleep terror is usually seen in children and occurs in slow wave sleep with no memory of dreaming. The person awakens in terror, with intense fear and autonomic arousal. Hypnopompic hallucinations are hallucinations that occur just as a person awakens.

2. C In patients with PTSD, there is hyperresponsivity to the negative feedback of cortisol. This can be demonstrated using exogenous steroids (such as dexamethasone), which cause exaggerated suppression of cortisol. This is probably related to an increase in receptor sensitivity because of the low levels of circulating cortisol.

3. B Hypervigilance is a criterion of PTSD and is part of the "hyperarousal" cluster of symptoms. The criteria for PTSD include having experienced a trauma with re-experiencing, avoidance, and hyperarousal. A trauma is an event that involved actual or threatened death or serious injury or a threat to the physical integrity of oneself or others. Substance abuse is not a criterion for PTSD, although it is not uncommonly a comorbid diagnosis. Paranoid delusions are symptoms of a psychotic disorder, such as schizophrenia. Worthlessness is a symptom of depression. Nightmares are an example of re-experiencing phenomena, but night terrors occur in stage IV sleep, delta sleep (not REM sleep) in the first third of the night. The prevalence is about 3% in children and less than 1% of adults. In children, it is more common in boys, usually begins between the ages of 4 and 12 years, and resolves spontaneously. In adults, it usually begins between 20 and 30 years of age, is more chronic, and may be associated with psychiatric disorders such as PTSD and borderline personality disorder. It is not a criterion for PTSD.

4. B Individuals with PTSD have elevated levels of catecholamines (e.g., norepinephrine and dopamine), and this is associated with increased levels of their metabolites in urine (5-hydroxy indoleacetic acid [5-HIAA] and homovanillic acid [HVA], respectively). Circulating levels of cortisol are decreased in PTSD. Imaging studies show statistically decreased hippocampal size and increased reactivity of the amygdala (which is an important component of the fear circuit). Marked frontotemporal atrophy is associated with Alzheimer's disease.

Case 25

1. D Exposure and response prevention constitute the basic underlying principle behind behavioral therapy, which has been shown to be beneficial in clinical trials for the treatment of obsessive

compulsive disorder (OCD). As this is a psychiatric disorder, and not just excessive worry about a real-life problem (he is spending more than 8 hours washing per day), rationalizing with him or educating him is unlikely to affect his behavior or symptoms.

2. A Serotonin has been most consistently implicated in OCD. This is mainly gleaned from the differential treatment response between serotonergic medications and medications affecting other transmitter systems.

3. E Using behavioral therapy. Strategies in treating OCD include maximizing the dose of serotonergic medications (SSRIs or clomipramine), augmenting with antipsychotic medications, and using behavioral therapy in addition to pharmacologic management. Although lithium augmentation of antidepressants may have a role in treating refractory depression, and lithium is effective in treating bipolar disorder, there is no literature that suggests it is beneficial in OCD. Stimulants (e.g., methylphenidate) may be used to augment antidepressants in the treatment of major depression. Clozapine is used primarily for treating refractory schizophrenia.

4. B Occasionally, even with adequate pharmacotherapy and/or behavioral therapy, patients may still experience intractable incapacitating symptoms. In these cases neurosurgery has been used. Obviously, the symptoms must be very severe, and the patient must have proven resistant to multiple psychological and somatic therapies over the course of many years. The success rate is about 50% to 70%. In general, the surgical procedures used—anterior capsulotomy, cingulotomy, and limbic leukotomy—aim to interrupt the connection between the cortex and the basal ganglia and related structures. Frontal lobotomy is a procedure that was common in the 1940s, with approximately 18,000 lobotomies performed in the United States. It was a fairly nonspecific procedure that caused a great deal of morbidity. Occipital lobe ablation would cause cortical blindness and is not used as a psychiatric treatment. Neither desipramine (a tricyclic antidepressant causing primarily norepinephrine reuptake inhibition) nor acetylcholinesterase inhibitors are efficacious in this disorder.

Case 26

1 D. Hyperthyroidism is also associated with tremor, hyperreflexia, increased sweating, warm and moist skin, and so on. Peptic ulcer disease can cause some symptoms that are seen in a panic attack, namely, nausea or GI discomfort, not palpitations. The side effects of caffeine affect primarily the cardiovascular and CNS. They include increased heart rate, left ventricular output, and stroke volume irritability, restlessness, and jitteriness. Alcohol withdrawal is associated with hypertension and tachycardia. Hypocalcemia is associated with paresthesias, neuromuscular irritability, arrhythmias, and so on. Hypercalcemia is associated with confusion, obtundation, renal insufficiency, myopathy, weakness, and bone pain.

2. A Hyperventilation causes a decrease in bicarbonate, hypocapnea, respiratory alkalosis, and ionized calcium. This causes paresthesias and muscle excitability. In severe case of respiratory alkalosis, tetany and seizures may be seen.

3. C Sodium lactate infusions are associated with panic in those prone to the disorder. Sodium bicarbonate, sodium lactate, and breathing 5% CO_2 mixed with room air have all been experimentally shown to induce panic attacks in people who are prone to them. α_2-Antagonists increase anxiety and may cause panic attacks. α_2-Agonists, such as clonidine, do not provoke panic attacks, nor do beta-blockers, or oral sodium bicarbonate used as an antacid. Thirty minutes of 100% CO (carbon monoxide) would most likely cause death. CO is a common cause of poisoning, often intentional (i.e., suicide attempts with car exhaust). It is associated with elevated carboxyhemoglobin levels, flulike symptoms, altered mental status, syncope, and cardiac ischemia. Needless to say, it has not been used experimentally to induce panic attacks.

4. C The other symptoms are all consistent with a panic attack. The symptoms as listed in *DSM-IV* include palpitations or tachycardia; nausea or abdominal distress; derealization or depersonalization; sweating; chest pain or discomfort; chills or hot flashes; trembling or shaking; feeling dizzy, light-headed, or unsteady; shortness of breath; sensation of choking; paresthesias (numbness, tingling); fear of dying; and fear of losing control or going crazy.

Case 27

1. C The symptoms described are consistent with an anticholinergic agent. The only medication on the list that has significant anticholinergic activity is diphenhydramine. Physical symptoms from anticholinergic medications result from postganglionic parasympathetic blockade (antimuscarinic action). They include dilated, poorly reactive pupils; warm, dry skin; facial flushing; dry mouth; tachycardia; GI slowing with constipation; and urinary retention.

2. B The symptoms of ataxia, ophthalmoplegia (lateral gaze paralysis), and confusion are the classic triad seen in Wernicke's encephalopathy. The cause is low thiamine, and it is usually seen in alcoholics. The emergent treatment is IV thiamine, before anything else, especially glucose.

3. E The symptoms and time frame are classic for alcohol withdrawal delirium, which usually begins 24 to 72 hours after the last drink. Although individuals may be confused or delirious after general anesthesia, alcohol withdrawal does not classically cause mania. Antibiotics can also cause delirium but are unlikely to cause the autonomic hyperarousal seen in this patient. Cocaine intoxication is associated with hypertension and tachycardia but is unlikely to cause visual hallucinations or significant confusion. Binge cocaine use may be associated with paranoia.

4. B This gentleman was delirious on admission. Given that 1 month after the event he is no longer delirious but still has cognitive problems (short-term memory, orientation to time, remembering the name of the street), he probably has an underlying dementia; thus A is incorrect. B is the correct answer, describing someone with mild dementia (difficulty with memory and executive functioning) who had a superimposed delirium. C is incorrect, as it describes someone who is much more impaired at baseline (probably moderate to severe dementia) and does not explain the delirium or the improvement in symptoms. D is incor-

rect because he does not have the symptoms of dementia pugilistica (which include masked faces, tremor, bradykinesia), and E is incorrect because he has no neurologic signs of a large middle cerebral artery (MCA) stroke (which would be associated with contralateral hemiparesis).

Case 28

1. C Vitamin B_{12} deficiencies, syphilis (the causative agent being *Treponema pallidum*), hypothyroidism, and various things that can be identified on MRI (strokes, tumors, subdural hematomas, etc.) can all cause the clinical syndrome of dementia. Vitamin C deficiency is not associated with late-life dementia; it causes scurvy, which is characterized by weakness, anemia, mucocutaneous hemorrhage, spongy gums, and brawny induration of the leg muscles. Vitamin K controls the formation of coagulation factors II, VII, IX, and X in the liver. Although there is the possibility that a total body CT scan would reveal a cause of dementia (e.g., a primary malignancy), it is an inappropriately broad test. Ceruloplasmin is tested for Wilson's disease. Wilson's disease is a progressive and uniformly fatal disorder of copper metabolism that affects one person in 30,000. Unless treated with lifelong uninterrupted treatment with chelating agents, it is always fatal, generally before age 30. This woman is too old to have new-onset symptoms. It is an autosomal recessive disorder caused by mutation in gene chromosome 13. In about 40% to 50% of patients, the disease first affects the CNS, and can cause tremors, dystonia, dysarthria, dysphagia, chorea, drooling, and lack of coordination; grossly inappropriate behavior; sudden deterioration of schoolwork; or, rarely, psychosis indistinguishable from schizophrenia or manic-depressive illness.

2. C The APOE-ϵ_4 allele has been found in 50% of patients with Alzheimer's disease (AD). The rare ϵ_2 allele is probably protective against AD. Although mutations on chromosomes 1, 14, and 21 have been associated with AD, they are rare and are more frequently seen in patients with early-onset disease with strong family histories. Trinucleotide CAG repeats on chromosome 4 are seen in Huntington's chorea.

3. E The findings are associated with AD and include tangles (intracellular paired helical filaments of hyperphosphorylated tau protein, plaque [extracellular aggregations of beta amyloid that form the core and are surrounded by many things, including microglia, reactive astrocytes, and dystrophic neuritis], atrophy, ventricular enlargement, and decreased choline acetyl transferase). Alpha synuclein is the main component of Lewy bodies. When found diffusely in the cortex, they are associated with Lewy body dementia. When they are found in the substantia nigra, they are associated with Parkinson's disease. Astrogliosis, neuronal loss, and spongiform change are seen in spongiform encephalitis, such as Kuru or Creutzfeld-Jakob. Ischemic periventricular leukoencephalopathy is seen in Binswanger's disease.

4. A In general, the frontal lobes are markedly involved in personality, emotions, and executive functioning. They are also inhibitory in terms of controlling behavior. The classic example of a person with a frontal lobe syndrome is Phineas Gage, a foreman of a railway construction gang who, in an accidental explosion, had a tamping iron blown through his head. Before the accident he was capable and efficient. Afterward, he was impatient, profane, and unable to make a plan and execute it. Temporal lesions may cause the inability to encode new memories (e.g., with bilateral hippocampal lesions), whereas occipital lesions are known to cause visual defects, and in severe cases, cortical blindness. Parietal lobe lesions may be associated with anosognosia, not recognizing a part of one's body as one's own. Brainstem lesions may be associated with ipsilateral cranial nerve involvement with contralateral weakness or sensory deficit.

Case 29

1. C DP is perfectionistic, obsessed with order and detail; he also sounds emotionally rigid and inflexible. He sees this as completely ego syntonic (part of himself). This cluster of symptoms is most consistent with obsessive-compulsive personality disorder (OCD). In OCD there needs to be intrusive obsessions, compulsions that often feel excessive or ego dystonic, and the compulsions usually exist to try to counteract the obsessive thoughts. There is no evidence that this man has any of those symptoms. Although people with avoidant personality disorder or schizoid personality disorder may avoid social interactions or want to work at home, they do so for different reasons. Avoidant persons feel inadequate and are hypersensitive to criticism. Schizoid persons are just disinterested in social relationships and are affectively flat ansd socially withdrawn. Antisocial personality refers not to people who avoid social contact, but to those who have a disregard for the rights of others; are exploitative and aggressive, impulsive, and remorseless; and are often involved in illegal behavior.

2. B She meets criteria for schizotypal personality disorder, with her ideas of reference, odd beliefs, magical thinking, paranoia, and lack of close social relationships. Correlates of central nervous system dysfunction seen in schizophrenia have been observed in schizotypal personality disorder (PD), including performance on tests of visual and auditory attention and smooth pursuit eye movement. People with this disorder see their eccentricities as being ego syntonic (i.e., compatible with their sense of self), not ego dystonic. The prevalence of schizotypal PD is increased in the families of schizophrenics, and there is an increased risk of schizophrenia in families of people with schizotypal PD. Although there is an increased risk of schizophrenia, in schizotypal PD, only approximately 10% to 15% will go on to develop schizophrenia. This disorder may be seen slightly more often in men than women, although the M:F ratio may be 1:1.

3. E ZC displays a pervasive pattern of grandiosity, need for admiration, and lack of empathy, which is consistent with narcissistic personality disorder. People with narcissistic PD are often quite vulnerable to threats to their self-esteem, and they may react defensively with rage, disdain, or indifference but are actually struggling with feelings of shock and humiliation. His feelings of insecurity may be masked by arrogance. He probably has difficulty in sustaining long-term intimate relationships and in accepting feedback. Narcissistic PD is seen in males more often than in females. Histrionic PD is characterized by needing to be the center of attention, being inappropriately seductive, having rapidly shifting shallow emotions, using appearance to draw attention, having an impressionistic style of speech, displaying excessive theatricality, being suggestible, and considering relationships to be more intimate than they are. It is most often diagnosed in women.

4. B This patient has antisocial personality disorder. He has a long-standing pervasive disregard for and violation of rights of others; he lies, engages in illegal behavior, and is impulsive, aggressive, and remorseless. Antisocial PD is seen in 3% of men, 1% of women, and 20% to 50% of forensic/prison populations. It is associated with childhood abuse and neglect, but is not associated with particular abnormalities on an EEG.

Case 30

1. D His presentation is classic for the Münchausen's type of factitious disorder. He seems to be estranged from his family or contacts, has a strange and intriguing disorder, is getting a great deal of attention from the staff, and is probably feigning his symptoms. There is no hint of secondary gain from this history, which would suggest malingering. Somatization disorder does not involve the intentional feigning of symptoms. Confronting the patient about his symptoms will likely make him flee from care. Because he does not have any clear evidence of a mood or anxiety disorder, there is no indication for SSRIs.

2. E Somatization disorder. This woman has had multiple symptoms in multiple areas of the body that are required for a diagnosis of somatization disorder. These include pain in multiple body areas, GI symptoms besides pain, sexual symptoms, and neurologic symptoms. The complaints have lasted for years, and they started before age 30. The work-ups were on the whole unrevealing and could not explain her symptoms. Her neurologic symptoms of sensory and motor changes in her hand could well be a conversion symptom, but her overall symptomatology is much broader. Conversion symptoms are relatively common, and apparently account for 1% to 3% of neurologic visits. They are thought to represent a physical manifestation of a psychiatric symptom and seem to be more common in people who have difficulty verbalizing their distress. Hypochondriasis refers to being fearful of having a serious illness without objective evidence. It often may be associated with misinterpreting normal physiologic sensations as being indicative of a terrible disease. Approximately 5% of patients in primary care practices may meet criteria for this disorder. Body dysmorphic disorder refers to a disorder where the patient inappropriately believes that some aspect of his or her appearance is grossly abnormal, and becomes incapacitated in some way by this belief. Factitious disorder requires the intentional creation of symptoms, of which there is no evidence in this patient.

3. D In factitious disorder, and other somatizing disorders, illness may bring a socially isolated person into contact with support systems. Physical illness may be *less* stigmatizing than psychiatric illness, and illness may be an excuse for not succeeding. Childhood trauma, especially sexual or physical abuse, may predispose people to somatize. It is possible that pain and illness are associated with nurturing. Certain parenting styles may encourage or discourage using the sick role by the attention given to illness or physical complaints. These disorders, unlike malingering, are not due to a direct desire for financial gain or avoiding legal consequences.

Malingering, on the other hand, is the intentional production of signs or symptoms for that express purpose.

4. D Patients with this disorder are at risk for iatrogenic complications. For instance, they may have multiple intra-abdominal procedures to evaluate pain, which may lead to adhesions that may cause pain. But an important consideration is that patients with these disorders also do have various medical and psychiatric diseases. An evaluation should be made for comorbid anxiety, depression, OCDs, delusional disorder, dissociative disorder, and so on. Invasive testing and consultation to specialists should be reserved for significant signs and symptoms of disease but need to be considered in the continued evaluation of the patient. All caregivers, though, should work together as a team, and communication is extremely important. Telling the patient that the symptoms are "in your head" will probably serve to alienate him or her, and will not foster greater insight into the illness.

Case 31

1. A The prevalence of schizophrenia is 1%. Schizophrenics are more commonly born in the winter months, whether in the Northern or Southern Hemisphere. This suggests that there may be an association with viral infection or other intrauterine exposure during pregnancy. Approximately 50% of monozygotic and 15% of dizygotic twins are concordant for schizophrenia. This suggests a genetic component to schizophrenia, as well as an interplay between genetic vulnerability and some psychological, social, and/or environmental factors. First-degree relatives have a significantly higher risk than the general population.

2. B This patient most likely has the disorganized subtype. The five subtypes are

a. **Disorganized.** Prominent disorganized speech, behavior, inappropriate affect, poor grooming.

b. **Paranoid.** Prominent delusions and/or auditory hallucinations, without significant disorganization of speech or behavior. This is associated with better social functioning.

c. **Catatonic.** Motor immobility, excessive purposeless activity, abnormal voluntary movements (posturing, "waxy flexibility" in which the person will maintain any posture, as a wax figure would), echolalia.

d. **Undifferentiated.** The criteria for schizophrenia are met but do not fit into any of the above subtypes.

e. **Residual.** There is a history of an acute episode of schizophrenia, but the patient does not currently manifest significant positive symptoms. The person may have either low-grade psychotic symptoms or prominent negative symptoms.

Grandiosity is a symptom, often associated with mania. People can have grandiose delusions, but this does not define a subtype of schizophrenia.

3. C About 50% of all patients with schizophrenia attempt suicide at least once in their lifetime, and 10% to 15% die by suicide during a 20-year follow-up. Male and female schizophrenic patients are equally likely to commit suicide. The major risk factors for suicide include depressive symptoms, young age, and high levels of premorbid functioning (especially a college education). Individuals with schizophrenia have serious economic, social, and psychological effects: unemployment, disrupted education, limited social relationships, isolation, legal involvement, substance abuse, and significant family stress. Such sequelae form the most distressing aspects of the illness for many people and contribute to the increased risk of suicide among those diagnosed with schizophrenia.

This patient will most likely not return to his previous level of functioning. Although approximately 33% either undergo a remission or are left with mild residual symptoms, 20% may require long-term hospitalization. Most schizophrenics continue to have symptoms. Both because of their positive symptoms and, even more significantly, because of the negative symptoms, they have significant deficits in functioning. The negative symptoms of avolition (reduction or inability in initiating and persisting in goal-directed behavior) and alogia (impoverishment in thinking) significantly impair the ability to function. Cognitive problems associated with schizophrenia include difficulty in processing information, abstraction, attention, memory, and executive functions (e.g., planning and carrying out goal-directed behaviors).

4. D The course of schizophrenia can be divided into three sections, the prodrome, which may span months to years before the onset of active symptoms; the active phase; and finally the residual phase. The prodrome may be characterized by an insidious onset of subtle behavioral changes, social withdrawal, inappropriate affect, impairment in work or school performance, avolition, and/or strange ideation. The acute phase of the illness is characterized by hallucinations, delusions, disorganized speech and/or behavior; it may have exacerbations and remissions, and may last for many years. In the residual phase, the active phase symptoms are not very active or prominent, but the person frequently has prominent negative symptoms with role impairment.

Case 32

1. C Thioridizine is a low-potency medication, associated with sedation and orthostatic hypotension. Haloperidol is a high-potency medication. Typical antipsychotics have their effect through blockade (antagonism) of the D2 receptor. Akathisia refers to an internal sense of restlessness. Parkinsonian symptoms are referred to as *extrapyramidal symptoms*.

2. B Clozapine is associated with a number of significant side effects, including lowered seizure threshold and agranulocytosis. Perphenazine is a typical mid-potency antispsychotic. Atypical agents usually do have some effect on dopamine receptors, although they may be more potent antagonists at dopamine receptor subtypes (such as D4) rather than the D2 receptors targeted by the typical antipsychotics, or at the 5-HT$_{2A}$ receptor. Antipsychotics do not have their primary action at cholinergic (either nicotinic or muscarinic) receptors.

3. A In general, all antipsychotic medications, except probably clozapine, can cause the serious side effect of tardive dyskinesia (TD). The typical antipsychotics (e.g., chlorpromazine, haloperidol) have been the most studied. The atypical agents may have a lower frequency of TD. TD is an often permanent movement disorder caused by the long-term use of antipsychotic drugs. It is characterized by repetitive, involuntary, purposeless movements, including grimacing, tongue protrusion, lip smacking, rapid eye blinking, and movements of the arms, legs, and trunk. Decreasing the dose of a medication may make the movements more pronounced. Treatment is mainly to switch to an atypical agent and attempt to decrease the medication dose. Akathisia is defined as a subjective sense of restlessness, inability to sit still. The term *extrapyramidal symptoms* (EPS) refers to a number of medication side effects that are thought to be associated with antipsychotic blockade of the D2 receptors in the basal ganglia. In general, they include parkinsonian symptoms, acute dystonias, and akathisia. Clozapine causes fewer of these symptoms.

4. C Neuroleptic malignant syndrome (NMS) is a rare, severe complication of antipsychotic treatment consisting of muscular rigidity, dystonia, obtundation, hyperpyrexia, diaphoresis, tachycardia, hypertension, increased WBC count, creatinine phosphokinase (CPK), and liver function tests (LFTs). The mortality is approximately 20%. It can be seen at any time in antipsychotic treatment and is usually treated supportively in an intensive-care setting. It has a frequency of 0.02% to 2.4%. Treatment includes rapid external cooling, intravenous benzodiazepines to decrease muscle rigidity, and discontinuation of the antipsychotic. If antipsychotic medication is necessary, one of a different class can be introduced after 1 or 2 weeks.

Malignant hyperthermia is typically a fulminant life-threatening syndrome that occurs when a person with a susceptibility trait is exposed to triggering factors, which include most inhalational anesthetics and succinylcholine. Classic malignant hyperthermia is characterized by hypermetabolism, muscle rigidity, muscle injury, increased sympathetic nervous system activity, and extreme hyperthermia. Death can result from cardiac arrest, brain damage, internal hemorrhaging, or failure of other body systems.

It is unlikely that this man has an infectious meningitis.

Case 33

1. B Stimulants (e.g., amphetamines, methylphenidate) are the most effective treatment for ADHD and have been extensively studied. They have been shown to be safe in children, to be not addictive, to carry little medical risk, and to be effective in 75% to 90% of cases. Their primary effects are to increase task performance, vigilance, attention, organization, and social appropriateness. Other medication options include drugs that affect catecholamines, such as the tricyclic antidepressants, bupropion, and α2-agonists. Benzodiazepines are not used in this disorder.

2. C The rates of comorbid anxiety and of learning, mood, and behavior disorders are significantly higher than those of the general population. Psychotic disorders are not significantly increased in persons with ADHD.

3. C Amphetamine increases extracellular dopamine by promoting the reverse transport of intracellular dopamine into the extracellular compartment. In short, it increases dopamine release into the synapse. Cocaine and methylphenidate have reuptake-blocking effects. Dopamine is broken down by monoamine oxidase, not acetylcholinesterase (which breaks down acetylcholine). Most antipsychotic medications block postsynaptic receptors.

4. E The possibility of a psychological explanation (e.g., understimulation of an extremely bright child) should always be considered. It is unlikely that his symptoms result from hypothyroidism, Crohn's disease, or dissociative fugue. All these are associated with psychiatric symptoms, but not in this hyperactive, aggressive manner. Dissociative fugue is a psychiatric disorder in which there is sudden unexpected travel with inability to recall one's past. If some of these symptoms were present prior to age 7 and if on interview he met full criteria (see text for full symptoms list), they might be due to attention deficit disorder. If this were a new-onset behavior, the important things to consider in the differential would be the possibility of a substance-induced behavioral change or a new onset of bipolar disorder. Organic etiologies such as hyperthyroidism should also be considered.

Case 34

1. A This presentation is consistent with withdrawal tremors and seizures, which occur within 48 hours after the last drink. Delirium tremens is unlikely, as this condition usually occurs after 48 hours and usually is accompanied by severe autonomic instability and vital sign fluctuations. TN did not report visual hallucinations and therefore is not experiencing hallucinosis. Wernicke's encephalopathy is an alcohol-induced organic brain symptom characterized by the classic triad of ataxia, ophthalmoplegia, and altered mental status. Korsakoff's syndrome is a persistent amnesia with confabulation (*mnemonic: K* is for *k*onfabulation). Both Wernicke's and Korsakoff's syndromes are caused by thiamine deficiency. These syndromes are usually present in the stable alcoholic patient. Given TN's apparently normal mental status, these conditions are unlikely etiologies for his presentation.

2. D Given the recent appearance of black stool and her normal mean corpuscular volume (MCV), it is likely that her anemia is caused by an acute event such as a Mallory-Weiss tear in her mucosa at the gastroesophageal junction caused by severe retching from excessive alcohol intake. Such a mucosal tear would produce moderate upper gastrointestinal hemorrhage that appears as melena (black stool). Chronic etiologies of anemia include iron, folate and vitamin B_{12} deficiency as well as anemia of chronic disease. Since her mean corpuscular volume is normal, it is unlikely that she has an iron deficiency anemia or anemia of chronic disease, which produce microcytic anemias. Folate or vitamin B_{12} deficiency would produce a macrocytic anemia. Lastly, although retching can rupture gastric varices, this would present with more profuse bleeding with frank hematemesis as well as a more fulminant clinical course.

3. B Ingestion of large amounts of alcohol during college hazing rituals has been associated with CNS depression severe enough to completely depress respiratory drive and result in death. Such severe intoxication must be treated with respiratory support until the patient can metabolize the alcohol. Heroin intoxication is less likely in this case, given the lack of stigmata like pinpoint pupils and track marks, although he can be given naloxone empirically. Benzodiazepine overdose is also possible but less likely. His vital signs and physical exam are inconsistent with a cocaine overdose. Lastly, his glucose level does not suggest an insulin overdose.

4. E Vitamin K deficiency is associated with coagulopathy due to inability to produce sufficient coagulation factors. Such coagulopathy can predispose an individual to hemorrhagic strokes. Thiamine deficiency can produce altered mental status along with paresthesias. Long-term organic brain syndromes such as Korsakoff's syndrome can cause amnestic symptoms with confabulation. Chronic liver disease can predispose someone to hypoglycemic events, which can manifest as syncope. Lastly, chronic liver insufficiency can produce high levels of serum ammonia, which can produce a hepatic encephalopathy and decreased sensorium.

Case 35

1. E This clinical scenario emphasizes the difficulty in diagnosing the varied clinical manifestations an opiate-dependent person can present with. Given his fever, murmur, and track marks, bacterial endocarditis is possible, with valve vegetations producing a tricuspid stenosis murmur. This is an important consideration in an injection drug user. Acute gastroenteritis is also possible with his 1 day of diarrhea and tender abdomen at the periumbilical region. Viral upper respiratory infections can also produce rhinorrhea, cough due to postnasal drip, *and* concurrent diarrhea. Heroin withdrawal is also possible, given all the symptoms mentioned earlier. This emphasizes the tricky nature of detecting a withdrawal episode in an opiate-dependent person without proper history taking and cooperative disclosure from the patient.

2. D Although it may seem tempting to give morphine to someone screaming in agony, the appropriate step in this situation is to quickly assess the patient, treat with a non-opiod (like IV netorolac), and contact her primary physician. In the emergency room, the most appropriate medications for pain are nonopioid analgesics, which decrease pain from true inflammatory causes (remember the arachidonic acid pathway and the inhibition of cyclo-oxygenase by NSAIDs and acetaminophen). Ultimately, a single primary physician should be responsible for prescribing opiods, as it will avoid overprescription and increasing opiate tolerance and dependence. Increased dependence only worsens the pain syndrome when opiate treatment becomes insufficient. Thus it is inappropriate to administer intravenous morphine immediately without careful assessment, as it may do a disservice to the patient in the long run.

3. A Necrotizing fasciitis is a rapidly spreading and rapidly fatal staphylococcal skin infection that can be a complication of injection drug use. Unfortunately, it has a very nonspecific clinical picture. The skin infection may be of any size or morphology, and

the only clues that might lead one to suspect necrotizing fasciitis are tenderness out of proportion to exam, fever, other abnormal vital signs, and a general appearance of distress. This man otherwise has a cellulitis and a possible abscess, which are important but less concerning than the diagnosis of necrotizing fasciitis. These infections are usually not life-threatening and can be treated with incision and drainage (for abscesses) and antibiotics. Given his recent heroin injection, he is unlikely to be having withdrawal symptoms. Lastly, given the absence of a murmur, he is unlikely to have bacterial endocarditis, although it is important to keep on your differential in any injection drug user with a fever.

4. E It is important to remember that a person who appears to be a typical heroin user can have other causes of decreased level of consciousness. Benzodiazepines are also available on the streets and can produce a very similar clinical picture. Unlike heroin, this will respond to flumazenil, not naloxone. Given his lack of response to glucose, hypoglycemia is unlikely to be the cause of his decreased sensorium. Other metabolic abnormalities, such as hyponatremia, can cause altered level of consciousness but mostly present as seizure. Alcohol intoxication is another possible cause of his clinical picture, but given the lack of stigmata and negative Breathalyzer exam, it is highly unlikely.

Case 36

1. A PCP intoxication. This case of acute drug intoxication is a stereotypical presentation of intoxication with a stimulant. It is difficult to pinpoint the drug used from the physical presentation alone, and it is thus important to try to elicit this information so that one can anticipate the duration of action and the therapeutic needs of the patient. However, most cases of acute stimulant intoxication are managed in the same way, with stabilization of vital signs monitoring, and other supportive measures. The stigmata of vertical nystagmus and moist oral mucosa or hypersalivation lead one to suspect intoxication with PCP. Proper measures to secure the safety of the patient as well as the staff are necessary to counter the hypervigilance and threat of violence that may be induced by this drug.

2. E All the preceding cases can result in the above presentation. The first three cases of withdrawal emphasize the fact that all three drugs act on the $GABA_A$ receptor, and therapy with lorazepam, a $GABA_A$ receptor agonist, will suppress withdrawal symptoms. Methamphetamine overdose may also present in such a manner, emphasizing the dichotomous nature of physical dependence. Withdrawal generally produces symptoms that are opposite to the effects produced by the drug. Thus sedative withdrawal can also look like stimulant intoxication. Lastly, just because a person has no stigmata of alcoholism does not mean he is not experiencing alcohol withdrawal.

3. D Given her unique presentation of severe coma with an intact respiratory drive, she is likely presenting with an acute gamma hydroxybutyrate (GHB) overdose. This is a relatively new drug and has been used by sexual offenders as a sedative and amnestic for would-be victims. It is in liquid form and can be slipped into a drink. Moderate doses produce agitation, hallucinations, miosis, drowsiness, vomiting, and dizziness. Higher doses can produce seizures and coma. Such symptoms usually resolve within 8 hours of ingestion. Benzodiazepine, barbiturate, and alcoholic overdose can produce severe coma but always with accompanying respiratory depression. Lastly, ketamine is a stimulant and would rarely present in this manner.

4. B The classic drug of abuse that is associated with chest pain is cocaine, which produces an unstable angina (Prinzmetal's angina) thought to be due to acute coronary vasospasm. Any sympathomimetic drug can produce chest pain, which can be exacerbated by the tachycardia and hypertension associated with such intoxication. Although asthma can produce chest pressure, her clinical picture is inconsistent with asthma. Given her age, she is unlikely to have hypertension and associated coronary artery disease (although it still should be asked). The hypertension and tachycardia she has now are most likely due to some sort of sympathetic stimulation, most likely due to intoxication with a sympathomimetic. Although family history of early myocardial infarction is a cardiac risk factor and should be inquired about, she is unlikely to have atherosclerosis associated with familial types of myocardial infarction, given her age. Lastly, while exogenous estrogen use is theoretically associated with hypercoagulability, intravascular thrombosis, and increased cardiac risk, current low-dose oral contraceptives with combination estrogen and progesterone are not associated with increased cardiac risk. Therefore this is less concerning than a possible history of drug use.

Case 37

1. C Many long-term smokers started smoking when they were teenagers. Thus it is particularly important to address this issue with all teenagers in the clinical setting as well as in schools. Some effective methods of discouraging smoking are public service announcements that address the issues regarding peer pressure and self-confidence that teenagers may be dealing with. High costs of cigarettes due to taxation may make buying cigarettes difficult for teenagers. Schools can also have significant influence by addressing the issue early, particularly during the elementary school years, while children are still very impressionable. In addition, after-school programs that promote teenagers' positive self-image can help keep them from succumbing to peer pressure to smoke. Lower-tar cigarettes, nicotine patches, clonidine, and bupropion are not helpful to teenagers or adults in preventing tobacco use.

2. D Smoking cessation is the single most effective therapy in preserving this man's lung function and reducing mortality in chronic obstructive pulmonary disease (COPD). Oxygen therapy also has benefits in slowing down the decline of respiratory function and reducing mortality, although not as much as smoking cessation. Beta-agonists, atropine, and ipratropium are helpful for counteracting bronchoconstriction in the acute setting of COPD exacerbation but have no long-term benefits with regard to reducing mortality.

3. D Pulmonary embolism is the most concerning diagnostic possibility in this woman with acute-onset shortness of breath. She has multiple risk factors, including exogenous estrogen use, a recent

episode of prolonged stasis, and current cigarette use. All women taking estrogen-containing oral contraceptive pills should be advised to not smoke and should in fact be offered other modes of contraception if they are smoking, given the risk of developing deep venous thrombosis and pulmonary embolism. Chronic bronchitis and emphysema produce more gradual onset shortness of breath. Pneumonia is unlikely, given her lack of fever and normal chest x-ray. Asthma is unlikely, given her normal lung exam.

4. C Bupropion is the most useful antidepressant in this clinical situation, given his motivation to quit smoking as well as its medical necessity. He has many risk factors for having a recurrence of a major cardiac event and needs optimal treatment of all these conditions, *including* his smoking addiction. Answers A, B, and D are good antidepressant medications but do not have any effects on nicotine cravings. Olanzapine is an atypical antipsychotic, which will address neither his depression nor his smoking addiction.

Case 38

1. D It is rare to have a disorder of written expression without another learning disorder, and the specific prevalence of this disorder is unknown. Approximately 60% to 80% of those diagnosed with reading disorder are males, and about 4% of schoolchildren have this disorder. It has been estimated that approximately 1% of schoolchildren have mathematics disorder. Learning disorders are often found in association with medical disorders such as fetal alcohol syndrome or lead poisoning.

2. E Down syndrome may also be called mongolism and has several characteristic features, which include epicanthic folds; cataracts; strabismus; small, round head with high cheekbones; small nose and ears; high arched palate; protruding tongue; short neck and limbs; single palmar creases; ulnar loops; and hypotonic muscles. Umbilical hernias are common, as is deafness. Associated medical complications include congenital heart defects in 40% (atrial septal defects [ASD], ventral septal defects [VSD], tetralogy of Fallot [TOF], and patient ductus anteriosus [PDA]), congenital cataracts, nystagmus, GI abnormalities such as duodenal atresia, pyloric stenosis, imperforate anus, Hirschsprung's disease, hypothyroidism, leukemia, epilepsy, and the neuropathologic changes of Alzheimer's disease in their 30s, with onset of dementia in their 40s. In 95% of cases it is caused by trisomy-21(22) but can be caused by a translocation in 5% of cases. Prognathism (the jaw and facial skeleton jutting forward), a large, long head, floppy ears, hypertelorism (increased distance between two orbits), blue eyes, single palmar creases, hyperextendable joints, and macroorchidism (post puberty) are associated with fragile X syndrome in males. It is the most common inherited cause of mental retardation and is a triple repeat expansion. It occurs in 1 in 1200 males and in 1 in 2400 females. The fragile site is at Q27–28 on the X chromosome.

3. B The life expectancy of those with mental retardation is directly related to their level of intellectual functioning and the etiology of their impairments. Those with mild mental retardation have increased mortality rates of twice that of the general population. However, this rate increases drastically with the increases in mental impairment. Prevalence rates of psychiatric disorders among those with mental retardation range from 30% to 70%. Disorders seen may include the full spectrum of psychiatric disorders, particularly mood disorders, autism, and schizophrenia. Impulsive aggressive behaviors may be common. Those more severely impaired individuals may not present with symptoms like hallucinations and delusions. Self-injurious behavior may occur. Most individuals with mild mental retardation function quite well in the community either with their families or in a group care setting.

4. C Rett's syndrome has only been reported in females and is thought to be fatal in males. The onset is after a period of normal postnatal development around the age of 5 months. Head growth slows down, causing microcephaly. Previously acquired purposeful movements are lost, and these girls develop characteristic stereotypic hand-wringing or hand-washing movements. They lose social engagement early in the illness but may make some progress as an adolescent. Coordination of the limbs and gait, impaired receptive and expressive language, and severe psychomotor retardation develop. These girls tend to suffer from moderate to severe mental retardation.

Case 39

1. C Brain tumors may present with nonfocal symptoms caused by raised intracranial pressure; these include nausea, vomiting, headaches, lethargy, and confusion. Patients may also present with more focal signs or symptoms, such as cranial nerve palsies, hemianopia, hemiparesis, or focal seizure. But focal and nonfocal signs and symptoms may occur together. Headaches are early symptoms in approximately one-third of patients with a brain tumor. Vomiting occurs also in approximately one-third of patients; it may not be related to meals and may occur on wakening. Seizure, either generalized or focal, may occur in 20% to 50% of patients.

2. B Most cognitive effects found in long-term survivors of brain tumors are reported to be caused by radiation treatment. Acute effects of radiation include nausea, vomiting, headache, and fatigue. Delayed effects may include somnolence syndrome, neurologic deficits and cognitive dysfunction. These effects may be caused by transient demyelination and resolve usually spontaneously or with steroid treatment. Late effects of radiation may include necrosis, progressive global cognitive decline, and unstable gait. This may be caused by vasculopathy or neuronal/glial injury. These late effects may be helped with corticosteroids, antioxidants, anticoagulants, or pentoxifylline. Endocrine abnormalities may be caused by damage to the hypothalamus or the pituitary. Chemotherapy may also cause neurotoxic effects (e.g., methotrexate is reported to cause leukoencephalopathy). Corticosteroids are used to control symptoms caused by cerebral edema, but they may also cause unwanted side effects of myopathy, opportunistic infections, GI upset, osteoporosis, cataracts, glucose intolerance, and mood and cognitive changes. Mood changes may include depression, insomnia, hypomania, irritability, hyperactivity, or euphoria and may require treatment with neuroleptics. Progression of the tumor may cause further cognitive dysfunction, depending on its location.

3. E In conduction aphasia there is fluent language output, impaired repetition, but preserved comprehension. These patients can comprehend while reading but cannot read out loud. Their writing may also contain paraphasic errors. This type of aphasia is associated with a lesion of the arcuate fasciculus in the left parietal region. Schizophrenia, depression, and OCDs are all associated with frontal lobe dysfunction.

4. A Cognitive outcomes are related to the Glasgow Coma Scale (GCS) scores and the level of posttraumatic amnesia. Cognitive deficits occur in between 20% and 80% of head injury patients. Recovery from diffuse injury is related to diffuse axonal injury, not hypoxia in head injuries. Approximately 30% of those with an open head injury will develop seizure disorders, whereas 5% of those with a closed injury will develop seizures. Most neuropsychiatric disturbances after head injury are of the behavioral decontrol type. Other neuropsychiatric disturbances include mood disorders, anxiety disorders, apathy, and psychotic disorders. The risk of developing a neuropsychiatric condition after head injury is increased most by the following factors: poor premorbid social functioning, prior psychiatric illness, alcohol dependence, arteriosclerosis, and increased age. About 50% of head injuries are caused by motor vehicle accidents; the next most common cause is falls, followed by violence and sports. Traumatic brain injuries are the leading cause of disabilities in individuals less than 45 years of age. Physical problems may improve but changes in personality, behavior, cognitive function, and mood disorders are common and may be chronic.

Case 40

1. D Given the set of numbers {1,2,4,6,7,8,9}, the sum of these numbers is 37 and there are seven values, so the mean is 37/7 = 5 2/7, or 5.28. The median, which is the center of an odd number of values, is the number 6, with 1, 2, and 4 below and 7, 8, and 9 above.

2. D Given the set of numbers, {1,1,1,1,2,3,5,5,6,6,7,7,9,9}, there are 14 numbers, and their sum is 63. Thus the mean is 4.5; clearly, the median is 5; and the mode is 1. Thus the answer is D, which is a mode of 1 and a mean of 4.5.

3. E What a 95% confidence interval (CI) tells you is that if you repeated the same experiment that you did to get your summary statistic (e.g., the mean or proportion), an infinite number of times, 95% of the time you would get a value that falls within the 95% CI. It does not tell you that the true value you are seeking is going to fall within your confidence interval, particularly because your experiment may be faulty or biased; thus the true value may be missed by the CI. Even with a perfectly performed experiment, the CI is not used to tell you about the true value; it gives just the results of that particular experiment.

4. B The question asks, "In what type of distribution is the mean greater than the median?" The mean will equal the median in normal and uniform distributions. In a symmetric bimodal distribution this will also be true. In a skewed-to-the-left distribution, the median will be greater than the mean, whereas in a skewed-to-the-right distribution, the mean will be greater than the median.

Case 41

1. B A type II error is made when you do not reject the null hypothesis when it should be rejected. This a false-negative study result. The ability to avoid a type II error is statistical power, in this case 0.96. Thus the probability that a type II error was made is $1 - 0.96 = 0.04$.

2. D In this study design, you are attempting to determine whether there is a difference in any of these groups of patients with respect to the risk for type 2 diabetes. The test that is needed must be able to compare proportions between multiple groups. The only one that can do that is the chi-square test. The student's *t* test is to compare two means; the *z* test is to compare the proportions of two groups. A power analysis is performed to measure the power of a particular study to reject the null hypothesis. A Bonferroni correction is performed when making more than one comparison using, for example, a student's *t* test. Using a cutoff of the test that allows a 5% chance of type I error goes awry when you make many comparisons of outcomes in the same study. For example, if you compared 100 different means, on average you would expect five of them to meet the $p = .05$ requirement. Thus a Bonferroni or, more commonly, the student-Newman-Keuls test, can be used to adjust the cutoff when making multiple comparisons.

3. A From the Thumbnail in this case, you can see that a type I error is that of a false-positive test as described by answer choice A. Answer choice D describes a false-negative result, which is that of a type II error. Answer choices B and C are true positive and true negative results, respectively.

4. E Type I error is that of having a false-positive result. So type I error equals the number of false-positive results over the total number of patients with true results that are negative or not diseased. Type II error is the false-negative mistake. Thus type II error equals the number of false negatives over the total number of patients with disease, or with true results that are positive (see Table A-41).

Case 42

1. E For the disease described there is actually only the benefit of knowledge of disease to be gained from diagnosis. Thus the goal for a screening program would be to have as few false-positive test results as possible. This would happen with the greatest specificity. Although it is often difficult to measure the tradeoff between sensitivity and specificity, in this particular case, it is likely that increasing the specificity to 99% is worth the drop in sensitivity.

2. A We only know three of the four boxes in the 2×2 table. We know that there are six false positives. Thus the remaining four positive tests must be true positives. Since there are exactly 10 people with disease, there must be six false negatives. Using this information we can calculate the sensitivity, but not the specificity. Sensitivity is $a/(a + c) = 4/10 = 0.4$, or 40%.

3. E In the diabetes screening test we only know three of the four boxes in the 2×2 table as well. Ninety of the 100 positive screens have diabetes, so they must be true positives. The remaining 10 must be false positives. Since there are 100 people with diabetes, there must be 10 false negatives as well. So we can calculate positive predictive value (PPV), but not negative predictive value (NPV). The PPV is equal to $90/100 = 0.9$.

4. C Remember that

$$LR(+) = \frac{\text{Prob(pos test given disease)}}{\text{Prob(pos test given no disease)}} = \frac{a/(a + c)}{b/(b + d)}$$

$$= \frac{\text{sensitivity}}{1 - \text{specificity}}$$

So to determine the positive likelihood ratio [LR(+)] one must calculate the sensitivity and specificity first. In this screening test, 90 of the 100 diabetics were identified, giving a 0.9 (or 90%) sensitivity. The specificity is all of the true negatives over the nondiabetics; that would be 890 divided by $900 = 0.9889$ (or 98.89%). Thus the likelihood ratio is $0.9/0.0111 = 81.081$

Case 43

1. C Sampling bias occurs when the subjects chosen to be involved in the study are chosen for some reason unrelated to the study (e.g., those who volunteer may differ from the general population). This can be a problem for both cross-sectional and interventional studies. Selection bias occurs when either the investigator or study subject can choose participation in either treatment groups or the placebo group leading to bias; this is reduced by using randomization. Blinding of both the subjects and the investigators (double blind) to the assigned treatment also minimizes bias in intervention studies. If the randomization is not performed properly, the study can be biased.

Table A-41

True Results		
Study Results	**Positive**	**Negative**
Positive	True Positive—85	False Positive—50 Type I error = 50/1000 = 0.05
Negative	False Negative—15 Type II error = 15/100 = 0.15	True Negative—950

2. B This is the correct definition of incidence. Prevalence ratio refers to the specific number of individuals with a disease at a specific point in time (e.g., on January 1, 2002) divided by the total population at the mid-point of that year. The prevalence of a disease equals the incidence of the disease multiplied by the average duration of the disease. If the disease is chronic or long-lasting, the prevalence is greater than the incidence. If a disease resolves quickly or is rapidly fatal, then the incidence and prevalence are approximately equal.

3. D This study could also be accomplished as a retrospective case–control or cohort study. However, there are a number of reasons why a retrospective design for this study would be inferior to a prospective study. Information on diet and exercise obtained retrospectively is likely to be a poor substitute for information gained in a prospective study. Further, the study may be biased, since patients with heart disease may die at a different rate than those without, so the sample at any point in time will not be representative of the individuals who were available in the past. These concerns are also true of a cross-sectional study. A prospective case–control study does not make sense, unless you are examining whether diet and exercise can treat heart disease. To study how these risk factors affect the probability for developing heart disease, a prospective cohort study should be performed.

4. A For a rare disease, it is much more efficient to use a case–control study. If the purpose of the study is to examine risk factors for the development of disease, then the study should be retrospective. A cohort study would work to study this disease; however, it would take much more time to collect information on the 10,000 people who do not have the disease than to collect it for just a handful of control patients. A case series could be used to describe the disease in question, but would not examine the same risks in control patients, so it could not be used to examine associations with risk factors. Finally, a prospective randomized, controlled trial (RCT) would be useful to examine a treatment of the disease but would not apply in this setting.

Case 44

1. C Despite wanting to form a supportive relationship with this patient, allay her fears, and answer her questions, as a physician it is important to be able to prioritize seriously ill patients above less ill patients. In this scenario, the patient with possible appendicitis is top priority, despite patient number 1 having been in the emergency department the longest. Thus when radiology pages you regarding this patient, you should answer this page as soon as possible to determine whether this patient needs surgery. However, there are better ways to excuse yourself from your third patient. If you tell her, "I will be right back" and then do not come back for a long time, she is likely to become annoyed. However, if you acknowledge her concerns by consulting plastic surgery and explain quickly that you have another sick patient who requires your care, she is likely to understand and to feel that her waiting is justified. Telling her, "no one will notice this scar" does not acknowledge her concerns about scarring and is inappropriately paternalistic.

2. B In this setting of an emergent procedure needing to be performed, rapid, efficient action is the most important thing. While in most cases it is best to document events as they occur, a physician in this case should act first and worry about documentation second. Further, there is never an indication to change prior documentation or adjust timing on notes to make it seem as if they were being written prior to when they actually were. It is useful to communicate the plan of action to the nurse, who is likely to document at some point what that plan was. However, you cannot rely on other practitioners to do your documentation, as everyone may have a different viewpoint on how events occurred. The best way to document an event of this sort is to deal with the emergency, perform the cesarean section, and move the patient to recovery. Once there, discuss the timing of events with nursing and anesthesia and write a note that reflects your best understanding of what occurred.

3. D It is unclear why this patient has changed physicians. He may have already undergone an extensive work-up for his chronic back pain that you do not need to repeat. If this was a first visit for this symptom, ibuprofen and an x-ray would be a reasonable way to begin management. However, for this patient, who has likely already used ibuprofen and had x-rays, it is unlikely to contribute to his care. It is also folly to assume that a patient has had the appropriate work-up thus far, as he may have switched providers a number of times and not had good continuity of care. Thus the most important thing to do is to acknowledge his prior care and attempt to assemble a plan of care with his prior practitioner that is acknowledged as workable by you and the patient.

4. D Answer A is the only one that has malpractice. However, because this action did not result in any harm, it is unlikely to lead to a lawsuit. Answers B, C, and E all involve the physician communicating in an ongoing way with the patient and her family. Although answer D results in excellent care, because the physician does not follow up with the patient during her acute event, she may feel abandoned. Furthermore, by waiting to follow up with patient after discharge, if she ends up in a nursing home, goes to a rehabilitation facility, or dies, the physician will not have the opportunity to see the patient at all.

Case 45

1. C and 2. B Moral hazard is consuming more of something than you would have if you had to experience the full costs and consequences of consumption. An insured patient who wants an extensive work-up that is not medically indicated is one classic example of moral hazard. Adverse selection occurs when the healthy opt out of health insurance and only the sick purchase it. This leads to increasing costs of insurance, driving the healthy out of the market. The diabetic patient who pays for better drug coverage is an example of consumption of an appropriate amount of insurance based on need (though this could have been interpreted as a component of adverse selection). The patient who only buys half the medication prescribed is an example of the complications of the uninsured or underinsured—the flip side of moral hazard. Finally, the patient with chest pain who goes to the emergency room probably provides an example of an appropriate action.

3. E Any modification to 100% coverage for health care may diminish moral hazard. Three standard ways this is done include copayments and/or coinsurance for the use of services and having a deductible to pay before services are used.

4. D Answers A, B, and C are ways to decrease moral hazard and would not affect adverse selection. Providing health insurance at the same price to everyone is exactly what causes adverse selection, because on average, healthier individuals will not pay the same premium as the sick. However, if premiums were risk-adjusted based on health status, this would decrease adverse selection, since the healthier individuals would actually pay less than the sicker individuals.

Case 46

1. E Assuming that this patient has gone to a hospital out of her network, health maintenance organizations (HMOs) will not cover care out of network unless it is truly an emergency. CC has a common cold, which does not qualify as an emergency; thus she is likely to bear the full $500+ cost of the emergency room visit. If she had a standard indemnity plan, she would be fully covered. The other managed care plans will provide partial coverage, though they may give her trouble, since she did not get preapproval.

2. E Although HMO care has been criticized widely in the media, of all managed care plans, group and staff model HMOs actually are easier to navigate by health care providers. These HMOs are designed so that the providers have incentives to provide cost-effective health care and thus face less red tape in order to get patients services. The other forms of managed care often require preapproval for hospital admissions, surgery, and expensive outpatient therapy.

3. B Although there are other factors that govern the provision of health care by physicians, such as paternalism, professionalism, and tort law, how physicians are reimbursed has been shown to change the way they provide care. In general, physicians who are paid fee-for-service (FFS) are more likely to see more patients and do more procedures. Physicians who are paid on a prospective, capitated (per head) basis are less likely to utilize expensive services. Physicians who are paid a salary are less likely to be productive. However, they have no incentive to provide less expensive care and in fact may replace their own efforts with those of specialists and expensive diagnostic tests. A bonus for seeing more patients would just lead to increased expenditures on seeing these extra patients.

4. C Health insurance and health plans began first as indemnity plans, the largest of these being the "Blues"—Blue Cross and Blue Shield. The concept of HMOs was introduced in the 1940s but was not in the mainstream of medical practice until the late 1960s. Preferred provider organizations (PPOs) were introduced by indemnity plans to cut costs in the 1980s, and finally independent practitioner associations (IPAs)were assembled in the 1990s to compete with group and staff model HMOs.

Index

Index note: page references with a *b, f,* or *t* indicate a box, figure or table.